Psychiatric Neurology

A Clinical Approach

Psychiatric Neurology

A Clinical Approach

Edited by

Sheldon Benjamin, M.D.

Kathy Niu, M.D.

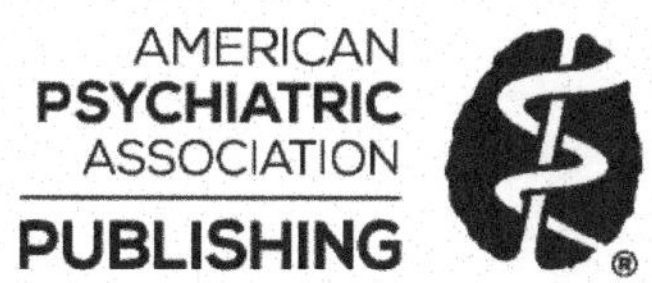

First Edition

Manufactured in the United States of America on acid-free paper
29 28 27 26 25 5 4 3 2 1

American Psychiatric Association Publishing
800 Maine Avenue SW, Suite 900
Washington, DC 20024–2812
www.appi.org

ISBN: 978-1-61437-474-8
eBook ISBN: 978-1-61537-475-5
Online ISBN: 979-8-89455-112-8

Library of Congress Control Number: 9781615374748

British Library Cataloguing in Publication Data: A CIP record is available from the British Library.

EU GPSR Authorized Representative: LOGOS EUROPE, 9 rue Nicolas Poussin, 17000, LA ROCHELLE, France; E-mail: Contact@logoseurope.eu

To my spouse and life partner, Miriam, for humoring me during the lengthy gestation of this book and everything else in life, and to the residents, fellows, and medical students who inspire me to teach neuropsychiatry.

—S.B.

To my mentors, colleagues, and family from whom I have learned so much, and to the students, trainees, and patients who motivate me to learn ever more.

—K.N.

Contents

List of Videos

Number	Title	Time (minutes)
1.1	Examination for Internuclear Ophthalmoplegia (INO)	0:21
1.2	Doll's Eyes Maneuver	0:14
1.3	Test for Optokinetic Nystagmus (OKN)	0:20
1.4	Anti-saccades	0:15
1.5	Examination Safety	0:32
1.6	Muscle Tone Activation	0:32
1.7	Glabellar Tap	0:15
1.8	Forced Grasping	0:17
1.9	Dysmetria Test	0:21
1.10	Finger-Nose-Finger Test with Finger Chase Component	0:23
1.11	Circumducting Gait	0:15
1.12	Pull Test	0:22
1.13	Test for the Romberg Sign	0:20
1.14	Nonphysiological Hemianopia	1:09
1.15	Test for Nonphysiologic Upper-Extremity Hemisensory Loss	0:33
1.16	Test for Nonphysiological Lower-Extremity Hemiparesis	0:31
1.17	Luria 3-Step Task	0:43
1.18	Fist-Ring Test	0:38

Acknowledgments

The authors acknowledge the many people who helped make this book possible: Terrence Flotte, M.D., Provost of UMass Chan Medical School, for generously providing a writing sabbatical for SB; Stephan Heckers, M.D., Chair of Psychiatry at Vanderbilt University School of Medicine, the institution where KN wrote a portion of this book; Timothy Nicholson, MBBS, MSc, PhD, King's College Institute of Psychiatry, Psychology and Neuroscience, for hosting SB's writing sabbatical; Kyle Blackburn, M.D., at University of Texas Southwestern, for providing neuroimaging examples; Elizabeth DeGrush, D.O., and Miriam Rosenblum for their assistance in video production; and Alexis George, for her help with the headache chapter. Finally, we acknowledge the guidance and tremendous patience of the editors of American Psychiatric Association Publishing, as this book slowly came together.

Contributors

Oluwatosin Akintola, M.D.
Assistant Professor of Neurology, Larner College of Medicine at the University of Vermont; University of Vermont Medical Center, Burlington, Vermont

Deepti Anbarasan, M.D.
Associate Professor, Departments of Psychiatry and Neurology, NYU Grossman School of Medicine, New York, New York

X. Michelle Androulakis, M.D., M.S.
Staff Neurologist, Ralph Johnson VA Health Care System, Charleston, South Carolina

Miya R. Asato, M.D.
Associate Professor, Department of Neurology, Johns Hopkins School of Medicine; Vice President of Training, Kennedy Krieger Institute, Baltimore, Maryland

Sheldon Benjamin, M.D.
Professor Emeritus of Psychiatry and Neurology, University of Massachusetts T.H. Chan School of Medicine, Worcester, Massachusetts

Shamik Bhattacharyya, M.D.
Anne Finucane Distinguished Chair in Neurology, Program Leader for Autoimmune Neurology, and Associate Professor of Neurology, Harvard Medical School; Department of Neurology, Brigham and Women's Hospital, Boston, Massachusetts

Ankur Butala, M.D.
Movement Disorder Specialist and Assistant Professor of Neurology, Psychiatry, and Behavioral Sciences, Johns Hopkins University, Baltimore, Maryland

L. Nicolas Gonzalez Castro, M.D., Ph.D.
Assistant Professor of Neurology, Harvard Medical School. Brigham and Women's Hospital; Center for Neuro-Oncology, Dana-Farber Cancer Institute, Boston, Massachusetts

Mattia Wruble Clark, M.D.
Instructor in Neurology, Harvard Medical School; Department of Neurology, Brigham and Women's Hospital/Massachusetts General, Boston, Massachusetts

Elizabeth DeGrush, D.O.
Assistant Professor of Psychiatry and Neurology; Program Director, Combined Neuropsychiatry Residency, Departments of Psychiatry and Neurology, UMass Chan Medical School, Worcester, Massachusetts

Bradford Dickerson, M.D., M.M.Sc.
Professor of Neurology, Frontotemporal Disorders Unit, Department of Neurology, Harvard Medical School, Boston; Tommy Rickles Chair in Progressive Aphasia Research and Director, Frontotemporal Disorders Unit and Laboratory of Neuroimaging, and Athinoula A. Martinos Center for Biomedical Imaging, Department of Radiology, Massachusetts General Hospital, Charlestown, Massachusetts

Brigid C. Dwyer, M.D.
Assistant Professor, Department of Neurology, Boston University School of Medicine, Boston, Massachusetts; Encompass Health Braintree Rehabilitation Hospital, Braintree, Massachusetts

Mark Eldaief, M.D., M.M.Sc.
Assistant Professor of Neurology, Frontotemporal Disorders Unit, Division of Neuropsychiatry and Neuromodulation, Harvard Medical School, Boston; Director, TMS Core and Staff Physician, Center for Brain Sciences, Harvard University, Cambridge; Department of Psychiatry, and Athinoula A. Martinos Center for Biomedical Imaging, Department of Radiology, Massachusetts General Hospital, Charlestown, Massachusetts

Lindsey Gurin, M.D.
Assistant Professor, Departments of Neurology, Psychiatry, and Rehabilitation Medicine, NYU Grossman School of Medicine, New York, New York

Susan Hutchinson, M.D.
Director, Orange County Migraine & Headache Center, Irvine, California

Andres M. Kanner, M.D.
Professor of Clinical Neurology and Director, Comprehensive Epilepsy Center, and Head, Epilepsy Division, Department of Neurology, Miller School of Medicine, University of Miami, Miami, Florida

Douglas I. Katz, M.D.
Professor, Department of Neurology, Boston University School of Medicine, Boston, Massachusetts; Encompass Health Braintree Rehabilitation Hospital, Braintree, Massachusetts

Khurshid A. Khurshid, M.B.B.S.
Professor of Psychiatry, University of Massachusetts T. H. Chan School of Medicine, Worcester, Massachusetts

Howard S. Kirshner, M.D.
Professor of Neurology, Vanderbilt University Medical Center, Nashville, Tennessee

Kevin Kyle, M.B.B.Ch.
Instructor, Department of Neurology, Massachusetts General Hospital, Harvard Medical School, Boston, Massachusetts

Mia T. Minen, M.D., M.P.H.
Chief of Headache Research and Associate Professor, Departments of Neurology and Population Health, NYU Langone Health, New York, New York

Kathy Niu, M.D.
Director, Combined Neurology/Psychiatry Residency Program, Assistant Professor of Psychiatry and Neurology, University of Texas Southwestern Medical Center, Dallas, Texas

Ashley Paul, M.D., M.Ed.
Movement Disorder Specialist and Assistant Professor of Neurology, Johns Hopkins University School of Medicine, Baltimore, Maryland

David L. Perez, M.D., M.M.Sc.
Associate Professor of Neurology and Psychiatry, Harvard Medical School; Mass General Brigham Departments of Neurology and Psychiatry, Massachusetts General Hospital, Brigham and Women's Hospital, Boston, Massachusetts

Scott W. Powers, Ph.D.
Professor of Pediatrics, University of Cincinnati College of Medicine; Co-Director, Headache Center, Cincinnati Children's Hospital, Division of Behavioral Medicine and Clinical Psychology, Cincinnati Children's Hospital, Cincinnati, Ohio

Matthew Schrag, M.D., Ph.D.
Assistant Professor of Neurology, Vanderbilt University Medical Center, Nashville, Tennessee

Sonali Sharma, M.D.
Assistant Professor, Department of Neurology, Medical University of South Carolina, Charleston, South Carolina

Huma U. Sheikh, M.D.
Assistant Professor, Icahn School of Medicine Mount Sinai; CEO, NY Neurology Medicine, PC, New York, New York

Clay E. Smith, M.D.
Assistant Professor, Department of Neurology, Johns Hopkins School of Medicine; Neurology Faculty, Kennedy Krieger Institute, Baltimore, Maryland

Alexandra M. Stillman, M.D.
Instructor, Department of Neurology, Harvard Medical School; Cognitive Neurology Unit, Beth Israel Deaconess Medical Center, Boston, Massachusetts

Melinda A. Thiam, M.D.
Staff Psychiatrist, New Mexico VA Health Care System, NWMetro CBOC, Rio Rancho, New Mexico

Taylor Young, M.D., M.A.
Assistant Professor, Departments of Psychiatry and Neurology, UMass Chan Medical School, Worcester, Massachusetts

Disclosures

The following contributors have indicated a financial interest in or other affiliation with a commercial supporter, manufacturer of a commercial product, and/or provider of a commercial service as listed below:

Sheldon Benjamin, M.D.

- Author for and partner in Brain Educators LLC, publishers of The Brain Card®, a neuropsychiatry examination pocket card reference;
- Honorarium: Psychiatry Director, American Board of Psychiatry and Neurology (ABPN);
- Speaking honoraria: various grand rounds lectures

Shamik Bhattacharyya, M.D.

- Consultant, Alexion Pharmaceuticals
- Grant/research support, Alexion Pharmaceuticals, National Institutes of Health, Roche, UCB
- Speaking honoraria, American Academy of Neurology, UpToDate
- Publication/writing honoraria, American Academy of Neurology
- Expert testimony, Merck

Mattia Wruble Clark, M.D.

Grant/research support, Alexion Pharmaceuticals

Bradford Dickerson, M.D., M.M.Sc.

Consultant, Acadia, Alector, Arkuda, Biogen, Eisai, Lilly, Merck, Quanterix

Susan Hutchinson, M.D.

- Consultant/advisory board, AbbVie, Astellas, Biohaven, Impel, Lilly, Lundbeck, Pfizer, Teva, Theranica, Upsher-Smith
- Speaker's bureau, AbbVie, Astellas, Impel, Lilly, Lundbeck

Andres M. Kanner, M.D.

- Consultant, Epilepsy Foundation, Neurelis
- Speaking honoraria, Jazz Pharmaceutical

Douglas I. Katz, M.D.

Co-editor, Springer/Demos Publishing

David L. Perez, M.D., M.M.Sc.

- Honoraria, *Brain and Behavior*
- Royalties, Springer Nature
- Speaking honoraria, Harvard Medical School

Matthew Schrag, M.D., Ph.D.

Consultant, Guidepoint Consulting

The following contributors stated that they had no competing interests during the year preceding manuscript submission:

Oluwatosin Akintola, M.D., Deepti Anbarasan, M.D., X. Michelle Androulakis, M.D., M.S., Miya R. Asato, M.D., Ankur Butala, M.D., L. Nicolas Gonzalez Castro, M.D., Ph.D., Elizabeth DeGrush, D.O., Brigid C. Dwyer, M.D., Mark Eldaief, M.D., M.M.Sc., Lindsey Gurin, M.D., Khurshid A. Khurshid, M.B.B.S., Howard S. Kirshner, M.D., Kevin Kyle, M.B.B.Ch., Mia T. Minen, M.D., M.P.H., Kathy Niu, M.D., Ashley Paul, M.D., M.Ed., Scott W. Powers, Ph.D., Sonali Sharma, M.D., Huma U. Sheikh, M.D., Clay E. Smith, M.D., Alexandra M. Stillman, M.D., Melinda A. Thiam, M.D., Taylor Young, M.D., M.A.

Foreword

Clinical and academic textbooks have great value as milestones in the development of a field and the organization of emerging information for practitioners and academicians. *Psychiatric Neurology*, edited by Sheldon Benjamin and Kathy Niu, fulfills our highest expectations. Textbooks are most important when a field has undergone transformative changes, and that is the case with psychiatric neurology. Advances in therapies across CNS disorders, the emergence of new imaging and fluid biomarkers, and progress in understanding the relationship between behavior and brain function all demand an update of the state of the field. The editors and authors of *Psychiatric Neurology* have risen to the challenge and are to be applauded for updating the science while maintaining a patient focus.

Beginning with the basics of psychiatric evaluation (including history, examination, and formulation) and proceeding to the neuropsychiatric workup, the first two chapters of *Psychiatric Neurology* build a strong foundation of clinical expertise informed by emerging neuroscience including imaging, biomarkers, and therapeutics. The volume transitions from fundamentals to a detailed discussion of psychiatric presentations of neurological disease in Chapter 3, including visual hallucinations, delusions, catatonia, apathy, effective liability, aggressive behavior, and pain. Each of these represents a significant challenge for the clinician. The emphasis is on the differential diagnosis and evaluation of commonly observed syndromes presenting in the clinic. The interface between the clinician and the patient is at the heart of these discussions.

Psychiatric Neurology presents in detail the major neurological disorders, beginning with dementia in Chapter 4. There has been tremendous progress in understanding Alzheimer disease and other dementia syndromes. Biomarkers are now available for the diagnosis of Alzheimer. The recognition of Parkinson disease dementia, dementia with Lewy bodies, and frontotemporal dementia depends on clinician expertise and careful examination. These key areas are emphasized, and tools are provided to the clinician reader.

Traumatic brain injury, both civilian and military, represents an evolving area of psychiatric neurology and is covered in Chapter 5. Head trauma occurs in a variety of circumstances, such as battlefield exposures, contact sports, domestic violence, and vehicle accidents. The injury may be a one-time event with gradual recovery or part of a history of repetitive head injury and possible evolution into chronic traumatic encephalopathy. All of these areas of traumatic brain injury have unifying and distinguishing features addressed in this chapter.

Toxins, substances, and nutritional conditions, the subject of Chapter 6, are increasingly recognized as sources of neuropsychiatric symptoms and are well presented in *Psychiatric Neurology*. Evaluation and treatment of alcohol, cannabinoids, opioids, and nutritional disorders are discussed.

Chapter 7 delves into neurodevelopmental disorders, among the most challenging of clinical conditions with neuropsychiatric syndromes. These include a wide variety of genetic disorders as well as early-occurring brain insults. Expert management requires recognition of the disorder, characterization of the neuropsychiatric symptoms, and accommodation for the developmental context of the child. The overlap of Down syndrome with Alzheimer disease, the recognition of increased dementia risk with a variety of childhood-onset disorders, and the management of neurodevelopmental disorders that continue in adulthood such as autism have added new complexities and new opportunities for the care of individuals with this group of disorders.

Epilepsy is among the main disorders evaluated by the neuropsychiatric practitioner. As presented in Chapter 8, the many manifestations of focal epilepsy and the neuropsychiatric complications of focal seizures are both common and challenging. Generalized seizures add complexity to considerations of epilepsy diagnosis and management. A repertoire of anti-epileptic therapies and treatments for disorders accompanying epilepsy is presented in detail.

Movement disorders are common in neuropsychiatric practice. Diagnosis of both the movement disorder and the associated neuropsychiatric symptoms is reviewed in Chapter 9. Cognitive impairment is often present, and psychosis with delusions and hallucinations is among the drug-related disorders seen in Parkinson disease. Dementia with Lewy bodies has a diverse repertoire of neuropsychiatric symptoms, including delusions, visual hallucinations, auditory hallucinations, and depression. REM sleep behavior disorder is overrepresented among patients with movement disorders.

Functional neurological disorders, the subject of Chapter 10, are challenging and rewarding for the expert clinician. Patients are disabled and commonly have both psychiatric and neurologic manifestations of their illnesses. Substantial expertise is required in the management of these patients to optimize their function. A number of helpful diagnostic maneuvers are discussed.

Evaluation and treatment of headaches (Chapter 11) can be subtle, and the clinical diagnoses are complex. The chapter authors have broken down the necessary diagnostic challenges and included multiple tables for clarity.

Neuroinfectious diseases (such as HIV-related syndromes) are part of the practice of any neuropsychiatric clinician and are covered in Chapter 12. Treatments for the infections and neuropsychiatric symptoms are available and require expert management. The challenges associated with the neuropsychopharmacology of infectious disorders are well presented, putting new tools into the hands of the clinician.

Progress in neuro-oncology is making its way into neuropsychiatric practice, as shown in Chapter 13. Even severe brain tumors such as glioblastoma have new therapies appropriate under some circumstances. Meningiomas presenting with seizures and childhood tumors represent a specialized area of neuropsychiatric practice for which *Psychiatric Neurology* provides guidance.

Neuroimmunological syndromes are another mainstay in the practice of neurologically informed psychiatry and are covered in Chapter 14. Multiple sclerosis (MS) is among the most common neuropsychiatric disorders encountered and may present or cause depression, psychosis, anxiety, and other rarer behavioral syndromes. Disorders such as lupus affect brain function and must be managed with care and expertise. There has been substantial progress in disease-targeted therapies as well as symptom management for MS and other immunological disorders. Expert application of these new treatments changes the lives of patients and restores quality of life. Psychiatric consultants will appreciate the up-to-date coverage in this chapter.

Sleep disorders (Chapter 15) are manifestations of many types of neurologic disorders. They are particularly common in patients with Parkinson disease and dementia with Lewy bodies but also occur in Alzheimer disease and many other CNS conditions. Disorders such as REM sleep behavior disorder may present a physical threat to the bed partner; sleep disorders such as excessive daytime sleepiness and insomnia compromise patient function and require expert management. Consultants will find this chapter particularly useful.

Neurovascular disorders and stroke present with focal neurological syndromes such as aphasia, apraxia, and agnosia, or sometimes with more generalized cognitive decline, such as vascular cognitive impairment or vascular dementia. Imaging is an important tool for the management of cerebrovascular disease, and both symptomatic and preventive management of brain ischemia have important effects on patient outcomes. Chapter 16 guides the clinician through decision-making for these disorders.

Altogether, *Psychiatric Neurology* represents a terrific update on neuropsychiatric disorders and provides the clinician and academician with a wide variety of diagnostic and management tools. Psychiatrists, neurologists, neuropsychologists, geriatricians, and others engaged in the care of patients with neuropsychiatric syndromes will find *Psychiatric Neurology* to be a valuable resource. Clinicians will benefit from this organized presentation of current information, and patients and families will benefit from the application of lessons learned from this important text.

Jeffrey L. Cummings, M.D., Sc.D.
Joy Chambers-Grundy Professor of Brain Sciences
Director, Chambers-Grundy Center
for Transformative Neuroscience
Kirk Kerkorian School of Medicine
University of Nevada, Las Vegas

Preface

Why psychiatric neurology? The practice of psychiatry has evolved. Psychiatrists increasingly care for large populations via allied health professionals, consulting on outlier cases as needed. They are called on to provide consultation to increasingly ill medical patients during shorter hospitalizations. More than ever, psychiatric clinicians must be able to recognize neurologic diseases that cause psychiatric and behavioral symptoms, often ordering or suggesting the tests that will lead to diagnosis. The increasing precision of neurodiagnostic testing means that psychiatric clinicians are consulting on patients with neurological disorders that may have eluded diagnosis a decade ago. These disorders may co-occur with cognitive or psychiatric conditions, or they themselves may present as neuropsychiatric disorders.

Psychiatric trainees are now required to achieve competency in clinical neuroscience (Benjamin et al. 2014), and several authors have suggested approaches to neuropsychiatric education in support of those milestones (Benjamin 2013; Cooper and Walker 2021; Cooper et al. 2024; Jacoby et al. 2023; Schildkrout et al. 2016, 2023). In past years, U.S. psychiatrists seldom had more experience than the 2 months of neurology required for board certification, because this knowledge was considered to be of little practical use in psychiatry. Now, however, neuropsychiatry and neurology knowledge are among the hallmarks of a well-trained general psychiatrist. This book adds to the tools available for the neurological and neuropsychiatric education of psychiatric clinicians.

It is precisely because of the evolving role of psychiatric clinicians that we have created *Psychiatric Neurology*. The book begins with the basics: how to perform the neuropsychiatric examination; how to use the neurodiagnostic laboratory; and how to think through the differential diagnosis of problems commonly seen by psychiatric clinicians: visual hallucinations, new-onset psychosis, catatonia, apathy, affective lability, aggression, and pain syndromes. For the remainder of the book, the editors have invited content experts to prepare chapters that summarize both neurological diagnoses and their neuropsychiatric manifestations.

The book is not comprehensive. Its focus is on accurate evaluation and diagnosis rather than treatment. When treatment is discussed, it is done with attention to basic strategy rather than specific details of biological or psychotherapeutic methods. The editors have chosen to omit chapters on myelopathies, neuropathies, and myopathies, focusing instead on the neurological disorders most likely to be seen by psychiatric clinicians: dementia, traumatic brain injury, substances of abuse and related nutritional deficiencies, neurodevelopmental disorders, epilepsy, movement disorders, functional neurological disorder, headache, CNS infections, brain tumors, neuroimmunology, sleep disorders, and neurovascular disorders. Each chapter is framed by an example case vignette, starting with a case presentation and ending with case resolution; the body of the chapter contains the core content. A few summary points and review questions are included at the end of each chapter.

The editors came to know one another when one of them (KN) entered combined neurology/psychiatry training at UMass Chan Medical School under the direction of the other (SB). The editors completed residencies and board certification in both psychiatry and neurology out of a conviction that increased skill at neurological diagnosis would make them better psychiatrists and that people with neuropsychiatric disorders deserve physicians with specialized training at the interface of the two fields. They have both focused their careers on neuropsychiatric education to make the kind of knowledge represented in this textbook more widely available to clinicians.

Several of the chapters (substances and nutrition, epilepsy, movement disorders, functional neurologic disorders, neuroinfectious disease, and sleep disorders) were coauthored by neuropsychiatrists who similarly were trained in both fields and certified in both specialties by the American Board of Psychiatry and Neurology. Many of the authors are also certified in Behavioral Neurology and Neuropsychiatry by the United Council on Neurological Subspecialties. Five of the chapter authors (Drs. Anbarasan, Benjamin, DeDrush, Gurin, and Niu) are or have been psychiatry or combined neurology/psychiatry residency directors in addition to having been trained in both fields.

Although there are many neuropsychiatry and behavioral neurology textbooks, this book—written by clinician-educators—focuses on relevant basic neurology for the psychiatric clinician. We hope the passion expressed by the authors in this volume may lead the reader to explore more deeply the interface of these two fields, increase their neurodiagnostic skills, and stimulate curiosity about the universe of brain-behavior relationships.

References

Benjamin S: Educating psychiatry residents in neuropsychiatry and neuroscience. Int Rev Psychiatry 25(3):265–275, 2013 23859089

Benjamin S, Widge A, Shaw K: Neuropsychiatry and neuroscience milestones for general psychiatry trainees. Acad Psychiatry 38(3):275–282, 2014 24715675

Cooper JJ, Walker AE: Neuroscience education: making it relevant to psychiatric training. Psychiatr Clin North Am 44(2):295–307, 2021 34049650

Cooper JJ, Valencia VA, Niu K: Neuroimaging education in psychiatric training. Neuropsychopharmacology 50(1):298–304, 2024 39025952

Jacoby N, Gullick M, Sullivan N, et al: Development and evaluation of an innovative neurology e-learning didactic curriculum for psychiatry residents. Acad Psychiatry 47(3):237–244, 2023 36918470

Schildkrout B, Benjamin S, Lauterbach MD: Integrating neuroscience knowledge and neuropsychiatric skills into psychiatry: the way forward. Acad Med 91(5):650–656, 2016 26630604

Schildkrout B, Niu K, Cooper JJ: Clinical neuroscience continuing education for psychiatrists. Acad Psychiatry 47(3):297–303, 2023 37106262

1

The Neuropsychiatric Evaluation

History, Examination, Formulation

Sheldon Benjamin, M.D.

Neuropsychiatric evaluation, like other medical evaluations, includes the patient's history, a physical examination, and relevant laboratory findings. The neuropsychiatry formulation, however, is adapted to demonstrate brain-behavior relationships and synthesizes data from the history; physical, mental, and cognitive status examinations; available laboratory data; neuroimaging; and neuropsychological data. In this chapter, I address the neuropsychiatric history, examination, and formulation. For a guide to the use of laboratory tests and neuroimaging in neuropsychiatric evaluation, see Chapter 2, "The Neuropsychiatric Evaluation: Work-Up." Diagnosis-specific examination tips are also included in each chapter of this book.

Approach to Patients With Neuropsychiatric Symptoms

The neuropsychiatric examination is adapted according to the purpose of the evaluation, the patient's cognitive level, and the evolving diagnostic hypotheses being considered by the examiner. The consultant uses different examination approaches for patients who are unresponsive, uncooperative, demented, acutely ill, highly intelligent, intellectually disabled, autistic, violent, or catatonic, as well as for children or elderly patients. For example, asking a highly intelligent individual to perform single-digit addition or asking an individual with intellectual developmental disorder to interpret complex proverbs may not make sense. When examining the limb of a violent individual, it may be prudent to ask a staff member to hold the opposite limb for safety and approach the person from an oblique angle. When evaluating a person suspected of memory loss, the examiner can include cues to help the patient recall the examiner's name when introducing themself. Examinations for forensic evaluation, risk assessment, rehabilitation planning, or vocational assessment are also each structured differently. Sitting at the patient's eye level is preferred for the interview. The examiner should sit in the patient's "good" hemifield in the case of hemianopia, hemi-neglect, or hemi-inattention.

The Neuropsychiatric History

Gathering the neuropsychiatric history is an opportunity to begin building an alliance by understanding symptoms from the patient's perspective. Table 1.1 enumerates areas to include in a neuropsychiatric history and review of systems.

A skilled examiner forms a diagnostic hypothesis at the outset of each patient interaction and uses the examination to refine the hypothesis in real time. The history addresses whether the symptoms are acquired or pre-existing, single-episode or recurrent, and progressive or static. Behavior patterns consistent with known syndromes are noted, and evidence of neurological, medical, or psychiatric causes of the chief complaint or consultation question is used to further refine the history. Any hint of risk to self or others in the past is followed up with detailed inquiry. A good practice for avoiding omissions is to perform the examination in the same order as it is recorded and presented. While gathering the history, the examiner should be alert to

Table 1.1 Areas of inquiry in the neuropsychiatric history

Psychiatric/behavioral history	• Psychiatric disorders (hospitalizations, psychopharmacology and psychotherapy) • Aggressive behavior (age at onset, description/type, episode length, time of day, clear onset/offset, prodrome, precipitant, pattern, purpose, environmental factors) • Past danger to self or others
Medical history	• Medical and surgical history • Allergies, medication reactions
Neurological history	• Traumatic brain injuries (length of loss of consciousness, retrograde/anterograde amnesia, initial Glasgow Coma Scale, deficits, description of any hemorrhages or surgical intervention) • Seizures (cause if known; age at onset; frequency; longest seizure-free interval; details of semiology, including aura, automatisms, peri-ictal, post-ictal, and interictal behaviors; incontinence; injuries; EEG and MRI findings; antiseizure medication history) • Stroke (age, etiology, location, sequelae) • CNS infection/HIV-associated neurocognitive disorder • Pre-existing neurological deficits • Dementia (onset; rate of progression; risk factors; cognitive/personality deficits; motor involvement; contributions from sensory deprivation; genes/biomarkers) • Demyelinating diseases • Autoimmune disorders • Sleep disorders • Pain syndromes
Family history	Psychiatric, neurological, medical disease
Neurodevelopmental history	• In utero exposure, birth history • Known congenital or developmental syndromes • Handedness • Developmental milestones • Intellectual developmental disorder/learning disorder

Table 1.1 **Areas of inquiry in the neuropsychiatric history (*continued*)**

Social history	• Housing • Substance history • Education (highest level attained, best and worst subjects in school, grades, support needed) • Occupational history (description, longest-held jobs, environmental exposures) • Special skills • Household members • Partner(s), children • Means of support, disability income • Legal history (arrests, lawsuits, incarceration) • Military history (years of service, highest rank, combat exposure, injuries, service-connected disability) • Access to firearms • Trauma history
Neuropsychiatric review of systems	• Behavior changes • Motor symptoms and involuntary movements • Paroxysmal and periodic symptoms • Sleep symptoms • Cognitive symptoms • Neurovegetative functions • Endocrine symptoms • Rheumatological symptoms • ADLs and iADLs

ADLs = activities of daily living; CNS = central nervous system; EEG = electroencephalogram; HIV = human immunodeficiency virus; iADLs = instrumental ADLs; MRI = magnetic resonance imaging.

any aspects that do not fit their hypothesis and pursue those leads. It is helpful to have ready differential diagnoses of common neuropsychiatric presentations available, such as those listed in Table 1.2.

The examiner should be alert not only to the patterns of common neurological disorders but also to patterns characteristic of rare conditions. Rare disorders, taken together, affect approximately 1 in 15 people worldwide. These patterns include the following (Lauterbach et al. 2016):

- First presentation of a major psychiatric disorder with onset outside the usual age for that disorder

Table 1.2 Common neuropsychiatric presentations

Condition	Variations
Delirium	
Catatonia	Catatonic excitement Neuroleptic malignant syndrome Serotonin syndrome Autoimmune limbic encephalitis
Aggressive behavior	New-onset aggression in nonverbal individuals Self-injurious behavior Aggression related to cognitive deficits
Posttraumatic brain injury syndromes	
Autism or autistic features	
Intellectual developmental disorder with dysmorphic features	
Dementia	Dementia with extrapyramidal features Dementia with weakness or incoordination Dementia with prominent behavioral changes Dementia with prominent language changes Dementia with seizures
Stereotyped paroxysmal phenomena	
Alcohol-related conditions	
Sleep disorders (insomnia, hypersomnia, parasomnia)	
Frontal/dysexecutive syndromes	
Multiple CNS deficits	

- Major personality change
- Sudden symptom onset in a previously asymptomatic individual
- New psychiatric symptoms in the context of a steep decline in cognitive or functional level, especially in adolescence or young adulthood
- Stereotyped behavioral episodes
- Onset in proximity to or in the context of a medical or neurological condition
- Presence of dysmorphic features, birthmarks, or focal signs on neurological examination
- Family history of a rare disease

The Neuropsychiatric Examination

General Examination

After the clinician has checked vital signs, the examination may take different forms depending on the purpose of the examination and the person being evaluated. Preparation of specialized examinations for the types of evaluations listed in Table 1.2 is helpful. Note any face or limb asymmetry or abnormally large or small head size. In the setting of intellectual developmental disorder or autism spectrum disorder, the clinician should become familiar with frequently occurring phenotypes and observe for dysmorphic features as listed in Chapter 7, "Neurodevelopmental Disorders." Midline defects such as hypertelorism, for instance, are occasionally found in partial agenesis of the corpus callosum. The Face2Gene.com smartphone app, online rare disease databases such as OMIM and Orphanet (Amberger 2019; Rath 2012) and genetic references (Firth and Hurst 2017; Hamosh et al. 2005; Jones et al. 2013) can be helpful in evaluating neurodevelopmental syndromes. A differential diagnostic approach to psychotic syndromes can be found in Chapter 3, "Neurological Approach to Psychiatric Presentations."

The clinician should note the presence of alopecia, hirsutism, rashes, and birthmarks. The common ectodermal origin of the skin and brain gives rise to the dermatological abnormalities of the neurocutaneous syndromes. These syndromes commonly include seizures and learning disorders but also occur in the absence of neurological symptoms, especially in the carrier state. The most common neurocutaneous syndromes are described in Chapter 7.

The clinician should note risk factors for obstructive sleep apnea (see Chapter 15, "Sleep Disorders"), including small oropharyngeal opening and large neck and upper torso size. Atrophic glossitis, if seen, may be a clue to B_{12} deficiency. Arrhythmias or cardiac murmurs on cardiovascular examination may indicate an increased risk for stroke or vascular dementia (see Chapter 16, "Neurovascular Disorders"). The combination of rash and joint pain, swelling, or deformity can be seen in rheumatological disease (see Chapter 14, "Neuroimmunology").

Neurological Examination

Cranial Nerves

Table 1.3 provides instructions for the cranial nerve examination. Videos 1.1, 1.2, 1.3, and 1.4 illustrate aspects of the oculomotor examination. (To access all videos mentioned in this book, go to https://www.appi.org/Benjamin.)

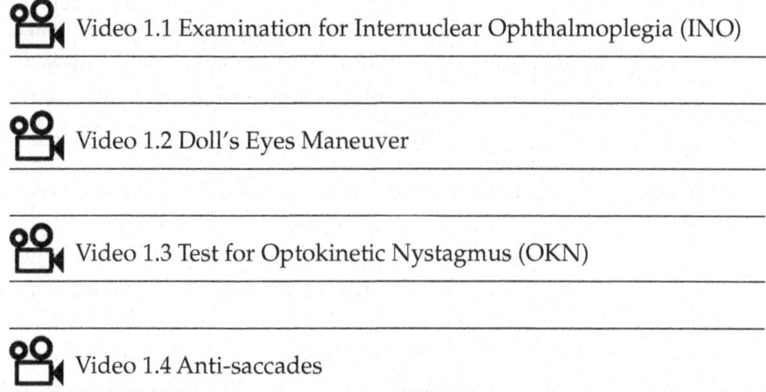

Video 1.1 Examination for Internuclear Ophthalmoplegia (INO)

Video 1.2 Doll's Eyes Maneuver

Video 1.3 Test for Optokinetic Nystagmus (OKN)

Video 1.4 Anti-saccades

Diminished olfaction in the absence of cigarette smoking or chronic rhinitis may be seen in traumatic brain injury, viral syndromes, neurodegenerative diseases, demyelinating disease, and orbitofrontal tumors. The combination of decreased vision and anosmia is seen in Foster Kennedy syndrome caused by unilateral compressive frontal tumors. In the presence of memory loss, fundoscopic signs of vascular pathology such as arteriovenous nicking, arteriolar narrowing, or hemorrhages may raise suspicion of vascular dementia.

Table 1.3 Examination of cranial nerves and associated structures

Nerve and test	Technique
I Olfactory	
Olfaction	Use tube of scented lip balm, scratch-and sniff cards (Doty 2015), or Sniffn' Sticks (Rumeau et al. 2016) for each nostril.
II Optic	
Retina	Direct visualization with fundoscopy: check for central venous pulsations, retinal hemorrhages, yellow refractile Hollenhorst plaques, arteriovenous nicking, arteriolar narrowing, and disc pallor.
Light perception (pupils)	Shine a flashlight first at one pupil then at the other while observing for direct and consensual pupillary responses. Afferent pupillary defect is diagnosed if the pupil constricts when light is shined in the opposite eye, then dilates when the light swings over it. Record pupillary diameters in mm for future comparison, commenting on amount of ambient light at time of observation.
Visual acuity	Use a Snellen card held 14 inches from each eye.
Visual fields to confrontation	With both eyes open, the patient indicates when they see the examiner's wiggling finger moving in from the periphery in each quadrant. Follow with detailed testing of each eye if findings are abnormal. If hemianopia is detected, test for macula involvement by holding a red-tipped stimulus (e.g., a pen top) behind a white stimulus (e.g., applicator stick) and moving the red stimulus laterally just outside the edge of the white stimulus. Failure to detect the red stimulus indicates macular involvement.
Double simultaneous stimulation	Patient indicates which finger is moving as examiner moves fingers on both sides simultaneously.

Table 1.3 Examination of cranial nerves and associated structures (*continued*)

Nerve and test	Technique
Color blindness	Assess by using Ishihara plates or a smartphone app such as Color Test containing pseudochromatic test stimuli.
Dysconjugate gaze	In addition to asking about diplopia during eye movement examination, shine a light obliquely at both eyes to see if it aligns on both pupils at the same "o'clock" location.
III Oculomotor, IV Trochlear, VI Abducens	
Ocular muscles	Patient follows examiner's finger as the shape of an H is traced in the air to isolate functions of the ocular muscles. If the eyes do not smoothly follow the examiner's finger, saccadic pursuits or square wave jerks may indicate cerebellar dysfunction or parkinsonism.
Nystagmus	Observe for sustained nystagmus on lateral gaze.
Internuclear ophthalmoplegia (INO)	Direct the patient to look quickly from one of the examiner's laterally outstretched hands to the other and back. An INO is diagnosed if the adducting eye does not move beyond the midline and the abducting eye develops nystagmus. See Video 1.1 for INO examination.
Supranuclear palsy	Supranuclear palsy is diagnosed if the patient cannot move their eyes to command but moves them in response to vestibulo-occular reflex (doll's eyes) testing. See Video 1.2 for doll's head maneuver.
Ptosis	Describe ptosis in relation to the pupil (e.g., ptosis to midpupil). Prolonged upgaze is included to screen for myasthenic eyelid fatigue.

Table 1.3 Examination of cranial nerves and associated structures (*continued*)

Nerve and test	Technique
Optokinetic nystagmus (OKN)	Pass a cloth with wide stripes horizontally in front of the patient's eyes while instructing the patient to count the stripes silently as they pass by. Failure to direct one's gaze to the approaching stripe (quick component) may indicate ipsilateral frontal dysfunction; failure to follow the moving stripe (slow component) may indicate ipsilateral dysfunction at the temporo-parieto-occipital junction. The OKN test may be used to estimate vision in infants or to demonstrate vision in visual loss due to FND. OKN may also be tested with a rotating OKN drum or a smartphone app such as OKN Strips. See Video 1.3 for a demonstration of OKN testing.
Antisaccades	After testing ocular movements, instruct the patient to move their eyes in the direction opposite the movement of the examiner's finger. Failure on this task indicates stimulus-bound behavior seen in frontal dysfunction. See Video 1.4 for demonstration of antisaccade test.
Visual grasp	Observe for prolonged visual fixation on a target as seen in posterior cortical atrophy and occasionally in Alzheimer disease.
V Trigeminal	
Light touch/pin prick	Touch (not stroke) soft stimulus and pointed stimulus in the three facial dermatomes. In an unresponsive or delirious patient, the afferent arc of V1 can be assessed by testing the corneal reflex, V2 by tickling the inner nares, and V3 by eliciting the jaw jerk.
Motor	Palpate the jaw as the patient clenches the jaw and grinds side to side. Tap a finger on the chin with a reflex hammer. Exaggerated jaw jerk may indicate upper motor neuron lesion.

Table 1.3 Examination of cranial nerves and associated structures (*continued*)

Nerve and test	Technique
VII Facial	
Upper division	Instruct the patient to raise their eyebrows while testing vertical gaze to command and then ask them to tightly shut their eyes. If skin wrinkles, resistance testing is not needed.
Lower division	Instruct patient to smile and puff out their cheeks.
Cortical vs. limbic control	Cortical: Check patient's smile to command. Limbic: Check patient's spontaneous smile (e.g., after hearing a joke).
VIII Vestibulocochlear	
Acoustic	Assess patient's perception of finger rubs, a 512 Hz tuning fork, or whisper in each ear.
	Weber test: In a quiet room, touch a lightly vibrating 512 Hz tuning fork to the forehead and ask whether the sound seems to come from one side more than the other. Sound appears louder on the side with conductive loss or contralateral to the side with unilateral sensorineural hearing loss. Follow with Rinne test.
	Rinne test: In a quiet room with the opposite ear covered, touch a vibrating 512 Hz tuning fork stem to the mastoid process and instruct the patient to state immediately when the sound ceases. At that moment, move the tuning fork over the ear canal. If the sound is still heard, the test is positive (normal). If the sound is not heard, the test is negative and suggests a conductive hearing loss on that side.
IX Glossopharyngeal, X Vagus	
Swallow/gag	Touch the back of the throat with an applicator stick. Have the patient drink a tumbler full of water without stopping (to assess aspiration risk).

Table 1.3 Examination of cranial nerves and associated structures (*continued*)

Nerve and test	Technique
XI Accessory	
Shoulder shrug/head turn	Ask the patient to shrug their shoulders and turn their head against resistance.
XII Hypoglossal	
Tongue	Observe the tongue for deviation at rest and on protrusion. Strength can be tested by pushing tongue into cheek against resistance.

FND = functional neurological disorder.

In addition to testing oculomotor function by following the examiner's finger, assessment for supranuclear gaze palsy is easily added. Inability to move eyes vertically on command despite preserved doll's eyes phenomenon with passive head movement (Video 1.2) is consistent with supranuclear gaze palsy, seen in progressive supranuclear palsy (PSP), most common in middle-age males; in Niemann Pick disease type C, typically occurring in young people; and in Whipple's disease. Internuclear ophthalmoplegia is seen in demyelinating disease and brainstem strokes affecting the medial longitudinal fasciculus. Sustained nystagmus on lateral gaze is seen in metabolic disorders, medication toxicity, and brainstem and cerebellar lesions.

Facial strength is tested in both the upper and the lower face because the upper face receives bilateral facial nerve innervation and the lower face receives crossed unilateral innervation. An intact smile on command coupled with an asymmetric spontaneous smile has been associated with lesions in the contralateral limbic system, basal ganglia, or supplementary motor area (Hopf et al. 1992). Lower motor neuron facial weakness may have many causes, including autoimmune disease or prior Bell's palsy, that typically result in a widened palpebral fissure and drooping of the corner of the mouth on the affected side.

To differentiate whether unilateral hearing loss is conductive or sensorineural, the examiner can perform the Weber test, followed by the Rinne test (these tests do not replace audiological testing).

If the patient's speech is dysarthric, weakness of the labial, lingual, or guttural speech muscles can be identified by having the patient repeat the sounds "pa," "ta," and "ka," respectively, over and over separately and together as "pa-ta-ka." Scanning speech due to cerebellar dysfunction may be elicited by having the patient say a prolonged "ahh" and listening for variability in volume and pitch.

Although the gag reflex is commonly used to test the ninth and tenth cranial nerves, a more useful test is watching the patient drink a full tumbler of water without pausing, to see if they cough. Dysphagia is a common source of morbidity in patients with neuropsychiatric movement disorders. An upper-motor-neuron hypoglossal lesion causes deviation away from the side of the lesion when the tongue is protruded. A lower-motor-neuron lesion would cause the tongue to deviate toward the side of the lesion and result in fasciculations and lateralized atrophy. Upper- and lower-motor-neuron hypoglossal weakness can be seen in bulbar amyotrophic lateral sclerosis (ALS).

Bilateral corticobulbar tract lesions can result in *pseudobulbar palsy*, named for their simulation of damage to the cranial nerve nuclei. Pseudobulbar palsy includes dysarthria, dysphagia, hyperactive jaw jerk and gag reflex, and affective lability. The affective lability of pseudobulbar palsy is also known as pseudobulbar affect, pathological laughing and crying, or emotional incontinence. Pseudobulbar palsy is commonly seen in ALS, demyelinating disease, traumatic brain injury, neurodegenerative disorders, and stroke.

Motor Examination

When examining someone who presents a risk of physical assault, it is preferable to perform the elemental neurological examination while remaining beyond the reach of the patient's arm or leg. Set up the examination space to allow sufficient room to approach the patient obliquely, bending forward to perform the motor and sensory components as illustrated in Video 1.5. It may be necessary to ask an assistant to hold the opposite extremity during the examination. Parts of the examination that cannot be performed safely may be postponed until the patient is better able to cooperate.

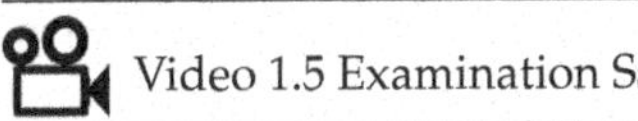
Video 1.5 Examination Safety

Muscle tone may be decreased in cerebellar or peripheral nerve dysfunction and increased in corticospinal tract damage or basal ganglia dysfunction. Increased tone can be described as lead pipe, cogwheel, or clasped knife. *Lead pipe rigidity*, consistently increased resistance to flexion regardless of force applied or speed of extremity movement, is seen in extrapyramidal dysfunction. *Cogwheel rigidity* is caused by the combination of tremor and rigidity and is characteristic of parkinsonian syndromes. The rigidity of catatonia is discussed later in this section. *Clasped knife rigidity,* in which resistance to flexion varies with the force and speed of contraction against resistance and may include the sudden give way of the flexed extremity, is a sign of chronic corticospinal tract damage. Paratonia refers either to the *gegenhalten rigidity* of diffuse frontal dysfunction or catatonia in which there is involuntary resistance to passive flexion in proportion to the force applied, or to *mitgehen* (overcooperation with limb movement), as seen in catatonia. Increased tone may be brought out by an activating maneuver such as having the patient move the contralateral extremity in a broad arc while the examiner flexes the ipsilateral extremity, as shown in Video 1.6.

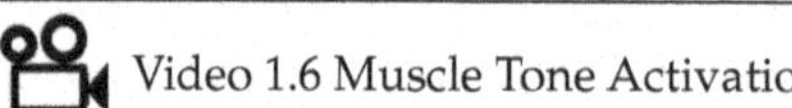

After examining the extremities for bulk, muscle tone, strength to resistive testing, deep tendon reflexes, and fine finger movements, the clinician should attempt to elicit pathological reflexes that can indicate upper motor neuron damage (Figure 1.1). The Babinski sign or extensor plantar response is obtained by stroking the sole of the foot with a blunt stimulus along the length of the lateral aspect of the sole and turning medially below the base of the toes. The Babinski sign is present if the big toe extends and the other toes flex or fan out. If the plantar response is equivocal or elicits marked withdrawal, the examiner may use alternative maneuvers such as the Gordon (squeeze the calf muscle), Chaddock (stroke the lateral aspect of the foot), or Oppenheim (stroke the tibia between two knuckles) maneuvers. Inability to suppress eye blinking after five glabella taps (from above and outside the visual field) is known as Myerson's sign and may be seen in Parkinson disease or diffuse frontal dysfunction (Video 1.7). Forced grasping, and the related groping response toward objects within the visual field, have been associated with dysfunction of the medial prefrontal and supplementary motor areas. The grasp response is elicited by lightly stroking the patient's outstretched palm between thumb and forefinger while reminding the patient not to hold on (Video 1.8). Forced grasping, typically seen in concert with paratonia, is diagnosed when the patient grasps increasingly more tightly onto the examiner's fingers as

Plantar reflex
Stroke the sole of the foot with a blunt stimulus such as the wooden end of an applicator stick as shown. The Babinski response occurs when the big toe extends and the other toes flare.

Gordon reflex
Squeeze the calf muscle and observe for movement of the big toe.

Chaddock reflex
Stroke the lateral aspect of the foot as shown and observe for movement of the big toe.

Oppenheim reflex
Stroke the medial aspect of the tibia by running the knuckles down the tibia bone as shown and observe for movement of the big toe.

Glabellar tap
Tap the area between the supraorbital ridges (the glabella) with a finger from outside the field of vision. An abnormal finding, known as Myerson's sign, consists of an inability to suppress eye blinking within a few taps.

Grasp reflex
Touch/stroke the patient's outstretched hand between the thumb and forefinger. An abnormal "forced" grasp occurs when the patient tightly grasps the examiner's finger and cannot let go when instructed not to hold on.

Foot grasp
Hold the reflex hammer in front of the patient's exposed foot in view of the patient. An abnormal response consists of the toes splaying out as if trying to grasp the object. If one then holds the hammer against the sole of the foot, the toes curl around the object in a frontal grasp response.

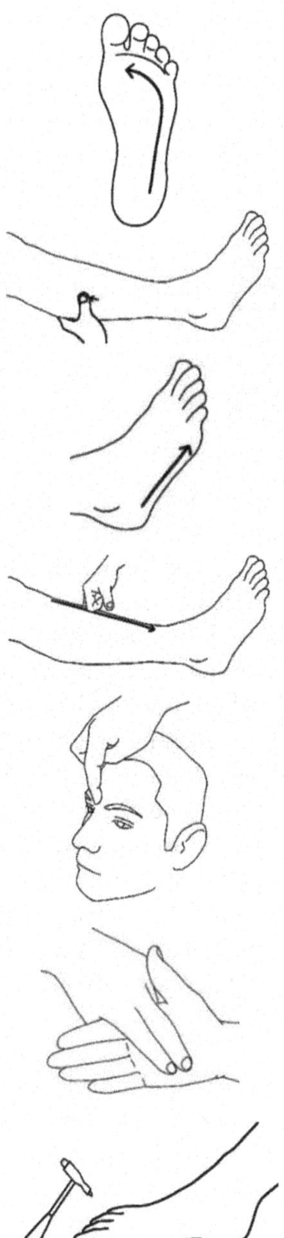

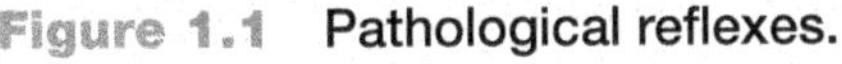

Figure 1.1 Pathological reflexes.

the examiner attempts to pull away. An analogous pathological reflex in the lower extremity, the *foot grasp,* may be elicited by stroking the sole of the foot of the seated patient with the side of the reflex hammer and then holding the hammer in front of the patient's foot. A positive response consists of the foot extending toward the hammer and the toes curling as if to grasp it.

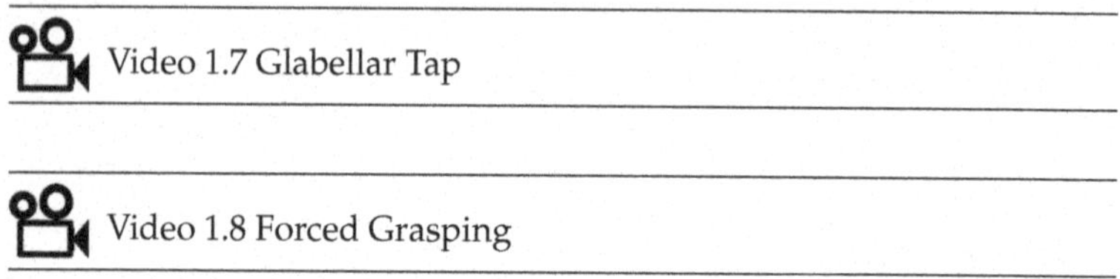

Primitive reflexes (Figure 1.2) are nonspecific indicators of brain dysfunction, so named because they also occur in infants. The *palmomental reflex,* elicited by stroking the thenar eminence of the palm and observing for ipsilateral mentalis muscle contraction under the lower lip, may be seen in both normal and abnormal brains. The *snout reflex* is elicited by tapping the philtrum with the reflex hammer; the *rooting reflex* is elicited by touching the corner of the mouth; and the *suck reflex* is elicited by touching an object to the lips.

Gegenhalten rigidity or paratonia, a release sign seen in catatonia and dementia, refers to variably increasing muscle resistance in proportion to the force or speed with which the examiner moves the patient's limb. An extreme form of Gegenhalten seen in the end stage of dementia is known as *paraplegia in flexion.* In this condition the patient's legs are permanently flexed.

Signs of cerebellar dysfunction include the following (Bodranghien et al. 2016):

- Saccadic intrusions and square-wave jerks when oculomotor movement is assessed
- Scanning speech
- Dysarthria on the "pa-ta-ka" test
- Decreased muscle tone
- Decreased check response during pronator drift and reflex testing
- Irregular performance on rapidly alternating movements
- End of movement dysmetria when reaching toward an object
- Difficulty smoothly following a target with a finger (Video 1.9)

Palmomental reflex
Stroke the palm with the wooden side of an applicator stick from the thenar eminence, beginning at the wrist and moving toward the base of the thumb, while watching the patient's mouth. The reflex, which can occur in both normal and neurologically impaired individuals, consists of ipsilateral wrinkling of the orbicularis oris and mentalis muscles.

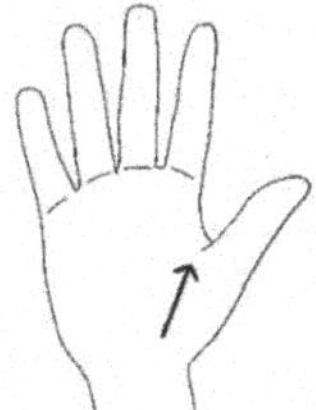

Snout reflex
Lightly tap the upper lip. The reflex consists of the two lips thrusting forward to form a snout.

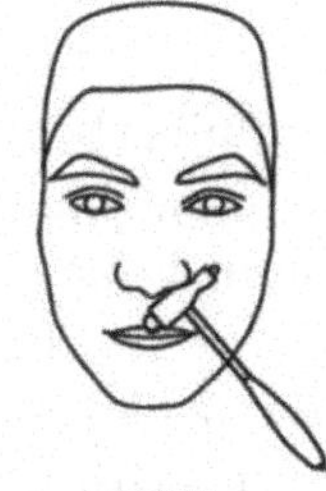

Rooting reflex
Touch the corner of the mouth. The reflex consists of the head turning toward the stimulus.

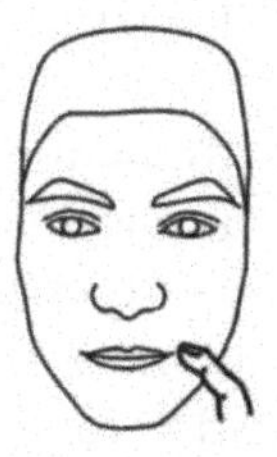

Sucking reflex
Lightly tap a tongue depressor laid vertically across the lips. In advanced dementia, the reflex may occur merely by approaching the lips with an object.

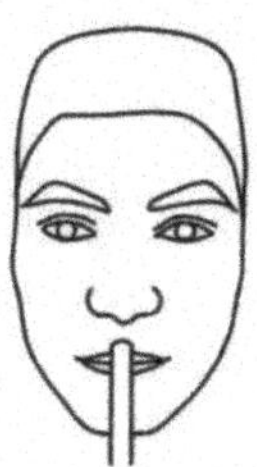

Figure 1.2 Primitive reflexes.

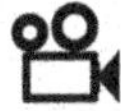 Video 1.9 Dysmetria Test

When performing the finger-nose-finger test for dysmetria, including a finger chase component brings out latent dysmetria. In this test, the examiner moves their finger in different directions, including movements that force the patient to extend their hand (Video 1.10). Cerebellar cognitive affective syndrome or Schmahmann syndrome (Bodranghien et al. 2016) features cognitive and affective equivalents of motor abnormalities (e.g., cognitive and affective dysmetria) and should be considered in patients with cerebellar motor findings and neuropsychiatric features (Schmahmann et al. 2007).

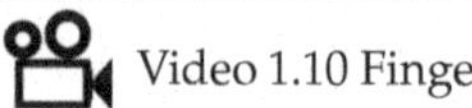 Video 1.10 Finger-Nose-Finger Test with Finger Chase Component

The examiner begins to assess for movement disorders from the moment they see the patient. Decreased movement may be due to depression, delirium, catatonia, stroke, basal ganglia lesions, metabolic disorders, drug side effects, or extrapyramidal disorders. Increased movement may be seen in psychomotor agitation, mania, ADHD, Tourette disorder,[1] tic disorders, OCD, delirium, catatonia, stroke, or other focal basal ganglia lesions, metabolic disorders, medication side effects, and extrapyramidal disorders. The most common hypokinetic movement disorder, parkinsonism, includes the triad of akinesia/bradykinesia, rigidity, and resting tremor. When examining a patient for parkinsonism, supranuclear gaze, cerebellar function, and orthostatic vital signs, observation for arm swing and en bloc turning during gait examination are included to facilitate diagnosis of Parkinson plus syndromes. Axial rigidity and akinesia form the core of the atypical parkinsonian syndromes such as PSP, corticobasal degeneration, and some frontotemporal dementias. Though not pathognomonic, the *applause sign* can be seen in patients with PSP who have difficulty stopping accurately when asked to quickly clap three times. The *alien hand sign*, seen in corticobasal degeneration and callosal disconnection, refers to the feeling that one hand is foreign or has a "mind of its own," and is often associated with involuntary hand movements (Doody and Jankovic 1992).

Tic, tremor, dystonia, choreoathetosis, hemiballismus, and myoclonus are hyperkinetic movements. A smartphone seismometer app can serve as an adjunct in recording tremor severity when an examiner is following a patient for tremor. Choreoathetoid movements, such as those seen in tardive dyskinesia, may be assessed using the Abnormal Involuntary Movement Scale (AIMS) (Munetz and Benjamin 1988). The AIMS examination is best done in a hard armless chair so as not to obscure subtle movements. The examination begins with the

[1] Tourette disorder was named for Georges Gilles de la Tourette. His correct surname is *Gilles de la Tourette.*

patient seated with arms at rest, then hanging at the sides, to observe for adventitious movements, which can be the earliest sign of a choreoathetoid movement disorder. Distracting maneuvers are done to accentuate movements with arms outstretched (piano-playing fingers) and during mouth opening, tongue protrusion, fine finger movement, standing, and walking. The patient's face, arms, trunk, and legs are observed during each distraction maneuver. The patient is observed for evidence of glottal movement or exploratory tongue movement with mouth closed (the *bonbon sign*) and sudden inhalation while speaking that may indicate diaphragmatic dyskinesia, a risk factor for aspiration. The *milkmaid grip,* elicited by having the patient sustain a steady grasp of the examiner's forefinger, is another sign of choreoathetosis. However, the presence of abnormal involuntary movements does not prove that the patient has tardive dyskinesia. Tourette disorder, Huntington disease, pregnancy, dopaminergic therapies and other conditions may also be responsible.

Dystonia refers to an involuntary muscle contraction associated with repetitive or twisting movements that can occur spontaneously or during a specific action such as writing or eating. Dystonia commonly occurs in the eyelids, neck, oromandibular area, vocal cords, and upper extremities. Cervical dystonia may be accompanied by a geste antagoniste or sensory trick (also known as an alleviating maneuver) in which the patient alleviates the dystonia by touching a particular place. Sometimes thought to be evidence of psychogenic origin, this feature actually supports the diagnosis of dystonia.

Tics are abrupt, nonrhythmic repetitive movements that involve discrete muscle groups, mimic normal coordinated movements, vary in intensity, and can be voluntarily suppressed temporarily. *Tourette disorder* involves motor and vocal tics and typically includes aspects of OCD. Motor tics are seen in OCD and in first-degree relatives of patients with OCD or Tourette disorder. Before the neuroleptic era, abnormal involuntary movements were also known to occur in individuals with schizophrenia. See Chapter 9, "Movement Disorders," for clinical features of movement disorders.

Catatonia, although typically hypokinetic, may also take the form of catatonic excitement with hyperkinesis. Components of the catatonic syndrome from the Bush-Francis Catatonia Scale are listed in Table 1.4 (Bush et al. 1996). DSM-5-TR (American Psychiatric Association 2022) criteria require the presence of 3 of 12 symptoms derived from this scale: stupor, catalepsy, waxy flexibility, mutism, negativism, posturing, mannerisms, stereotypy, agitation, grimacing, echolalia, and echo-

Table 1.4 Components of the catatonic syndrome from the Bush-Francis Catatonia Scale

Excitement	Waxy flexibility
Immobility/stupor	Withdrawal
Mutism	Impulsivity
Staring	Automatic obedience
Posturing/catalepsy	Mitgehen
Grimacing	Gegenhalten
Echopraxia/echolalia	Ambitendency
Stereotypy	Grasp reflex
Mannerisms	Perseveration
Verbigeration	Combativeness
Rigidity	Autonomic abnormality
Negativism	

praxia. Catatonia is treated as a neuropsychiatric emergency. When it is combined with seizures, anterograde amnesia, or medial temporal hyperintensities on fluid-attenuated inversion recovery (FLAIR) MRI, catatonia may also be a presentation of autoimmune limbic encephalitis. Elements of the syndrome may also occur in neuroleptic malignant syndrome or serotonin syndrome. See Chapter 3.

Sensory Examination

After primary sensory assessment of light touch, pinprick, vibration, and proprioception, cortical sensory loss due to contralateral parietal dysfunction is assessed by testing graphesthesia, two-point discrimination, stereognosis, and double simultaneous stimulation in a patient with intact primary sensory perception. Graphesthesia is tested by asking the patient to identify numbers traced on the fingertip or palm with an applicator stick. The two-point discrimination threshold may be assessed with metal calipers graduated in millimeters or with a note card in which pinholes have been made 5, 7, and 10 mm apart. Stereognosis is tested by asking the patient to close their eyes and name a small object placed in their hand. Inability to name objects placed in the left hand with preserved ability on the right is also seen in callosal disconnection. Double simultaneous stimulation tests hemi-neglect in the visual, somatosensory, or auditory spheres. In the visual sphere, the patient is asked to indicate the finger that is moving when the examiner moves fingers in both hemifields simultaneously. Somatosensory hemi-neglect is assessed by lightly touching both limbs at once and asking the patient to indicate the side being touched. Auditory hemi-inattention can be assessed at the bedside by simultaneously making different sounds in each ear (e.g., crinkling paper in front of one ear and jingling keys in front of the other) and asking the patient to identify the sound.

Gait Examination

During examination, note ease of gait initiation, stride length, step height, any aids or appliances used, gait-evoked involuntary movements, and arm swing. Observe the patient walking to assess for the presence of shortened stride length, circumduction, or antalgic (pain-induced) gait. An example of circumducting gait and decorticate rigidity indicative of corticospinal tract damage is seen in Video 1.11.

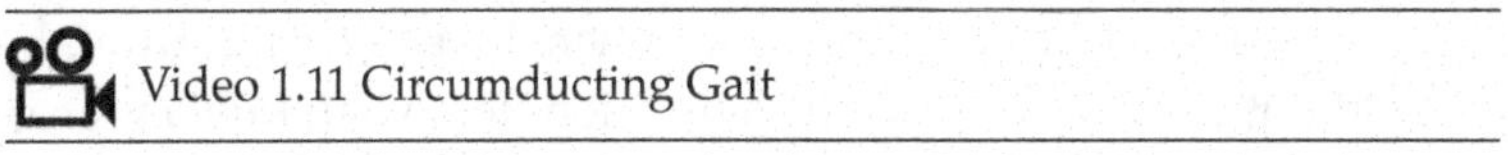

Video 1.11 Circumducting Gait

After this observation, ask the patient to walk on heels, toes, and in tandem (one foot in front of the other). If signs of parkinsonism are present, ask the patient to arise from a chair without using their hands, have them do an "about-face" turn to observe for en bloc turning, and include a "pull test" from behind to assess for retropulsion as seen in Video 1.12. When testing for the Romberg sign (Video 1.13), observe for signs of motor impersistence, seen in right frontal dysfunction. When asked to stand with feet together, eyes closed, and arms outstretched, the patient with motor impersistence requires repeated reminders to continue doing each of the three parts of the command.

Video 1.12 Pull Test

Video 1.13 Test for the Romberg Sign

Neurological "Soft Signs"

Neurodevelopmental or neurological "soft signs" (NSS), discussed in Chapter 7, are seen with increased frequency in individuals with neurodevelopmental disorders, schizophrenia, bipolar disorder, substance use disorders, OCD, or antisocial personality disorder, as well as in cases of prematurity, low birth weight, and malnutrition (Whitty et al. 2009). NSS are not associated with demonstrable abnormalities on brain imaging but may represent subtle brain dysfunction in the listed conditions, in early CNS damage, or in otherwise healthy patients. Those signs that are potentially lateralizing may reflect early CNS damage not seen on conventional imaging. NSS should therefore be considered a diagnosis of exclusion.

Functional Neurological Disorder, Embellishment, and Malingering

Neuropsychiatrists often examine people in whom there may be a question of functional neurological disorder (FND), symptom embellishment, or malingering. See Chapter 10, "Functional Neurological Disorder," for the FND examination. When investigating an embellished field cut or complaint of tunnel vision, test visual fields to confrontation at 14 inches, 3 feet, and 15 feet. Because visual fields expand in a conical fashion, the amount seen should increase with distance from the stimulus. An illustration of nonphysiological hemianopia is seen in Video 1.14. Similarly, hemisensory deficits to pinprick or light touch that precisely split the midline on the face or trunk or a hemivibratory loss on the skull are also physiologically inconsistent.

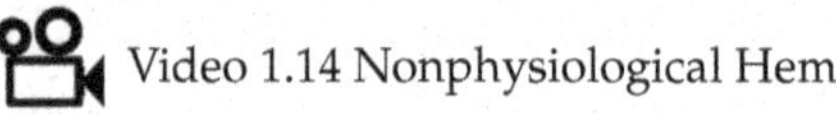
Video 1.14 Nonphysiological Hemianopia

Another technique that may be used to test for embellished or malingered hemisensory loss is to ask the patient to hold their hands out with thumbs down, then clasp, interdigitate, and rotate their hands upward before testing primary sensation on each finger as illustrated in Video 1.15. This makes it difficult for the patient to quickly track which of the interdigitated fingers are from the right versus the left hand. The Hoover sign is used to assess malingered or embellished leg weakness (see Chapter 10). Additional evidence of nonphysiological unilateral leg weakness may be obtained by having the patient walk around a chair with the weak leg out while using the chair back for support. Then have the patient switch hands on the chair back and walk the opposite way around the chair. The clinician should observe for inconsistency in gait circumduction. Video 1.16 illustrates this test.

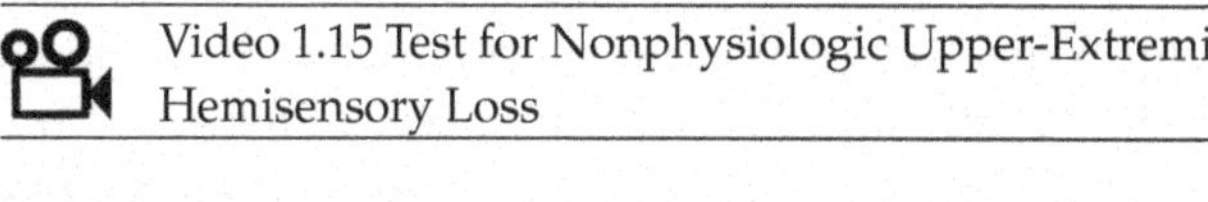

Video 1.15 Test for Nonphysiologic Upper-Extremity Hemisensory Loss

Video 1.16 Test for Nonphysiological Lower-Extremity Hemiparesis

Mental Status Examination

General Observations

The patient's level of consciousness can be described as alert, lethargic, stuporous, or comatose. Arousal may also be described in terms of response to verbal command or to pain. Idiosyncrasies of dress or behavior, unusual preoccupations or traits, mannerisms, and particular triggers of irritability (e.g., misophonia) should be noted. Compulsions, rituals, or stereotypies (repetitive, purposeless movements) should be described.

The ability to anticipate, plan, and self-monitor for errors is an indicator of executive function. In the presence of prefrontal dysfunction, patients may be unaware of their own behavior and may be unable to appropriately match their behavior to the environment or situation, missing social cues and failing to respect personal space. Denial of symptoms or deficits may be related to right hemisphere dysfunction. The examiner should note eye contact, cooperation, engagement, relatedness, degree of apathy or interest, attitude toward symptoms, and the degree of effort expended on cognitive tasks.

Mood and Affect

Mood can be described according to the subjective emotion reported by the patient, although in nonverbal individuals it must be inferred from affective cues. Affect is reflected in posture, facial expression, prosody, and gesture. The apparent emotion, range, amplitude, stability, mood congruency, and appropriateness of affect should be described. Common descriptors include depressed, dysphoric, euphoric, expansive, elated, anxious, hostile, and euthymic.

Verbal Production

Verbal production refers to speech and language, with language expanded further under the subsection "Cognitive Status Examination" later in this chapter. When describing verbal production, note fluency, phrase length, melodic line, and prosody of speech. Emotional prosody, which has more of a right hemisphere contribution than linguistic prosody does, can be noted separately. Note word-finding pauses, circumlocution, hesitation, paraphasic errors, pronunciation, and speech rhythm. Other important components of verbal production include volume, quantity, and rate of speech, ranging from mutism to tachyphemia (speech cluttering). Pressured speech is seen in mania.

Foreign accent syndrome is a particular type of dysprosody in which a person's pronunciation makes them sound as if they come from a foreign country. Foreign accent syndrome can be neurogenic and involuntary, caused by stroke, traumatic brain injury, or migraine, or it can be psychogenic and voluntary. Neurogenic cases have typically been reported following damage to left hemisphere sites, including Broca's area, the frontal operculum, the supplementary motor area, and the motor cortex, but they have also been reported as congenital abnormalities and following cerebellar lesions.

Dysarthria refers to a motor speech disorder as opposed to a language disorder. With dysarthria, muscles are flaccid in neuromuscular or lower motor neuron disorders, spastic in bilateral upper motor neuron and extrapyramidal disorders, ataxic in cerebellar disorders, hypokinetic in basal ganglia and parkinsonian disorders, hyperkinetic in basal ganglia disorders with abnormal involuntary movements, or mixed as in ALS with upper and lower motor neuron involvement. *Apraxia of speech,* typically seen accompanying Broca aphasia, describes problems correctly sequencing phonemic components, which result in effortful, poorly modulated speech, often with difficulty in initiation. *Stuttering,* the involuntary repetition of sounds or syllables, is more often developmental than acquired and appears to run in families. Acquired stuttering in adulthood is most commonly psychogenic but can occur rarely after traumatic brain injury (TBI) or stroke. In neurogenic cases, the stuttering is less likely to be limited to initial sounds; less likely to attenuate with adaptation to the situation; and more likely to occur across all types of speech output, including oral reading, repetition, conversation, and explanation (Cruz et al. 2018). *Palilalia,* the involuntary repetition of words, phrases, or even sentences, occurs in Tourette disorder, neurodegenerative disorders, and hypodopaminergic states. *Verbigeration* refers to obsessive repetition of words or phrases.

Unusual word production should be noted. Excessive punning or rhyming may be seen in psychotic disorders, mania, or frontotemporal dementia (Mendez et al. 2017). *Clang associations* describe connections between subsequent thoughts based only on rhyming words, a phenomenon seen in mania. *Witzelsucht* (excessive and pathological joking) and *moria* (excessive giddiness) may be seen in individuals with frontal dysfunction (Granadillo and Mendez 2016). The well-known phenomenon of *coprolalia*, seen in individuals with Tourette disorder, occurs in less than 10% of cases (Robertson et al. 2017). The presence of *malapropisms*, inappropriate uses of words that sound similar to the intended word, may indicate poor understanding of word meaning, or it may be an indicator of mania. *Neologisms* (made-up words) are seen in psychosis but also occur in fluent jargon aphasia and occasionally in focal seizures. One way to differentiate psychotic from aphasic neologisms is simply to ask the patient why they used that word. Aphasic neologisms are unintentional, whereas psychotic neologisms are used for a reason unique to that individual's thought process. Another language idiosyncrasy that may occur in schizophrenia is *metonymy*, the use of one word as a substitute for another, such as saying "I've lost my track of thought" instead of "I've lost my train of thought." Note that the mere presence of a language disorder does not signify neurogenic origin. Non-neurogenic language disorders such as non-aphasic misnaming are sometimes confused with neurogenic disorders (Mendez 2018).

Thought Process and Content

During the examination, the clinician attempts to understand whether the person's thoughts appear to flow logically from one another. The term *thought process* refers to the quantity, rate, organization, and connectedness of one's thoughts and is typically abnormal in psychosis. *Thought content* refers to the description of abnormal thoughts, including delusions, preoccupations, overvalued ideas, obsessions, phobias, depressive thoughts, and dangerousness to oneself or others. Patients with formal *thought disorder* exhibit disorganized, impoverished, or abnormally connected thoughts, including loose associations, derailment, thought blocking, circumstantiality, tangentiality, speaking in word salad, nonsequitur speech, and perseveration. Such individuals may exhibit *knight's move*, a discernible but unstated connection between loosely associated thoughts similar to the way in which a knight moves on a chessboard. In *Ganser syndrome*, seen in patients who are embellishing their symptoms, individuals provide approximate answers to questions (e.g., being consistently off by 1 on the day, date, or year).

Delusional misidentification and *reduplicative phenomena* can be seen in both psychiatric and neurological disorders. Delusional misidentification syndromes include the *Capgras delusion,* in which a familiar person has been replaced by an impostor, the *Fregoli delusion,* in which a persecutor is taking on the form of others, and the *intermetamorphosis delusion,* in which people are swapping identities without changing their outward appearance. *Reduplicative paramnesia,* the delusional belief that a place, event, or time has been duplicated or relocated, is seen in psychiatric disorders; following TBI; in delirium, focal seizures, or encephalopathy; and in other cases. Delusional misidentification syndromes of neurological origin often involve right frontal dysfunction.

Perceptions

Disorders of perception include dissociative symptoms, illusions, hallucinations, *pseudohallucinations* (recognized as hallucinations by the patient), and agnosia. *Derealization* and *depersonalization* are dissociative symptoms that can be seen in psychotic disorders, PTSD, focal seizures, or migraines. Hallucinations and illusions are common in neuropsychiatric conditions, including strokes, tumors, migraines, and focal seizures. *Autoscopic hallucination,* the perception of seeing oneself, has also been associated with migraines and focal seizures. *Formication,* the tactile hallucination in which one feels as if insects are crawling over one's skin, is seen in stimulant intoxication, substance withdrawal delirium, menopause, Parkinson disease, and occasionally in B_{12} or folate deficiency. Olfactory hallucinations are seen in depression and focal seizures, although olfactory hallucinations that last longer than about 3 minutes are unlikely to be seizures.

Hypnagogic and hypnopompic hallucinations, representing dysregulated rapid eye movement sleep, occur in narcolepsy. *Peduncular hallucinosis,* in which the patient sees vivid, well-formed images, mostly at night, also tends to occur in the context of sleep disorders (including insomnia and daytime sleepiness) or in thalamic, midbrain, or pontine pathology. The *Lilliputian hallucinations* of so-called *Alice in Wonderland syndrome* can occur in migraine, TBI, or CNS infection, but they are typically a form of peduncular hallucinosis.

Charles Bonnet syndrome refers to complex visual release hallucinations associated with diminishing vision, often in the elderly. Simple auditory hallucinations such as machine-like noises, as opposed to complex hallucinations of voices, are more likely of neurological origin. Musical hallucinations can be seen in temporal lobe pathology, seizures, migraines, psychiatric disorders, or as release phenomena with diminishing hearing, especially in the elderly. Commentary and command auditory hallucinations are experienced by people with schizophrenia.

Illusions (the misperception of sensory stimuli) are common in migraine sufferers but may also be seen in encephalopathy of any etiology. *Allesthesia,* the perception of a sensory stimulus applied to one side of the body on the contralateral side, occurs in right parietal lesions. Several visual illusions that have been described in migraine, including *micropsia, macropsia, teleopsia* (illusion of distance), *pelopsia* (illusion of nearness), *metamorphopsia,* and *chromatopsia,* also occur in other neurological conditions. *Palinopsia* refers to visual perseveration or afterimages. The trailing phenomenon is a related visual illusion reported by psychedelic drug users. *Hypoacusis* and *hyperacusis,* the perception of auditory stimuli as softer or louder than they are, are common auditory illusions seen in migraine and other disorders.

Certain illusions occur in healthy individuals. *Synesthesia,* the involuntary perception of a sensory or cognitive phenomenon when a different sense is stimulated, occurs in about 2% of the population (Ward 2013). *Pareidolia,* a common illusion, refers to the perception of a familiar pattern, shape, or sound when looking at or listening to an unfamiliar or ambiguous stimulus.

Agnosia, another disorder of perception, is the inability to recognize sounds, shapes, objects, or smells despite having intact primary sensory perception. Specific agnosias are listed in Table 1.5.

Insight and Judgment

Insight is best assessed by a person's awareness of their own symptoms and their effects on self and others. Insight may also include understanding diagnoses, etiology, and treatment options. Judgment is reflected in a patient's decisions and actions, such as their approach to medical treatment and their social behavior.

Cognitive Status Examination

Bedside Assessment

Bedside cognitive examination refers to interactive testing during neuropsychiatric evaluation that allows the clinician to form an opinion on the patient's attention, memory, language, visuospatial, executive, and other cognitive functions. These data may enable the clinician to form a cognitive hypothesis regarding a person's behavior. For example, a

Table 1.5 Specific agnosias

Agnosia	Definition
Akinetopsia	Inability to perceive motion despite intact ability to perceive objects
Alexia	Inability to read despite intact vision, language, and ability to write
Amusia	Loss of ability to recognize familiar melodies, read music, or identify notes
Anosodiaphoria	Minimization of importance of deficit despite acknowledgment of its existence
Anosognosia	Denial of deficit
Anton syndrome	Denial of blindness seen in bilateral occipital infarcts with cortical blindness
Astereognosis	Inability to recognize objects by feel (tactile agnosia) despite otherwise intact somatosensory perception
Auditory agnosia	Inability to discriminate sounds despite intact hearing, cognitive function, and language abilities
Autotopagnosia	Inability to recognize or point to parts of one's own body, an examiner's body, or a visual representation of a body despite intact vision (anosognosia may include corresponding hemi-autotopagnosia)
Color agnosia	Inability to recognize colors despite intact ability to match or group them
Environmental agnosia	Inability to recognize or give directions to familiar places
Finger agnosia	Inability to recognize fingers despite intact vision and sensation
Form agnosia	Inability to recognize objects despite ability to recognize their parts

Table 1.5 Specific agnosias (*continued*)

Agnosia	Definition
Phonagnosia	Inability to recognize familiar voices despite intact ability to understand language
Prosopagnosia	Inability to recognize familiar faces despite being able to describe and match them
Pure word deafness	Inability to understand spoken language despite intact hearing and otherwise intact language
Simultanagnosia	Inability to perceive more than one object at a time, which results in inability to recognize the whole of a picture or complex object despite ability to pick out some details
Social-emotional agnosia	Inability to understand body language, facial expressions, or emotional prosody (some overlap with emotional aprosodia and alexithymia) resulting in socially awkward interactions
Visual agnosia	Inability to recognize objects despite otherwise intact vision • Apperceptive: Inability to recognize, discriminate among, or copy objects • Associative: Inability to recognize objects despite intact primary sensory perception and ability to describe and copy them

patient who always becomes agitated and raises her voice when other patients are agitated and yelling near her may have stimulus-bound behavior related to frontal dysfunction or sensory hypersensitivity related to autism spectrum disorder.

Mental status rating scales are commonly substituted for more flexible and interactive cognitive assessment. General cognitive rating scales such as the Mini-Mental State Examination or the Montreal Cognitive Assessment allow for comparison of findings over time, at different venues, and as a tool in research. However, they are often not sufficient to determine the cognitive basis for a patient's complaint or to reach a precise neuropsychiatric diagnosis.

Bedside cognitive testing is not a substitute for neuropsychological testing. However, having determined the basic deficits and a cognitive hypothesis for symptoms, the clinician may order formal neuropsychological testing to obtain validated test results to confirm the findings, establish a cognitive baseline in neurodegenerative conditions, determine related deficits, assist in rehabilitation planning or occupational assessment, and chart recovery from neurological damage, among other reasons.

The examiner should adapt the tasks to the patient's educational level and to the cognitive complaint. Using a "screen and metric" approach increases examination efficiency, allowing less time to be spent on areas of relative strength and more time on areas of relative deficiency. For example, a patient who can readily solve a screening shopping problem may not need as much attention to metrics for auditory attention span, executive function, or arithmetic skills.

When presenting written tasks to the patient, plain, unlined paper in landscape mode is preferred. Presenting a clean sheet of paper for each task minimizes errors due to stimulus-bound behavior or perseveration. When explaining a cognitive task, the examiner should first minimize misinterpretation of performance errors by ensuring that the patient understands the instructions and that they are expected to do the task; this is referred to as *establishing set*. Cognitive status assessment includes assessing both deficits and strengths. The examiner should note not only the patient's response to each task but also the nature of the prompts needed to assist the patient in performing the task. These prompts may form the basis of instructions the examiner will later give to the clinical staff who will assist the patient in rehabilitation.

Convergent findings from different areas of the neurological and cognitive examinations increase the likelihood of dysfunction in the network or anatomical location implicated. For example, poor performance on a construction task does not necessarily indicate right parietal dysfunction. In combination with a left inferior quadrantanopia, however, a compelling case may be made.

Attention

Attention is assessed early in the examination because other cognitive findings are unreliable if attention is impaired. The degree of distractibility and any perseveration should be noted. *Perseveration,* classically associated with prefrontal dysfunction, is nonspecific and may be seen with other causes of brain dysfunction as well. It is a frequent concomitant of aphasia and can make the language examination difficult. Perseverance may be assessed with the ramparts task (Figure 1.3), the "mn" task (Figure 1.4), or the multiple loops task (Figure 1.5) (Benjamin and Lauterbach 2016).

All three tasks should be presented by the examiner drawing the target stimulus twice to indicate it is to be repeated. The patient is then instructed to make a copy of the target stimulus beneath it and continue across the paper without stopping. For the mn and ramparts tasks, the patient is told not to lift the pen from the paper.

Observation of the patient's performance may yield additional information about prefrontal function. In the setting of severely stimulus-bound behavior, the patient's pen may be magnetically drawn upward to trace the target stimulus or may incorporate a copy of whatever else is above the area of the page on which the drawing is being done. Some patients with right anterior dysfunction will produce drawings of increasing size or sloping diagonally as they proceed. The mn and ramparts tasks are reciprocal motor programs that emphasize language and visual-spatial functions, respectively. On the multiple

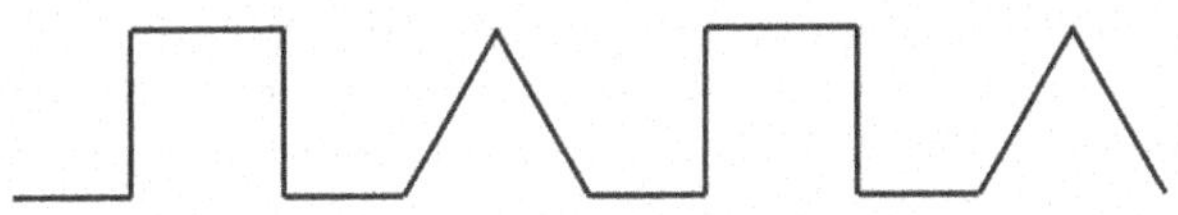

Figure 1.3 Perseverance task: ramparts task.

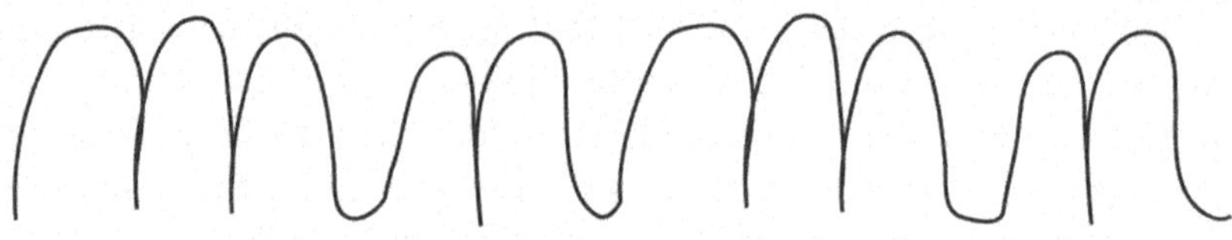

Figure 1.4 **Perseverance task: mn task.**

loops task, the stimulus-bound patient may draw the number 3 instead of the multiple loops.

Perseveration is defined as *continuous* if the patient fails to stop performing the task; it is defined as *stuck in set* if the patient is unable to switch from the previous command to the new command; and it is defined as *recurrent* if the patient returns to a task command given earlier in the examination (Sandson and Albert 1987). If perseveration is noted, the examiner may need to adjust the order of the examination or change to a different type of task (e.g., changing from written to oral responses) to "deblock" the patient to obtain the best response, especially for the aphasia examination.

There are several ways to assess for hemi-inattention or neglect. The clinician can simply ask the patient to look straight ahead and describe the things they see around the room, noting if fewer details are noticed on one side. The line bisection task is another simple method of assessing hemispatial attention. Draw a horizontal line across a sheet of paper presented in landscape mode and ask the patient to bisect it. Displacement of the bisection point to one side of the paper may indicate contralateral hemianopia or hemineglect. The multiple-line bisection task (Albert 1973) and the letter and symbol cancellation tasks (Mesulam 1985) are more accurate methods of assessing quadrantic inattention/neglect or hemi-inattention/neglect at the bedside.

Attention span is a determinant of how much information the examiner can convey to the patient at once. In non-aphasic individuals of average intelligence, attention span may be assessed by determining the number of digits a person can repeat, beginning with seven digits forward and adding or subtracting digits as needed. The examiner should then ask the patient to recite the digits in reverse order. Reversed digit span is typically about two digits fewer than forward digit span. In the presence of aphasia or other language impairment, object-pointing span may be used as a measure of attention span. Place five objects (e.g., pen, paper clip, key, comb, coin) on a table and verify that the patient can identify them. Cover the objects with a piece of plain paper and say (or

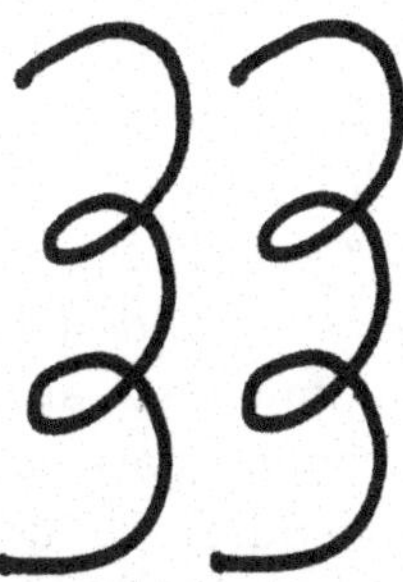

Figure 1.5 Perseverance task: multiple loops task.

indicate), "When I take away the paper, point to the objects in the order I say them," and establish how many objects the person can point to.

Reverse digit span is one measure of *working memory,* the temporary storage of information needed to complete a task. Other working memory tasks in order from simple to more complex include counting backward from 20, reciting the days of the week in reverse, reciting the months of the year in reverse, alphabetizing the letters in EARTH, and reciting the alphabet backward. The oral Trails B task, in which the subject is asked to verbally alternate letters and numbers beginning with A-1 until reaching M-13, is another measure of working memory (Daffner et al. 2015). The serial 7s task, in which the patient is instructed to subtract 7 from 100 and continue subtracting 7 from each result, is a measure of concentration but also assesses working memory. Another complex working memory task that includes elements of vigilance and executive function is to ask the patient to name the letters of the alphabet that rhyme with "key" or the capital block letters that have curves in them.

Auditory vigilance can be assessed with a continuous performance task. The examiner reads a long list of letters and instructs the patient to tap the table whenever they hear the letter A. Decreased auditory vigilance can occur in most types of attentional impairment.

Memory

Memory impairment may be caused by deficient memory storage or recall, impaired attention, or psychological factors. Memory assessment begins from the moment you encounter the patient. You can introduce yourself by associating your name with a phonemic or category cue to facilitate later inquiry. Recall tasks should be adjusted to estimated intellect and, if appropriate, may be associated with category cues when words for later recall are given. For example, you could tell the patient, "I'd like you to remember the flower daisy, the address 50 Belmont Street, and the color teal."

Difficulty recalling recent personal or news events may indicate problems with either memory or attention. Both verbal and nonverbal recall should be assessed with immediate and delayed recall conditions to help separate inattention from memory deficits. Verbal recall may be tested with three, four, or five stimuli, including less easily visualized objects for more than one of the stimuli. For example, include a color; a member of an object category (e.g., a particular type of flower); an address (with both number and street name); and an intangible word, such as a feeling or value. The number of repetitions required for the subject to register the items and repeat them back correctly is noted. After repeating the items until the patient can recall them immediately, the number recalled spontaneously at 5 and 15 minutes and the number produced when the patient is given category cues or phonemic cues (if necessary) are noted. If cued recall is incorrect, the patient may be read or shown a list of ten words and asked to select the ones that were in the original list. Poor spontaneous recall with improved performance on selecting from a word list is seen in frontal-subcortical retrieval-type memory deficits. Perseveration, intrusions, confabulation, or inconsistency are also noted.

Nonverbal recall is tested by having the patient copy an asymmetrical figure containing a distinct external shape and internal details (Figure 1.6), then removing the stimulus and having the patient draw the figure immediately and again at 15 minutes. The productions are compared to determine whether missing details were absent at immediate recall, implying an attention problem, or were lost only on delayed recall, implying a memory problem. If the patient is unable to copy or draw, nonverbal recall may be assessed with the hidden objects task. The examiner hides three objects within or under items in the patient's immediate surroundings in full view of the patient and then asks the patient what has been hidden and where. Immediate and delayed recall are again assessed.

Assuming intact arousal and attention, reciting the names of presidents of the country in reverse order can give a rough estimate of the temporal gradient of a patient's recall. In Korsakoff's psychosis, an abrupt falloff in memory may be traced to a particular era with further inquiry concerning historical events in past decades. People with Alzheimer disease may have some recall of distant historical facts but fewer and fewer approaching the present day.

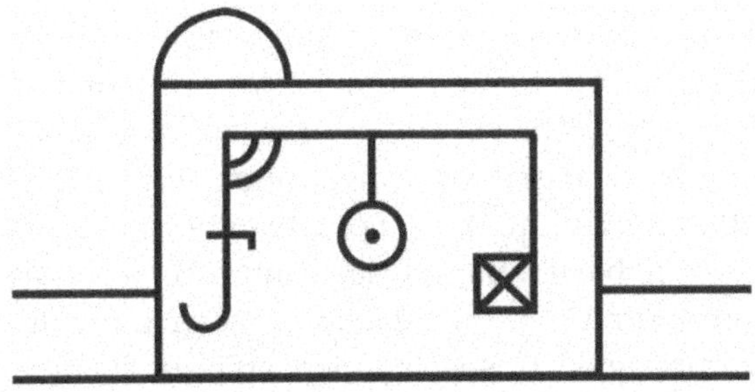

Figure 1.6 Nonverbal recall stimulus.

More detailed bedside assessment of learning and retention can be done with a 12-word list (Benjamin and Lauterbach 2016) or with a formal supraspan task such as the California Verbal Learning Test (Delis et al. 1987). Healthy individuals demonstrate a primacy and recency effect, recalling the initial and final words of a list most easily. Individuals with memory impairment do not show the primacy effect. People with attention deficit may recall different words on each trial. People with Alzheimer disease recall few words on the first trial and improve only modestly over all trials, with little word recall after a 15-minute delay and little improvement in selecting from a word list.

Other bedside memory tasks include paired associate learning and story recall. *Paired associate learning* involves presenting the patient with several easy word pairs (e.g., book-page) and several difficult word pairs (e.g., cabbage-elephant). The examiner then says one word and asks the patient to recall the paired associate word. *Story recall* involves reading the patient a story containing a known number of facts. The patient is asked to recall the story, and the number of facts correctly recalled is recorded.

Fund of Knowledge

Fund of knowledge is a measure of crystallized intelligence. It is composed of facts, understanding, and experience that a person has accumulated throughout life. An example is asking the reason why white clothing is cooler than dark clothing in the summer.

Language

The language examination is undertaken to determine whether aphasia is present and to ascertain that delirium, dysarthria, or psychiatric disorders are not the cause of the language abnormality. Complete descriptions of the most common aphasias are found in Chapter 16 (Tables 16.2 and 16.3). The examiner forms an initial opinion as to the presence of aphasia based on conversation with the patient. Short phrase length, effortful quality, and difficulty in articulation characterize nonfluent aphasias. Superficially intact sentence structure, ease of production, and normal articulation are seen in the fluent aphasias. Paraphasic errors, typically seen in fluent aphasia, are described as verbal or semantic when a real word is substituted for the intended word and literal or phonemic when the substitution is a nonsense word (often beginning with the same phoneme as the intended word). A common way to elicit a spontaneous speech sample for assessment of aphasia involves showing the patient the Cookie Theft Picture and asking them to describe orally or in writing what they see happening in the drawing (Goodglass and Kaplan 1983).

The script generation task elicits a sample of spontaneous speech to assess language function. The patient is asked to describe the steps in a common task (e.g., changing a tire, making scrambled eggs). Failure to recite the steps in order is seen in executive dysfunction.

Auditory comprehension may be assessed by giving a three-step crossed command, such as "close your eyes and touch your left shoulder twice with your right hand." The Marie 3 Paper Task (Marie 1906) also assesses auditory comprehension, with additional stress on attention span and working memory. The patient is given three pieces of paper and told, "Throw the large piece on the floor, hand me the medium-sized piece, and you keep the small piece."

Word-finding problems are assessed using naming and verbal fluency tasks. Naming is assessed by confrontation (pointing to objects and asking their name) or by responsive naming (describing an object and asking its name). Word list generation is a measure of verbal fluency: phonemic or letter fluency is assessed by asking the patient to name all of the words they can think of that begin with a given letter of the alphabet in 1 minute. To assess category fluency, ask the patient to name all of the members of a given category they can think of (e.g., animals, items in a grocery store). If phonemic fluency was just assessed, it is helpful to specify that the words can begin with any letter. The examiner transcribes the words listed, marking 15-second intervals. Frontal-subcortical pathology may result in a patient exhausting their ability to list words in the first 15–20 seconds. A patient with executive dysfunction might benefit from the increased structure of the category fluency task compared with the phonemic fluency task. Word list generation also provides information on self-monitoring (repeated words), rule following, and use of creative strategies. A high school graduate of average intelligence can usually produce 12 words in a phonemic task and 18 words in a category task.

Repetition ability is assessed by having the patient repeat progressively more complex phrases, including tongue twisters (e.g., "Methodist Episcopal" or "around the rugged rock the ragged rascal ran") and sentences laden with functor words that express syntactic relationships or connections or modify nouns or verbs (e.g., "No ifs, ands, or buts about it"). These types of sentences are particularly challenging for people with nonfluent aphasia. Oral reading and reading comprehension are assessed by having the patient read a paragraph and explain what they read. Gathering a writing sample allows the examiner to assess for aphasia by looking for similar deficits to those in running speech, with the addition of noting spelling errors. Suggesting that the patient focus the writing sample on something related to their treatment can be helpful.

Paralinguistic Functions

The paralinguistic functions of emotional prosody and comprehension of idiom, pun, and sarcasm require intact right hemisphere networks in addition to left hemisphere language functions. Gestural, intrinsic (the rhythm of speech such as that indicated by punctuation), and guttural (nonverbal sounds that convey meaning) prosody are left hemisphere functions. To assess spontaneous emotional prosody, ask the patient to say an intrinsically neutral sentence (e.g., "I am going to the movies") as if they are angry, sad, happy, and surprised. Then the examiner stands out of sight of the patient and asks the patient to identify the examiner's emotion while stating a neutral sentence as if angry, sad, happy, or surprised. Emotional prosodic repetition can also be tested.

Assessment of comprehension of idiom, pun, and sarcasm requires culturally appropriate stimuli and is difficult to assess in someone from a different culture or who requires an interpreter. For native English speakers, idiomatic comprehension can be assessed by asking what is meant by expressions such as "backseat driver," "cry wolf," or "go cold turkey." The ability to decode puns, sarcasm, and double entendre is an aspect of lexical processing that relates to humor comprehension. The examiner can ask the patient to explain a joke such as "What did the mayonnaise jar say to the refrigerator? Shut the door, I'm dressing" or "Did you hear about the fellow who swallowed the spoon? He didn't stir." The ability to decode sarcasm requires analysis of context in addition to denotative meaning. The examiner might, for example, tell the patient, "I told my partner I would have to miss our daughter's birthday party because I was on call for the hospital, and he said, 'Great, you're missing another family event.' How did my partner feel about my being on call that day?"

Failure to comprehend the paralinguistic aspects of language places one at a tremendous disadvantage. The paralinguistic functions are components of *pragmatics,* the use of language in social context. Pragmatic deficits can occur in the setting of right hemisphere dysfunction, intellectual developmental disorder, autism spectrum disorder, and other conditions. In some cases, they can lead to reinforcement of paranoid ideas in addition to causing social dysfunction.

Praxis

Apraxia refers to the inability to plan and carry out a motor command despite intact comprehension, muscle strength, and coordination. Patients with ideomotor apraxia can explain a movement but cannot act it out or pretend they are doing it. In ideational apraxia, the patient cannot perform a complex motor act in the correct sequence despite being able to perform parts of the task correctly in isolation. Praxis is assessed with buccofacial, axial, and limb commands. Buccofacial commands include asking the patient to pretend to blow out a match, sniff a flower, or cough. Axial commands include asking the patient to assume a boxing stance or pretend to swing a golf club. Limb praxis commands may be gestural ("pretend to stop traffic" or "wave good-bye") or transitive (pretend to use a tool such as a screwdriver, toothbrush, or comb). A common error in ideomotor apraxia is to use a body part as the object (e.g., pretend to brush teeth with a finger instead of an imaginary toothbrush). Apraxia tends to occur in left hemisphere lesions, especially in association with aphasia.

Constructional Praxis

Constructional apraxia involves the inability to draw simple shapes despite intact comprehension and motor function. Common bedside tests of constructional praxis include figure copying, clock drawing, drawing a three-dimensional cube or a simple house in perspective (showing the front and one side), and design fluency. Copying an asymmetrical figure for assessment of nonverbal recall also yields information about constructional praxis, hemi-attention, and learning style.

The clock drawing task is an excellent screen for construction ability, hemispatial attention, and prefrontal/executive function. Instruct the patient to "draw a big circle, put in the numbers so it looks like a clock, and draw the hands so the time is 10 past 11."

Design fluency is a measure of constructional ability and executive function. As with verbal fluency tasks, there is an unstructured version and a structured version. The patient is instructed to draw as many simple objects as possible in 1 minute in the unstructured task (normal is three to four). For the structured task, the patient is asked to make as many designs as possible in one minute using four straight lines (normal is five) (Jones-Gotman and Milner 1977).

Calculation

Attention, recall, working memory, and arithmetic skills are required to solve oral math problems. Doing simple arithmetic problems on paper avoids some of these issues. Spatial acalculia may impair oral or written performance when the patient must align digits, carry digits, or maintain the structure of a problem to solve it. Arithmetic functions per se are generally localized to the left hemisphere. Spatial acalculia, however, implies right hemisphere dysfunction. To assess for spatial acalculia, the examiner asks the patient to add, subtract, multiply, or divide two- to four-digit numbers using unlined paper.

Right-Left, Topographic, and Finger Orientation

Right-left orientation may have already been assessed with auditory comprehension. One can also simply ask the patient to touch the examiner's left hand. Topographic orientation requires familiarity by both the examiner and the patient of a topographic area being visualized. In a hospitalized patient, for example, the examiner may establish topographic orientation by asking for directions from the patient's bedroom to the nursing station. In case of difficulty with this screening task, the examiner should follow up as needed with tests of visual recall, right-left orientation, and working memory. Finger orientation, the most frequently disturbed body part orientation symptom, is assessed by naming the finger being pointed to and pointing to the finger being named. Finger agnosia, a component of Gerstmann syndrome, is diagnosed only if both hands are affected and a unilateral sensory deficit is absent. It may be due to dysfunction in either hemisphere but occurs most often in left parietal dysfunction.

Prefrontal and Executive Functions

The complex problem-solving or shopping problem task may be used as a screening test for prefrontal executive function. Ask the patient, "How much change should you expect from $5 if you buy four packs of peanuts at 89 cents per pack?" Solving this problem requires planning, working memory, sequencing, cognitive estimation, error checking, and basic arithmetic. If the patient cannot solve the problem orally, the examiner assesses the component functions of the problem to determine the source of error. Individual components of prefrontal and executive functions are easily examined at the bedside. Cognitive estimation may be assessed by asking the patient to guess the height of the examination room ceiling or the length of the average person's spine.

Inhibition and motor regulation may be tested using reciprocal motor programs and the go/no-go task. After establishing set for an imitation task in which you ask the patient to copy you by holding up either one or two fingers when you do, instruct the patient to do the opposite of what you do, holding up two fingers if you hold up one and one finger if you hold up two. Once the set is established for this reciprocal motor program, convert to the go/no-go task by explaining that the patient should continue to hold up two fingers when you hold up one but refrain from holding up any fingers at all when you hold up two fingers ("no-go"). Note any errors of omission or commission.

Cognitive flexibility can be assessed with the alternate uses, inferential reasoning, and headline tasks. The alternate uses task is an indicator of divergent thinking or the ability to come up with novel solutions to real-life problems, such as being locked out of one's apartment. The patient is asked to name all the uses they can think of for a common object (e.g., a paper clip, a toothpick). Normal individuals can generate at least 10 uses in 3 minutes (Dippo 2013).

Inferential reasoning and conceptual flexibility may be assessed by telling the patient, "Sally took a pen and notebook to meet a famous athlete. What do you think she planned to do?" After the patient responds, the examiner may then say, "Sally is a journalist writing an article about famous people's opinions on global warming. Now what do you think was Sally's plan?"

Another approach to the assessment of cognitive flexibility that also addresses connotative reasoning is the headline test, in which the examiner presents the patient with a double-entendre headline such as "Red Tape Holds Up New Bridge" or "Thief Gets Two Years in Violin Case" and asks the patient to explain the story that might have gone with that headline. A patient who comprehends the double entendre will generally smile immediately and explain that the headline is funny because of the double meaning, whereas a person who relies primarily on left hemisphere strategies will work through the meaning in serial order before realizing the humor in it. A related task is conceptual series completion, in which the patient is asked to fill in the blank to complete a series ranging from simple to difficult. An example of a simple conceptual series problem is AZ BY CX D_.

The capacity for abstract reasoning is typically assessed with the proverbs and similarities tasks, although the headline task and the assessment of paralinguistic functions just described assess related areas of cognitive flexibility and connotative reasoning. Like all cognitive tasks, the examiner ascertains that the patient has established a set before proceeding with the task. This can be accomplished by saying, "We sometimes use expressions to teach lessons. For instance, have you ever heard the expression 'Don't cry over spilled milk?'" Having established that the patient is able to provide an abstract explanation for simple proverbs, the examiner then asks for an interpretation of a more difficult proverb, such as "One swallow doesn't make a summer" or "The golden hammer breaks the iron door." Because proverbs are dependent on language fluency and cultural reference, this task is best used with native English speakers. For common proverbs from other countries, see https://creativeproverbs.com. In the similarities task, the patient is asked how two things are alike, beginning with simpler concepts (e.g., apple and orange) and moving to more abstract associations (e.g., watch and ruler, tree and fly). If the patient is slow to grasp what is meant by the task command, the examiner can say, "Into what category could the following items be placed?"

Sequencing is a basic function of the prefrontal cortex. Motor sequencing is assessed using Luria's three-step task (shown in Video 1.17), in which the patient is asked to mimic the examiner in performing three hand positions: fist, side, flat. The examiner demonstrates the move three times and then asks the patient to do it with their right and left hands. If the patient is unable to do so, the examiner can describe the three positions using action words while demonstrating them: "knock, chop, slap." If three positions appear too complex for the patient, the examiner decreases to two positions by asking the patient to alternately make a fist and then a ring with their thumb and third finger as shown in Video 1.18. A much more basic version of this task, using alternating fists, is shown in Video 1.19.

Video 1.17 Luria 3-Step Task

Video 1.18 Fist-Ring Test

Video 1.19 Alternating Fist Test

Verbal sequencing can be assessed by presenting the patient with cards containing the words right, hand, change, the, him (or police, car, found, the, alert) and asking them to unscramble the sentence. (The answers are "Hand him the right change" and "Alert police found the car.") Nonverbal sequencing can be assessed at the bedside with a series of picture cards that tell a story if arranged correctly.

Another basic prefrontal function is the capacity for independent behavior. Behavior that is entirely dictated by the most salient stimulus to which a person is exposed is called *stimulus-bound behavior.* Failure of behavioral independence may manifest in *echopraxia* or *utilization behavior.* If you suspect echopraxia, first place a finger over your closed lips to indicate silence, then extend your hands above your head, cross your arms, or assume other postures to see if the patient mimics your action.

The examination for utilization behavior is a bit more nuanced: Place various objects on a table to be positioned between you and the patient before bringing the patient into the room. The most salient objects would be those related to the patient's occupation, although common objects such as a notebook and pen, glasses, or a smartphone could be used. Utilization behavior describes the situation that occurs if the patient picks up the objects and starts to use them unbidden during the interview.

Concluding the Examination

The examination concludes with the examiner explaining the findings and their significance to the patient, outlining any plans for diagnostic testing (see Chapter 2), and answering the patient's or family's questions.

Neuropsychiatric Formulation

The history, behavior description, and neuropsychiatric review of systems, combined with the findings on neurological, mental status, and cognitive examination, and relevant ancillary tests, become part of the neuropsychiatric formulation. The neuropsychiatric formulation includes the following:

- A summary of the patient's signs and symptoms
- The anatomical localization or network dysfunction causing the neurocognitive findings
- The differential diagnosis of the symptoms
- One or more cognitive hypotheses for the symptoms (how a person's cognitive strengths and deficits lead to a particular presentation)
- A list of potentially reversible symptoms
- A treatment and rehabilitation plan that addresses the symptoms and diagnoses in the context of the cognitive hypothesis
- A prognostic statement

When the data from all ancillary testing and neuropsychological evaluation are available, the formulation may be updated.

Key Clinical Points

- The neuropsychiatric examination must be adapted to the clinical context and the abilities of the patient. Examinations for each of the neuropsychiatric disorders in this book include a basic examination drawn from this chapter and certain additional techniques particular to the disorder. Examinations for forensic purposes differ from examinations for clinical diagnostic purposes in some cases. The examination of nonverbal, neurodevelopmentally atypical, or uncooperative patients also must be adapted to the individual.
- Conducting the neurological examination in the same order as it is recorded and presented helps ensure that major areas are not omitted.
- Cognitive rating scales, useful in research, are often not sufficient for individualized diagnosis. The clinician must supple-

ment any general rating scale used with tasks tailored to the presenting complaint to attempt to understand the precise cause of the patient's concern.

- Convergent findings from different areas of the neurological and cognitive examinations increase the likelihood of localizing a patient's dysfunction.
- The neuropsychiatric evaluation concludes with a neuropsychiatric formulation. The formulation includes the salient findings from the history; behavioral description; review of systems; neurological, psychiatric, and cognitive examinations; neurodiagnostic and laboratory tests; anatomical or network localization of the dysfunction; differential diagnosis; cognitive hypotheses for behavior; potentially reversible symptoms; treatment and rehabilitation plan; and prognosis.

Review Questions

1. In a person with frontotemporal dementia, which of the following findings would be most likely when the patient is asked to draw a clock with hands set to 10 past 11?

   A. Inability to draw a circle.
   B. Crowding of the numbers on one side of the clock.
   C. Hands pointing to the 10 and the 11.
   D. Difficulty placing the numbers in the correct order.
   E. Drawing hands that extend beyond the boundaries of the circle.

2. A person with focal impaired awareness seizures has a symmetrical smile to command, but the left side of the mouth appears weaker than the right in response to a joke told by the examiner. Which of the following is the most likely location of the person's seizure focus?

   A. Left frontal lobe.
   B. Right pons.
   C. Left insula.
   D. Right temporal lobe.
   E. Left parietal lobe.

3. In assessing a person with serious and persistent mental illness for independent living, the treatment team has asked if the person could solve everyday problems of living, such as if they were to lose their prescription bottle. Which of the following cognitive tasks would best predict the patient's ability to solve these sorts of problems?

   A. Draw a clock task.
   B. Five-item recall task.
   C. Alternate uses task.
   D. Proverb interpretation.
   E. Verbal fluency.

Answers

Question 1: C. This is a classic finding in stimulus-bound behavior seen in dysfunction or degeneration of the dorsolateral prefrontal cortex. The patient hears the examiner say "10" and "11," and instead of drawing hands pointing to the 11 and the 2, the patient has difficulty overcoming the impetus to point to the numbers given in the task instruction.

Question 2: D. Asymmetry of the lower face in response to humor but with a symmetrical smile to command reflects dysfunction in the contralateral limbic system, basal ganglia, or supplementary motor area. The correct answer is the right temporal lobe, likely because of limbic seizure focus. A right frontal focus impacting the supplementary motor area could also cause this result.

Question 3: C. The alternate uses task evaluates divergent thinking or the ability to brainstorm various solutions to a problem. Although a person with serious and persistent mental illness might well have difficulty with any or all of the other task choices, this task most directly addresses this real-life problem that could come up in an independent living situation.

References

Albert ML: A simple test of visual neglect. Neurology 23(6):658–664, 1973 4736313

Amberger JS, Bocchini CA, Scott AF, Hamosh A: OMIM.org: leveraging knowledge across phenotype–gene relationships. Nucleic Acids Res 47(D1):D1038–D1043, 2019 30445645

American Psychiatric Association: Diagnostic and Statistical Manual of Mental Disorders, 5th Edition, Text Revision. Washington, DC, American Psychiatric Association, 2022

Benjamin S, Lauterbach M: The Brain Card®, 3rd Edition. Boston, MA, Brain Educators, 2016

Bodranghien F, Bastian A, Casali C, et al: Consensus paper: revisiting the symptoms and signs of cerebellar syndrome. Cerebellum 15(3):369–391, 2016 26105056

Bush G, Fink M, Petrides G, et al: Catatonia. I. Rating scale and standardized examination. Acta Psychiatr Scand 93(2):129–136, 1996 8686483

Cruz C, Amorim H, Beca G, et al: Neurogenic stuttering: a review of the literature. Rev Neurol 66(2):59–64, 2018 29323402

Daffner KR, Gale SA, Barrett AM, et al: Improving clinical cognitive testing: report of the AAN Behavioral Neurology Section Workgroup. Neurology 85(10):910–918, 2015 26163433

Delis D, Kramer J, Kaplan E, et al: CVLT: California Verbal Learning Test Manual. San Antonio, TX, The Psychological Association, 1987

Dippo C: Evaluating the Alternative Uses Test of Creativity, Proceedings of the National Conference on Undergraduate Research. La Crosse, University of Wisconsin, 2013, pp 427–434

Doody RS, Jankovic J: The alien hand and related signs. J Neurol Neurosurg Psychiatry 55(9):806–810, 1992 1402972

Doty RL: Olfactory dysfunction and its measurement in the clinic. World J Otorhinolaryngol Head Neck Surg 1(1):28–33, 2015 29204537

Firth HV, Hurst JA: Oxford Desk Reference: Clinical Genetics and Genomics, 2nd Edition. Oxford, UK, Oxford University Press, 2017

Granadillo ED, Mendez MF: Pathological joking or Witzelsucht revisited. J Neuropsychiatry Clin Neurosci 28(3):162–167, 2016 26900737

Goodglass H, Kaplan E: The Assessment of Aphasia and Related Disorders, 2nd Edition. Philadelphia, Lea & Febiger, 1983

Hamosh A, Scott AF, Amberger JS, et al: Online Mendelian Inheritance in Man (OMIM), a knowledgebase of human genes and genetic disorders. Nucleic Acids Res 33(Database Issue):D514–D517, 2005 15608251

Hopf HC, Müller-Forell W, Hopf NJ: Localization of emotional and volitional facial paresis. Neurology 42(10):1918–1923, 1992 1407573

Jones KL, Jones MC, Campo MD: Smith's Recognizable Patterns of Human Malformation, 7th Edition. Philadelphia, PA, Elsevier Saunders, 2013

Jones-Gotman M, Milner B: Design fluency: the invention of nonsense drawings after focal cortical lesions. Neuropsychologia 15(4–5):653–674, 1977 896022

Lauterbach MD, Schildkrout B, Benjamin S, et al: The importance of rare diseases for psychiatry. Lancet Psychiatry 3(12):1098–1100, 2016 27889002

Marie P: Révision de la question de l'aphasie. La Semaine Médicale 26:241–247, 1906

Mendez MF: Non-neurogenic language disorders: a preliminary classification. Psychosomatics 59(1):28–35, 2018 28911819

Mendez MF, Carr AR, Paholpak P: Psychotic-like speech in frontotemporal dementia. J Neuropsychiatry Clin Neurosci 29(2):183–185, 2017 27707194

Mesulam MM: Principles of Behavioral Neurology. Philadelphia, PA, FA Davis, 1985

Munetz MR, Benjamin S: How to examine patients using the Abnormal Involuntary Movement Scale. Hosp Community Psychiatry 39(11):1172–1177, 1988 2906320

Rath A, Olry A, Dhombres F, Brandt MM, Urbero B, Ayme S: Orphanet: a European database for rare diseases. Orphanet J Rare Dis 7(Suppl 1):S1, 2012 22422702

Robertson MM, Eapen V, Singer HS, et al: Gilles de la Tourette syndrome. Nat Rev Dis Primers 3:16097, 2017 28150698

Rumeau C, Nguyen DT, Jankowski R: How to assess olfactory performance with the Sniffin' Sticks test(®). Eur Ann Otorhinolaryngol Head Neck Dis 133(3):203–206, 2016 26344139

Sandson J, Albert ML: Perseveration in behavioral neurology. Neurology 37(11):1736–1741, 1987 3670611

Schmahmann JD, Weilburg JB, Sherman JC: The neuropsychiatry of the cerebellum: insights from the clinic. Cerebellum 6(3):254–267, 2007 17786822

Ward J: Synesthesia. Annu Rev Psychol 64:49–75, 2013 22747246

Whitty PF, Owoeye O, Waddington JL: Neurological signs and involuntary movements in schizophrenia: intrinsic to and informative on systems pathobiology. Schizophr Bull 35(2):415–424, 2009 18791074

2

The Neuropsychiatric Evaluation

Work-Up

Kathy Niu, M.D.

After the clinical interview and examination (see Chapter 1, "The Neuropsychiatric Evaluation"), the workup is tailored to the particular case to rule in or rule out disease or to monitor disease progression. In situations of low pretest probability and overly inclusive testing, there is a risk of false positives, costs, and undue side effects for the patient. On the other hand, many diagnoses are made only after specific laboratory tests, and results may be important for directing treatment. Understanding the differential and how test results may change management is important to consider prior to ordering the tests. In this chapter, I lay the foundation for the most common laboratory, neuroimaging, and electrophysiological studies, as well as some neuropathology studies, and the chapter is intentionally brief. The laboratory evaluation of specific neurological disorders is covered in their respective chapters.

Blood, Urine, and Cerebrospinal Fluid Testing

For most neuropsychiatric presentations, serum testing for complete blood count (CBC) and comprehensive metabolic panel (CMP) is helpful. Besides ruling out or assessing the degree of contribution from medical etiologies, baseline laboratory work includes hepatic and renal functioning to inform how medications will be metabolized as well as monitor for side effects. There is a very low threshold for ordering a thyroid-stimulating hormone (TSH) test with reflex-free T4 (thyroxine) for any presentation that may be due to a thyroid issue. When the clinician suspects poor nutrition or absorption, cyanocobalamin (B_{12}) ± methylmalonic acid (MMA), folate (B_9), vitamin D, thiamine (B_1), pyridoxine (B_6), and niacin (B_3) can be considered in neuropsychiatric presentations. An elevated MMA level is supportive of a B12 deficiency and is not abnormal in a folate deficiency. Depending on the presentation, infectious etiologies may need to be investigated with a treponemal immunoglobulin G (IgG) or rapid plasma reagin (RPR), HIV screening, and in endemic areas, Lyme testing. Given the extensive list of possible tests for various presentations, more specific advice is provided in subsequent chapters of this volume.

Genomic testing is becoming more widely available. Clues to a genetic etiology include family history, dysmorphic features, and younger than expected age at onset of symptoms. Referral to a genetic counselor can help guide optimal testing algorithms and orient the patient and family to the utility, limitations, and potential repercussions of the results. For example, cases of new variants or copy number variants of unknown significance are not uncommon when microarray or whole genome sequencing is used. Genetic panels are available for Alzheimer disease (both causative and risk factor genes) and frontotemporal dementia (causative genes). For autism spectrum disorder, chromosomal microarray and testing for fragile X syndrome is recommended. If a balanced translocation, aneuploidy, or mosaicism is suspected, a karyotype may also be added. Metabolic testing may also be considered in neurodevelopmental disorders with specific food intolerance, lethargy, hypotonia, dysmorphic features, intellectual disability, hearing or vision impairment, odd odors, early seizures, or lack of newborn screening. Metabolic testing evaluates for disorders involving amino acids, carbohydrates, purines, peptides, or mitochondria.

Common urine tests include pregnancy testing with human chorionic gonadotropin or toxicology screens for drugs of abuse. A lumbar puncture to examine the cerebrospinal fluid (CSF) should always include cell count, cell differential, protein, and glucose. An opening pressure can also be obtained when relevant. When the clinician is concerned about possible CNS infection, a gram stain, culture, and meningitis and encephalitis panel (polymerase chain reaction testing for the most common bacterial and viral pathogens) are included. When autoimmune or demyelinating conditions are suspected, oligoclonal bands and IgG index (both compared with serum) and specific antibodies or autoimmune panels can be ordered. CSF testing is also useful in testing for prion disease with real-time quaking-induced conversion or in seeking evidence for Alzheimer disease with amyloid β42 and total and phosphorylated tau levels.

Neuroimaging

Although many psychiatrists use neuroimaging only to rule out neurological causes rather than to diagnose psychiatric disorders, the ability to appropriately order and interpret neuroimaging is critical to the psychiatrist. Delirium and dementia are frequently encountered by consultation-liaison and geriatric psychiatrists, and the use of neuroimaging is debated less often in scenarios involving their patients. However, knowledge of neuroimaging is helpful to the general psychiatrist as well. First, the patient and other doctors may not know there is an underlying neurological cause, so the psychiatrist may be the one to determine the most appropriate imaging modality, the need for contrast, and any special image sequences or postprocessing. Second, radiology reports may not contain the level of detail desired (e.g., atrophy vs. localization of subtlely disproportionate atrophy), and the degree of pathology (e.g., mild, moderate, severe) is best appreciated by visualizing for oneself. Third, understanding the location and extent of a lesion helps the psychiatrist to determine whether the lesion is related to the presenting symptom or not. Comparison of current studies with prior neuroimaging side-by-side is helpful for demonstrating changes from baseline or disease progression. The importance of neuroimaging education for psychiatrists is described in more detail elsewhere (Cooper et al. 2024).

Neuroimaging techniques may be divided by technology (e.g., magnetic resonance imaging [MRI], computed tomography [CT]) or type of information (structural, functional, molecular). Ultrasound and infrared imaging are not reviewed in this chapter. Structural imaging includes CT and MRI. Common functional and molecular imaging techniques used clinically or in research include perfusion imaging, positron emission tomography (PET), single photon emission computed tomography (SPECT), magnetic resonance spectroscopy (MRS), and functional MRI (fMRI).

Structural Neuroimaging

When the architecture of the brain is suspected to be affected, an MRI or CT should be obtained. Factors to consider when ordering an MRI or CT are listed in Table 2.1. Contrast is used when one needs to visualize blood vessels (e.g., vascular malformations; aneurysms; atherosclerotic stenosis, vasculitis, vasospasm, occlusion, or thrombosis) or pathology in which the blood–brain barrier may be compromised causing contrast enhancement (e.g., inflammation, infection or abscess, active demyelination, neoplasm).

Computed Tomography

CT measures the degree of penetration of x-rays. This is quantified in Hounsfield units (HU) and visually presented on a scale from white/bright/hyperdense to black/dark/hypodense. Denser material such as metal and bone appears brighter, and less dense material such as air and fluid appears darker. Brain parenchyma generally lies on a gray scale. Examples of clinical scenarios in which CT is useful include detection of acute hemorrhage (hyperdense), acute ischemic stroke (hypodense), hydrocephalus (enlarged ventricles), presence of major or large lesions, and atrophy.

Magnetic Resonance Imaging

MRI uses a strong magnetic field to align hydrogen protons, applies radiofrequency pulses to move the hydrogen protons into a higher-energy state, and then measures the energy released as the protons relax or realign. MRI scans are also presented in a gray scale from black/dark/hypointense to white/bright/hyperintense, but this scale is more complex than that in a CT. The image produced by MRI depends on different standardized sequences that vary parameters such as the time between radio-frequency pulses to emphasize different tis-

Table 2.1 Comparison of CT and MRI

CT	MRI
More readily available	Less readily available
Less expensive	More expensive
Shorter scan duration	Longer scan duration
Lower image resolution	Higher image resolution
Better for assessing bone and calcium	Better for assessing most pathology (e.g., edema, acute ischemia, microhemorrhages, demyelination)
More artifact in posterior fossa	More artifact from motion (patient needs to be able to remain still)
No absolute contraindications, but uses ionizing radiation (need to minimize in children and pregnant patients)	Contraindicated with some metal (e.g., shrapnel near sensitive location) and incompatible implants/devices
Larger bore and more open	Smaller bore and more enclosed so may induce claustrophobia or may be too small for patients with very high body mass index (larger-bore or open MRI may be available)

sue types. The most common MRI sequences are outlined in Table 2.2, and examples of their clinical utility are given in Table 2.3. Although a particular image may be preferred to answer a clinical question, a different image may be ordered for practicality. For example, in a patient who is unable to stay still for an extended period for the MRI, a CT may be ordered instead.

Another MRI sequence that is becoming more clinically available is diffusion tensor imaging (DTI). It measures the direction and magnitude of diffusion of water molecules. Freely diffusing water is termed *isotropic;* water molecules constrained along the length of an axon are said to have *high fractional anisotropy*. Thus, DTI may have clinical utility for white matter tractography before tumor surgery and for assessing mild traumatic brain injury when more subtle white matter tract damage such as diffuse axonal injury may otherwise be missed. DTI

Table 2.2 Common MRI sequences and clinical uses

MRI sequence	Visualization	Clinical utility
T1	White matter (hyperintense) > gray matter (hypointense); CSF is black	Good resolution for structural anatomy, localization of atrophy, and presence of developmental abnormalities such as disorders of neuronal migration
T2	Gray matter (hyperintense) > white matter (hypointense); CSF is white	Most lesions/pathology (e.g., edema, ischemia, infection, inflammation, demyelination, tumor, gliosis) appear hyperintense.
FLAIR	T2 with CSF suppressed to black	Suppression of CSF allows better visualization of lesions close to CSF spaces such as those caused by periventricular microvascular disease or demyelination.
DWI	Restricted diffusion of water appears hyperintense	Identifies acute ischemic stroke, infection/abscess, dense cellular tumors, hypoxic ischemic changes, metabolic encephalopathies, seizure, CJD
ADC	Restricted diffusion of water appears hypointense	Match same area to hyperintensity on DWI for true restricted diffusion rather than "T2 shine-through"
SWI, GRE, SWAN	Deoxyhemoglobin, hemosiderin, ferritin/iron (e.g., blood products), or mineralization (e.g., calcium) appear hypointense/black	Can detect blood products that can be found in TBI and CAA, for example. Calcification can occur in various structures such as the choroid plexus (normal) and basal ganglia and within lesions. SWI is more sensitive (has more distortion) than GRE and SWAN.

Table 2.2 Common MRI sequences and clinical uses (*continued*)

MRI sequence	Visualization	Clinical utility
DTI	Water diffusion maps white matter tracks that can be color coded according to direction	White matter tractography before tumor operation guides the surgeon to minimize postoperative deficits. Even when other imaging is normal in mild TBI, DTI may detect loss of integrity of white matter to aid diagnosis and prognosis.

ADC = apparent diffusion coefficient; CAA = cerebral amyloid angiopathy; CJD = Creutzfeldt-Jakob disease; CSF = cerebrospinal fluid; DTI = diffusion tensor imaging; DWI = diffusion-weighted imaging; FLAIR = fluid-attenuated inversion recovery; GRE = gradient echo sequence; SWAN = star-weighted angiography; SWI = susceptibility weight imaging; TBI = traumatic brain injury.

Table 2.3 Selection of clinical neuroimaging method

Clinical presentation	Diagnostic question	Neuroimaging method
Acute symptoms		
Acute TBI	Are there fractures, subdural or epidural hematomas, intracerebral hemorrhages, subarachnoid hemorrhages, or contusions?	CT (I–)
Recent TBI with loss of consciousness and focal neurobehavioral syndrome but normal initial CT/MRI	Is there evidence of diffuse (traumatic) axonal injury?	MRI with GRE, SWAN, or SWI images to facilitate detection of iron in blood breakdown products from axonal injury
Delirium with focal signs	Is there a mass lesion, vascular pathology, hemorrhagic lesions, or increased intracranial pressure?	CT (I–) as initial screen, and if negative or need better resolution on finding, MRI (G+)
Acute-onset seizures or movement disorder, with amnestic syndrome	Is there evidence for lesion causing seizure or autoimmune limbic encephalitis (hippocampal enhancement on FLAIR images)?	MRI (G+) with seizure protocol
Acute febrile illness with seizures, amnestic syndrome	Is there evidence of herpes (or other) encephalitis?	MRI (G+) with seizure protocol

Table 2.3 Selection of clinical neuroimaging method (*continued*)

Clinical presentation	Diagnostic question	Neuroimaging method
Acute cortical neurologic deficits	Is there a stroke or metastasis? Is there hemorrhage? Evaluate candidacy for tPA treatment.	CT (I–) and CTA, CT perfusion if penumbra assessment is needed (for delayed endovascular treatment), MRI (G–) if CT is normal for stroke work-up, abbreviated hyperacute stroke MRI if needed, MRI (G+) if metastasis is suspected
Remote or chronic symptoms		
Remote head injury	Is there focal atrophy, gliosis, or an arachnoid cyst suggestive of prior hemorrhage?	MRI (G–)
Remote head injury with deterioration	Has hydrocephalus developed?	MRI (G–) or CT (I–); MRI offers better visualization of the aqueduct
Frontal lobe syndrome of unknown etiology	Is there focal frontal pathology (vascular, remote trauma, tumor, FTD)?	MRI (G+ if deterioration has occurred)
Seizures	Is there focal cortical pathology, evidence of past temporal lobe damage (focal atrophy), mesial temporal sclerosis, or heterotopias?	MRI with seizure protocol (including coronal T1, T2, FLAIR images with thin cuts through medial temporal lobe), preferably on a 3T magnet

Table 2.3 Selection of clinical neuroimaging method (*continued*)

Clinical presentation	Diagnostic question	Neuroimaging method
Dementia with history of stroke	Is there evidence for vascular dementia, small vessel disease (white matter), or combined AD and vascular dementia?	MRI (G–)
Dementia of unknown origin	Is there hydrocephalus, basal ganglia disease, vascular disease, tumor, focal atrophy consistent with FTD or AD, or white matter diseases?	MRI (G–), MRI (G+) if tumor suspected
Multiple lesions separated in time and space	Is there demyelinating disease, vasculitides, and other diseases?	MRI (G+)
Dyskinesia	Is there evidence for Huntington (caudate atrophy) or other basal ganglia disease?	MRI (G–)
Specific (focal) learning disorder	Is there congenital hemispheric damage (also see developmental disability)?	MRI (G–)
Developmental disorder with seizures, developmental regression, microcephaly, macrocephaly, dysmorphic features, or neurocutaneous signs	Is there agenesis of the corpus callosum, pachygyria, polymicrogyria, Dandy-Walker syndrome, cortical dysplasia, hydrocephalus, aqueductal stenosis, Arnold-Chiari malformation, neurocutaneous syndromes, arachnoid cysts, vascular malformations, evidence of congenital stroke, or leukodystrophies?	MRI (G–)

Table 2.3 Selection of clinical neuroimaging method (*continued*)

Clinical presentation	Diagnostic question	Neuroimaging method
Pseudobulbar palsy	Are there bilateral lesions of brainstem and/or hemispheres?	MRI (G+/–)
AIDS with neurological deterioration	Is there focal abscess, tumor, or progressive multifocal leukoencephalopathy?	MRI (G+)
Psychosis with signs of neurodevelopmental disorder or dysmorphic features	See developmental disorder	MRI (G–)

AD = Alzheimer disease; CT = computed tomography; CTA = CT angiogram; FLAIR = fluid-attenuated inversion recovery; FTD = frontotemporal dementia; G+ = with gadolinium contrast; G+/– = may or may not need gadolinium contrast depending on clinical concern; GRE = gradient recalled echo; I– = noncontrast; I+ = with iodine contrast; MRI = magnetic resonance imaging; SWAN = 3D T2 star-weighted angiography method used in GE scanners; SWI = susceptibility weighted imaging used in Siemens scanners; TBI = traumatic brain injury; tPA = tissue plasminogen activator.

Source. Adapted from Benjamin S: "Neuropsychiatric Assessment," in *Neuropsychiatry and Behavioral Neurology: Principles and Practice.* Edited by Silbersweig DA, Safar LT, Daffner KR. New York, McGraw Hill, 2021, pp. 171–196. Used with permission.

may also have a role in estimating white matter damage from stroke, neurodegenerative diseases, and other neuropathological processes.

Each MRI facility has its own menu of magnetic resonance sequences used for different diagnostic questions. It is helpful for clinicians to get to know their own radiology department's routine procedures and to formulate the referral question clearly for the radiologist. For example, for evaluation of focal seizures, ordering an MRI with seizure protocol will include a coronal FLAIR with thin cuts through the medial temporal lobe (common site for pathology causing seizures) and high-resolution T1 images for abnormal migration disorders.

Functional Neuroimaging

Many functional techniques are available to measure cerebral blood flow, metabolism, and network connectivity, and molecular imaging can label biomolecules in vivo. These techniques are frequently used in research; examples of clinical uses can be found in Table 2.4. PET scans may be of interest to psychiatrists for their utility in diagnosing and differentiating dementia types, in which decreased function or hypometabolism often precedes gross structural change. In cases of uncertainty or to ensure accurate diagnosis before committing to amyloid-clearing antibody treatment, a positive amyloid PET can support the diagnosis of Alzheimer disease. A DaT scan is a specific type of SPECT scan that uses a radioactively labeled ligand to detect dopamine transporters in the brain. Decreased dopamine transporter activity is typically seen in the putamen first and then additionally the caudate in Parkinson disease. The DaT scan may also be abnormal in Parkinson plus syndromes such as multiple-system atrophy, corticobasal degeneration, progressive supranuclear palsy, and dementia with Lewy bodies, but will be normal in essential tremor and drug-induced parkinsonism. In fMRI, changes in hemoglobin oxygenation (BOLD imaging) in specific brain areas correlate with increased or decreased activation, whereas magnetoencephalography (MEG) measures small magnetic fields produced by electric currents from neurons. Both may be used for presurgical localization of seizures and identification of task-specific eloquent cortex (e.g., location of language center).

Electrophysiological Testing

The most common electrophysiological tests that psychiatrists come across are electroencephalography, polysomnography, and autonomic

Table 2.4 Examples of functional neuroimaging techniques and uses

Neuroimaging modality	Content mapped	Clinical utility
Perfusion studies	Cerebral blood volume and blood flow in MRI or CT	Identification of the penumbra (salvageable brain tissue at risk) during acute ischemic stroke; grade aggressiveness of tumors
PET	Radioactively labeled glucose (FDG-PET) or other specific molecules	FDG-PET to differentiate dementia type; amyloid-PET for biomarkers of Alzheimer disease
SPECT	Radioactively labeled contrast for perfusion or specific molecules	Pattern of decreased blood flow to differentiate dementia type; dopamine transporter (DaT) scan to aid in diagnosis of Parkinson and Parkinson plus disorders
MRS	*N*-acetyl-aspartate, creatine, choline, glutamate and glutamine, and myo-inositol	Diagnosis and grading of tumors
fMRI	Task-based increase in oxygenated:deoxygenated hemoglobin ratio (BOLD signal) in MRI	Localization of eloquent cortex for presurgical evaluation in epilepsy and tumors
MEG	Magnetic fields generated by electrical activity of the brain	Localize seizure focus and identification of eloquent cortex, especially in presurgical planning

BOLD = blood-oxygen-level-dependent; DaT = dopamine transporter; FDG = fluorodeoxyglocuse; fMRI = functional MRI; MEG = magnetoencephalography; MRI = magnetic resonance imaging; MRS = magnetic resonance spectroscopy; PET = positron emission tomography; SPECT = single photon emission computed tomography.

testing. Sleep disorders are a common etiology of neuropsychiatric symptoms. Polysomnography is discussed in Chapter 15. Other tests, such as evoked potentials (EPs), electromyography (EMG), and nerve conduction studies (NCSs), are briefly reviewed in the subsection "Other Electrophysiological Tests."

Electroencephalogram

In obtaining an electroencephalogram (EEG), electrodes are placed on the scalp to measure electrical voltage differences between different standard points. The waveforms represent potential differences between electrodes or averages of electrodes, arrayed in configurations called *montages.* Several activating procedures, including sleep deprivation, strobe lights, and hyperventilation, may be included to increase the diagnostic yield for detecting epileptiform discharges. Extra temporal leads are sometimes applied to increase sensitivity, but nasopharyngeal leads are less often used because of discomfort and artifacts. EEGs are available in an office setting as a "spot" examination taking 20–30 minutes. Longer studies for seizure detection, taking hours to days, may be done at home or in the inpatient setting.

A normal EEG has a mix of different frequencies including a posterior dominant rhythm (PDR) in the alpha range (>8 and <13 Hz) when the patient is awake with eyes closed. This PDR may not form in severe encephalopathy and may slow with neurodegeneration and other pathologies. In a normal brain, there is an anterior-posterior gradient with faster frequency and lower amplitude anteriorly. The faster anterior beta frequencies (13–30 Hz) predominate in the setting of benzodiazepine, barbiturate, or alcohol use. Sharp waves, spikes, spike-wave complexes, and other paroxysmal changes are common findings in seizure disorders. Video EEG, the gold standard for the diagnosis of epileptic and nonepileptic seizures (Chapters 8 and 10), is often ordered in cases of recurrent, stereotyped neurological symptoms. EEG is sometimes used for unexplained altered mental status, in which diffuse slowing in the theta (4–8 Hz) and delta (<4 Hz) range are characteristic of encephalopathy. *Triphasic waves* are seen in hepatic and other encephalopathies. *Extreme delta brush* may be seen in anti-*N*-methyl-D-aspartate receptor encephalitis, and *periodic sharp wave complexes* may be seen in Creutzfeldt-Jakob disease. Asymmetry or focal differences may be seen in brain or skull structural abnormalities.

Autonomic Testing

Autonomic testing may be obtained in patients with otherwise unexplained dizziness, fatigue, syncope, paresthesia, abnormal sweating (too much or too little), bowel or urinary issues, or burning pain. Procedures during autonomic testing may involve deep breathing, Valsalva maneuver, a sweat test (quantitative sudomotor axon reflex test [QSART]; thermoregulary sweat test), and a tilt table test (controlled change in body position). Quantifying changes in heart rate, blood pressure, and sweat produced and correlating these with symptoms can help diagnose or monitor the severity of autonomic neuropathy, small-fiber neuropathy, and postural orthostatic tachycardia syndrome (POTS), which may have various etiologies. For example, the degree of autonomic dysfunction may differ in pure autonomic failure and parkinsonian syndromes. Tilt table testing of a person with POTS will reveal a sustained increase in heart rate of 30 bpm within 10 minutes in the upright (standing) position without an accompanying significant decrease in blood pressure.

Other Electrophysiological Tests

Evoked potentials measure electrical activity in the brain in response to different sensory modalities: visual, auditory, and somatosensory. The time it takes for a specific stimulus to reach the brain as measured by scalp EEG may be slowed for various reasons, including demyelination. A report of severe deficits with a normal EP might indicate a functional neurological disorder (e.g., blindness in a patient with a normal visual EP). Optical coherence tomography (OCT) may reveal thinning of the retinal nerve fiber layer indicative of optic nerve demyelination.

In cases of weakness, numbness, paresthesias, and neuropathic-sounding pain (sharp, shooting, burning), EMG and NCS may be helpful in the diagnosis of peripheral nerve disorders. NCS tests nerve conduction in a limb by applying an electric shock along a nerve and measuring the size and speed of transmission of the electrical impulse. EMG measures the activity of a motor unit and its muscle fibers by placing a needle inside a muscle and listening and watching both at rest and in contraction. The information can be synthesized to localize and identify the disorder as a neuronopathy, radiculopathy, plexopathy, polyneuropathy, focal neuropathy, neuromuscular junction pathology, or myopathy. The EMG/NCS can also be used to quantify severity of the dysfunction and its change over time.

Neuropathology

When diagnosis is unclear despite routine laboratory testing, biopsy, although more invasive, can often provide a definitive diagnosis. For example, if an MRI shows enhancement of brain tissue of unknown etiology, a biopsy may reveal the type of cancer, inflammation, or infection, each of which leads down different management paths. Patients with dementia may have overlapping symptoms or more than one pathology, and in some cases only receive diagnostic clarity in a postmortem examination. For example, the presence of amyloid plaques and neurofibrillary tangles points to Alzheimer disease; the presence of Lewy bodies points to Lewy body dementia and Parkinson disease; and so on. Postmortem brain examination may also reveal evidence of other undiagnosed neurodegenerative diseases, such as chronic traumatic encephalopathy or prion diseases. Diagnostic clarity offers closure for families or may have genetic implications.

Biopsy of other sites, such as muscle, nerve, or skin, can also be helpful. For example, small fiber neuropathy can be notoriously difficult to diagnose because it does not show up on neuroimaging or EMG/NCS. Even a skin biopsy may result in a false negative, but the presence of reduced intraepidermal nerve fiber density is diagnostic of small fiber neuropathy. A skin biopsy can also detect α-synuclein, which is supportive of Parkinson disease and related disorders. A muscle biopsy is used to confirm the diagnosis of myopathies and muscular dystrophies.

Key Clinical Points

- Given the cost and possible adverse effects of each diagnostic procedure, clinicians should have a clear diagnostic differential as well as know how they will use the results before ordering tests.
- Baseline and screening serum studies for most patients with neuropsychiatric disorders include complete blood count, comprehensive metabolic panel, and tests for thyroid-stimulating hormone and vitamin B_{12}. Additional testing is guided by the clinical question.

- CT scans are more accessible and faster and evaluate bone and calcium better than MRI. CT is also the better method for ruling out acute bleeding. MRI has additional potentially prohibitory considerations (metal in the body, claustrophobia, body habitus, inability to lie still) but offers higher-resolution images and more information through various sequences. Use of contrast may offer a better view of blood vessels or disruption of the blood–brain barrier in cases of infection, inflammation, and neoplasm.
- Diffuse slowing of the awake EEG is characteristically seen in encephalopathies. Paroxysmal bursts of sharp waves, spikes, or spike-wave complexes are seen in seizure disorders. Provoking factors such as sleep deprivation, photic stimulation, and hyperventilation increase the chances of finding epileptiform dischrages on EEG.

Review Questions

1. A patient's B_{12} level is 300 pg/mL, which is in the low normal range. Which of the following laboratory tests would confirm B_{12} deficiency?

   A. Homocysteine
   B. Methylmalonic acid
   C. Blood smear
   D. Complete blood count
   E. Mean corpuscular volume

2. Which of the following brain imaging procedures is the best for diagnostic clarification in a 70-year-old patient with insidious onset and slow progression of memory and visuospatial decline over 3 years?

   A. CT without contrast
   B. CT with and without contrast
   C. MRI without contrast
   D. MRI with and without contrast
   E. CT angiography

3. A patient's EEG results show an 11-Hz rhythm in the posterior region of the brain. Which of the following clinical scenarios is most consistent with this finding?

   A. Conscious patient with eyes closed
   B. Drowsy patient transitioning to sleep
   C. Intoxicated patient taking a benzodiazepine
   D. Delirious patient with hepatic encephalopathy
   E. Patient with epilepsy responding to photic stimulation

Answers

Question 1: B. Methylmalonic acid is elevated in B_{12} deficiency but not in folate deficiency. The elevation of homocysteine, macrocytic anemia, and hypersegmented neutrophils on blood smear can be present for both B_{12} and folate deficiencies.

Question 2: C. MRI offers better resolution than CT and will be more likely to detect findings of etiologic significance such as focal atrophy and vascular burden. Contrast is generally only needed if there is suspicion of breakdown of the blood–brain barrier, but the long timeline points to neurodegeneration as the most likely diagnosis. CT angiography may help with the diagnosis of vascular causes of dementia, but the case does not suggest a vascular etiology.

Question 3: A. The posterior dominant rhythm in the alpha range (8–13 hertz) is a normal finding for a conscious patient with their eyes closed. Drowsy patients may manifest slow eye movements; benzodiazepines create fast frequencies (excess beta). Delirious patients may have generalized slowing or triphasic waves. Photic stimulation in a patient with epilepsy might produce epileptiform discharges or provoke a seizure.

References

Benjamin S: Neuropsychiatric assessment, in Neuropsychiatry and Behavioral Neurology: Principles and Practice. Edited by Silbersweig DA, Safar LT, Daffner KR. New York, McGraw Hill, 2021, pp 171–196

Cooper JJ, Valencia VA, Niu K: Neuroimaging education in psychiatric training. Neuropsychopharmacology 50(1):298–304, 2024 39025952

3

Neurological Approach to Psychiatric Presentations

Kathy Niu, M.D.
Sheldon Benjamin, M.D.

This chapter serves as a guide for the evaluation of select common neuropsychiatric presentations: visual hallucinations, new-onset psychosis, catatonia, apathy, affective lability, aggressive behavior and pain syndromes. Each section starts with an introduction to review terminology and overarching principles used to organize the differential diagnoses. For example, outlining a clear timeline (onset and progression) is important to all diagnostic thinking. The introduction is followed by a table of the most common differential diagnoses along with their typical histories and examination findings, and some initial tests to consider.

This chapter is not intended to be comprehensive. For example, delirium can manifest with almost any neuropsychiatric symptom with a long list of possible etiologies, so delirium is intentionally not repeated throughout each section. The information is distilled for easy reference, with the assumption that the reader will apply their own clinical judgment in all evaluations.

Visual Hallucinations

Simple or *unformed* hallucinations are composed of light, lines, or geometric shapes, whereas complex or *formed* hallucinations are of people, animals, objects, or whole scenes. Some diagnoses—such as retinal pathology, optic nerve pathology, and almost all migraines with visual aura—exclusively feature simple hallucinations. Other diagnoses may feature either simple or complex hallucinations. An example descriptor of a complex hallucination is *Lilliputian*, which refers to miniature people or creatures.

Monocular hallucinations are experienced only through one eye and thus indicate pathology in that eye or optic nerve prior to the optic chiasm. For example, floaters on the right side of vision that disappears with closing the right eye indicates an issue in the right eyeball. However, many patients have difficulty knowing whether their experiences are monocular or binocular because they may not have tried closing one eye at a time, and some pathology isolated to one eye (e.g., retinal detachment) may produce flashing lights even with both eyes closed. Binocular hallucinations (present with either eye open) imply brain pathology but can also be secondary to bilateral eye issues. Knowing if the hallucination is always present in a certain quadrant or hemifield could be helpful for localization. For example, a visual hallucination in the right upper quadrant may indicate pathology in the left occipital lobe below the calcarine fissure.

Other organizing principles to note include the presence of hallucinations in other sensory modalities, level of insight, triggers, duration, and frequency (O'Brien et al. 2020). Evaluation of visual hallucinations is described in Table 3.1. Diagnoses not reviewed in the table include delirium, all neurocognitive disorders, and psychiatric disorders (e.g., schizophrenia spectrum and related disorders, mood disorders with psychotic features).

New-Onset Psychosis

The possible etiologies of new-onset psychosis vary by patient age. Psychosis due to inherited metabolic disorders often begins in childhood through young adulthood, with the most common causes listed in Table 3.2 (Benjamin et al. 2013). Idiopathic psychotic disorders tend to begin in adolescence or young adulthood through middle age. Psychotic disorders beginning in late middle age and later are more likely

Table 3.1 Evaluation of visual hallucinations

History and examination	Diagnosis	Investigation
History: Simple hallucination (e.g., flashing lights) lasting for seconds at a time, monocular > binocular, intact insight; may worsen with valsalva **Exam:** May have vision loss; fundoscopy may reveal retinal pathology	Retinal pathology (e.g., retinal tear or detachment, posterior vitreous detachment, retinopathy, cone dystrophies)	Ophthalmology referral
History: Simple hallucination, geometric shape (e.g., fortification spectra, scintillating scotoma), lasting minutes to hours, >1 minute to move across visual field, intact insight, usually binocular; often followed by headache **Exam:** Often normal unless headache is secondary to other CNS pathology; during aura, may have transient motor symptoms such as hemiparesis	Migraine with visual aura	Reassurance or brain MRI for secondary causes
History: Simple (e.g., colored circle) or complex (e.g., objects, people) hallucination lasting seconds to 2 minutes, moves across visual field in seconds, often binocular and hemifield, may have other ictal phenomena and postictal headache, insight usually intact **Exam:** Often normal between events unless seizures are secondary to other CNS pathology	Seizure	EEG, brain MRI with and without contrast

Table 3.1 Evaluation of visual hallucinations (*continued*)

History and examination	Diagnosis	Investigation
History: Simple or complex hallucination, stationary or with movement, binocular, variable duration and frequency, insight often intact, worse with less lighting or decreased arousal **Exam:** Poor visual acuity in one or both eyes	Visual release hallucination (i.e., Charles Bonnet syndrome)	If monocular vision loss, ophthalmology referral; if binocular, brain MRI
History: Simple or complex hallucination, binocular, may accompany auditory/tactile hallucinations, persists, ± insight, history of temporal relationship to discontinuation of alcohol or using new medication or substance **Exam:** Depends on substance, autonomic instability	Alcohol withdrawal, medication side effect (e.g., dopaminergic medications), substance use (e.g., stimulants, hallucinogens)	Urine or serum toxicology, drug levels, basic labs
History: Complex hallucination lasting seconds to minutes, binocular, full field, occurs during transition to sleep or awakening, insight intact; may accompany auditory or tactile hallucinations, cataplexy, sleep paralysis, and daytime somnolence **Exam:** Normal	Narcolepsy	Multiple sleep latency test

Table 3.1 Evaluation of visual hallucinations (*continued*)

History and examination	Diagnosis	Investigation
History: Complex hallucination, binocular, full field, variable duration but can be persistent, insight variable, associated with sleep disturbance, may accompany auditory or tactile hallucinations, may appear movie-like, as if hallucination is taking place all around them **Exam:** Focal examination depending on site of lesion in midbrain, pons, or thalamus	Peduncular hallucinosis	Brain MRI

CNS = central nervous system; EEG = electroencephalogram; MRI = magnetic resonance imaging.

Table 3.2 Evaluation of new-onset psychosis

Findings on evaluation	Diagnosis	Investigation
History: Delusions, hallucinations, or disorganized speech; negative symptoms or disorganized or catatonic behavior; at least two symptoms present; decline in function **Exam:** Normal or some choreoathetoid movements and/or soft neurological signs (Chapter 7), subtle deficits in executive function, working memory, and processing speed	Schizophrenia spectrum disorders: brief psychotic disorder, schizophreniform disorder, schizophrenia, schizoaffective disorder	Refer to DSM-5-TR (American Psychiatric Association 2022)
History: Manic or hypomanic behavior with or without depressive episodes; history of major depressive episodes; psychosis occurs only during mood episode	Mood disorders: bipolar I disorder, bipolar II disorder, major depressive disorder	Refer to DSM-5-TR

Table 3.2 Evaluation of new-onset psychosis (*continued*)

Findings on evaluation	Diagnosis	Investigation
History: Substance use, withdrawal symptoms, diplopia, muscle weakness, unsteady gait, new-onset seizures (Chapter 8) **Exam:** Attention and memory deficits, tremor, myoclonic jerks, extraocular muscle weakness, asterixis, proximal muscle wasting, dystonia, choreoathetosis, gait ataxia	Psychotic disorder due to substance use: intoxication, withdrawal, acute medication side effect, substance-induced psychotic disorder, Wernicke encephalopathy, Korsakoff psychosis, other nutritional deficiency	Toxicology screen, hepatic enzymes, bilirubin, B_1, B_{12}, folate levels
History: Memory loss or cognitive deterioration beginning in middle to old age, family history of dementia, behavioral disinhibition, spatial disorientation, psychotic symptoms (Chapter 4) **Exam:** Deficits in executive function, verbal or nonverbal recall, visual-spatial sense, language; behavior change; release signs, paratonia, parkinsonian signs, other movement disorder	Psychotic disorder due to neurodegenerative diseases: FTD (especially *C9orf72*), Alzheimer disease, Huntington disease, Parkinson disease, dementia with Lewy bodies, prion disease, corticobasal syndrome (multiple pathophysiological causes), other basal ganglia diseases	MRI; FTD genes (*C9orf72*, *GRN*, *MAPT*); if early onset or family history, Alzheimer genes (*APP*, *PSEN1*, *PSEN2*); HD gene (CAG repeats); PET or DaT scan; CSF 14-3-3 protein, QuIC; ceruloplasmin if indicated

Table 3.2 Evaluation of new-onset psychosis (*continued*)

Findings on evaluation	Diagnosis	Investigation
History: Cognitive deficits; mood disorder; movement disorder; seizures; motor, sensory, cerebellar symptoms; arthritis; dermatitis; neuropathy; subacute onset (Chapters 13 and 14) **Exam:** Variable motor, sensory abnormalities, and/or upper motor neuron deficits	Psychotic disorder due to autoimmune disease: autoimmune limbic encephalitis, other paraneoplastic syndromes, systemic lupus erythematosus, neurosarcoidosis, demyelinating disease, leukoencephalopathies	MRI; EEG; evoked potentials if indicated; C-reactive protein; serum ANA; urinalysis; CSF protein, oligoclonal bands, IgG synthesis; specific autoantibodies for suspected etiology or panel in serum and CSF (Chapter 14)
History: Adolescent, young adult, or early middle age; cognitive decline, psychosis, movement disorder; history of auditory, cardiovascular, dermatological, endocrine, gastrointestinal, genitourinary, hematological, hepatic, or visuospatial system abnormalities; neuropathy **Exam:** Cognitive deficits, with or without dysmorphic features, soft signs, variable neurological findings, and neurocutaneous signs (Chapter 7)	Psychotic disorder due to congenital genetic or metabolic disorder, acquired metabolic disorder: acute intermittent porphyria; autism spectrum disorder; Down syndrome; fragile X syndrome; Gilbert syndrome; glucose-6-phosphate dehydrogenase deficiency; XXX karyotype; Huntington disease; Klinefelter syndrome XXY; Marfan syndrome; neurofibromatosis type 1; oculocutaneous albinism; phenylketonuria; Turner syndrome; 22q11.2 deletion (velocardiofacial) syndrome; mitochondrial disorders	Genetic tests as appropriate, microarray testing with autism spectrum disorder, metabolic testing, heavy metal screen, porphyrins

Table 3.2 Evaluation of new-onset psychosis (*continued*)

Findings on evaluation	Diagnosis	Investigation
History: High-risk sexual behaviors or IV drug use, history of COVID-19 infection, tick bite, mosquito bites **Exam:** Skin rash, cranial mononeuropathy (Chapter 12)	Psychotic disorder due to infection: HIV-AIDS, COVID-19, neurosyphilis, Lyme disease, other infection	Specific antibody tests
History: Headache, seizures, focal neurobehavioral symptoms **Exam:** Focal neurological examination, upper motor neuron signs, disinhibition, apathy, frontal/executive dysfunction, frontal release signs (Chapters 11, 13)	Psychotic disorder due to migraine or neoplasm: migraine, neoplasm (especially frontal and limbic)	MRI
History: Known stroke, sudden onset, stepwise cognitive decline, recent vascular event **Exam:** Focal neurological or cognitive features depending on localization (Chapter 16)	Psychotic disorder due to neurovascular disease: vascular dementia, poststroke psychosis, CNS vasculitis	MRI, vascular imaging as indicated

Table 3.2 Evaluation of new-onset psychosis (*continued*)

Findings on evaluation	Diagnosis	Investigation
History: Recent increase or decrease in seizure frequency, recent change in antiseizure medication **Exam:** Visual and verbal recall deficits present during psychosis symptoms, Babinski sign may be present during seizure symptoms (Chapters 8 and 10)	Psychotic disorder related to seizure disorder: ictal psychotic symptoms, postictal psychosis, interictal psychosis, psychosis due to antiseizure medication	Antiseizure medication levels, EEG during symptoms
History: Description of head injury, duration of retrograde and anterograde amnesia, description of focal imaging abnormalities, seizures; dementia; unwitnessed TBI in care facilities; substance use **Exam:** Inattention, focal cognitive and/or neurological deficits (Chapter 5)	Psychotic disorder due to traumatic brain injury: contusions, hemorrhage, anoxic damage; hydrocephalus	MRI, EEG

ANA = antinuclear antibodies; CSF = cerebrospinal fluid; DaT = dopamine transporter; EEG = electroencephalogram; FTD = frontotemporal dementia; HD = Huntington disease; HIV = human immunodeficiency virus; IgG = immunoglobulin G; MRI = magnetic resonance imaging; PET = positron emission tomography; QuIC = quaking-induced conversion; TBI = traumatic brain injury.

to have medical etiologies. In each case, psychosis may be comorbid or part of the syndrome.

Visual hallucinations tend to occur more frequently in psychosis due to medical conditions (see previous section). Most medical conditions can result in delirium with psychosis; these are not extensively covered here. Examination findings refer to those seen in the diagnostic category, so they may not be present for each specific diagnosis. Prior to other specific investigations listed in Table 3.2, the usual baseline laboratory evaluation includes complete blood count (CBC), comprehensive metabolic panel (CMP), thyroid-stimulating hormone (TSH) level, syphilitic serology (rapid plasma reagin [RPR], serum or CSF Venereal Disease Research Laboratory [VDRL] test, treponemal antibody tests), and toxicology screen.

Catatonia

Catatonia is an urgent and potentially life-threatening psychiatric presentation that can be missed. *Catatonia* involves a psychiatric or medical deterioration with a progressive decrease or disorganization in communication combined with an increase or decrease in psychomotor activity. Decreased psychomotor activity may range from slowing to stupor. Increased activity can range from stereotypy or mannerism to extreme hyperkinesis. The development of autonomic instability with elevated blood pressure, temperature, and/or heart rate typically requires rapid intervention and treatment in an intensive care setting.

The Bush Francis Catatonia Rating Scale (BFCRS) and the DSM criteria for catatonia, found in Chapter 1, "The Neuropsychiatric Evaluation," are the basis of diagnosis requiring the presence of either two items on the BFCRS or three items in the DSM-5-TR criteria (American Psychiatric Association 2022). The differential diagnosis of catatonia includes psychiatric disorders, medical conditions, functional neurological disorders, and more volitional disorders such as malingering or factitious disorder.

The catatonic syndrome may be caused by or merely coincident with numerous medical and neurological syndromes, as illustrated in Table 3.3. Examples of reported causes include traumatic brain injury with encephalopathy, neurodevelopmental syndromes, brain tumors, autoimmune diseases, paraneoplastic syndromes, and autoimmune limbic encephalitis, CNS infection, demyelinating disease, neurodegenerative diseases, neurovascular disease, hepatic failure, renal fail-

Table 3.3 Evaluation of catatonia

Findings on evaluation	Differential diagnoses	Investigations
History: History of psychiatric disorder with superimposed catatonic syndrome	Primary psychiatric diagnosis: autism spectrum disorder, bipolar disorder, major depressive disorder, neurodevelopmental disorder, OCD, brief psychotic disorder with peripartum onset (postpartum psychosis), schizophrenia spectrum disorders	Refer to DSM-5 (American Psychiatric Association 2022)
History: Brief (seconds to minutes) stereotyped episodes or a co-occurring seizure disorder **Exam:** Automatisms, rhythmic movements, myoclonus, gaze deviation, series of 20-second to 2-minute stereotyped behaviors	Focal seizure	Video EEG for correlation of behavior with EEG, brain MRI with and without contrast (specify "epilepsy protocol")
History: History of substance abuse	Substance intoxication or withdrawal	Urine toxicology screen
History: Treatment with lithium or antipsychotic agents; recent changes in medications or medication dosage; combination of two or more serotonergic agents **Exam:** Tremor; rigidity of limb, trunk, or whole body (opisthotonos); elevated vital signs	Medication-related condition: lithium toxicity, lithium-induced hypothyroidism, neuroleptic malignant syndrome, neuroleptic dystonia, serotonin syndrome, tacrolimus toxicity	Serum lithium level, TSH, creatine kinase, urine myoglobin

Table 3.3 Evaluation of catatonia (*continued*)

Findings on evaluation	Differential diagnoses	Investigations
History: Acute catatonia with recent-onset subacute anterograde amnesia, movement disorder, and/or seizures **Exam:** Impaired attention and recall	Autoimmune limbic encephalitis	Brain MRI; EEG; serum neuronal autoantibody panel (see Chapter 14); CSF protein, IgG index and synthesis rate, oligoclonal bands, antineuronal antibodies; serum or CSF NfL levels may differentiate primary psychotic disorders from autoimmune causes
History: Acute catatonia with fever, headache **Exam:** Nuchal rigidity, confusion (Chapter 12)	Meningoencephalitis	CBC, cranial CT, CSF encephalitis panel
History: New-onset catatonia with headache **Exam:** Focal neurological signs, signs of increased CSF pressure (Chapter 13)	CNS neoplasm	Brain MRI with and without contrast

CBC = complete blood count; CNS = cerebrospinal fluid; CSF = cerebrospinal fluid; CT = computed tomography; EEG = electroencephalogram; IgG = immunoglobulin G; MRI = magnetic resonance imaging; NfL = neurofilament light chain, TSH = thyroid-stimulating hormone.

ure, hereditary metabolic disorders, hypothyroidism, and sepsis. The evaluation typically begins with a general medical laboratory workup, including CBC, CMP, TSH, RPR, HIV testing, B_{12} level, and evaluation of any of the patient's known metabolic conditions (Rogers et al. 2023).

Apathy

Apathy has been conceptualized as diminished motivation manifesting as an internal state and outwardly decreased voluntary behavior. Apathy can be divided into diminished initiative, interest, emotional expression, responsiveness, or other characteristics (Steffens et al. 2022). By definition, apathy should not be attributable to a decreased level of consciousness. Apathy may be considered the least severe presentation on a spectrum that runs to the more severe syndromes of abulia and *akinetic mutism*, the latter defined by the absence of volitional movement or speech. Apathy may be caused by disruption of frontostriatal, reward, salience, or executive pathways, and has many possible neurological causes. Distinguishing the anhedonia, low motivation, poor concentration, and low energy of major depressive disorder from apathy of a neurological disorder is not always easy, and the two can also co-occur. Accurate diagnosis is important because it may change management strategies. For example, a misdiagnosis of depression may result in the omission of necessary workup for a neurological etiology and can lead to prescribing a selective serotonin reuptake inhibitor, which may in turn worsen apathy owing to emotional blunting.

In reviewing the differential diagnosis of apathy (Table 3.4), the clinician should consider the presence of distress and any active avoidance of activities for a particular reason, both of which would argue for psychological or psychiatric reasons. The onset and progression of apathy may vary.

Affective Lability

Affective lability refers to instability of affect, the external cues to one's emotion. Key components of the history include triggers, duration, internal experience of the emotion, and associated features (Miller et al. 2011). The standard mental status examination makes the distinction between mood (internal emotion, as stated by the patient) and affect (external expression of emotion), and these tend to match (be congruent) in psychiatric diagnoses, although not always. When mood

Table 3.4 Evaluation of apathy

Findings on evaluation	Diagnosis	Investigations
History: Sadness; associated symptoms such as guilt, change in appetite, suicidal ideation; feelings of worthlessness or hopelessness; distress, anxiety; apathy feels ego-dystonic; active avoidance of activities **Exam:** May have psychomotor slowing, low verbal output, poor eye contact, and impaired attention and working memory on testing if symptoms are severe	Mood disorder (e.g., major depressive disorder, bipolar depression)	Refer to DSM-5-TR (American Psychiatric Association 2022)
History: Long-standing affective blunting, alogia, anhedonia, asociality, and avolition that may precede (prodromal) or follow (residual) the more positive symptoms of hallucinations and delusions **Exam:** Normal neurological exam other than neurological "soft signs" and more subtle cognitive deficits involving attention, executive function, or processing speed	Schizophrenia spectrum disorder	Refer to DSM-5-TR
History: Chronic apathy with insidious onset and generally slow progressive worsening **Exam:** Specific cognitive domains and exam findings depend on type of dementia (see Chapter 4)	Major or minor neurocognitive disorder (e.g., Alzheimer disease, behavioral variant frontotemporal dementia)	Brain MRI without contrast

Table 3.4 Evaluation of apathy (*continued*)

Findings on evaluation	Diagnosis	Investigations
History: Acute apathy with maximum symptoms at onset or more insidious progression **Exam:** Associated neurological signs depending on stroke location; if subcortical vascular disease, slowing of processing speed (see Chapter 16)	Stroke or chronic small vessel disease (e.g., stroke in prefrontal cortex, medial frontal, striatum, ventral basal ganglia, thalamus, or diffuse white matter)	Brain MRI without contrast
History: Chronic progressive symptoms with primary tumor and acute onset with metastasis; headache, seizure, focal deficits **Exam:** Associated neurological signs depending on tumor location; signs of increased intracranial pressure such as papilledema	Brain tumor (e.g., craniopharyngioma, meningioma involving frontal lobe)	Brain MRI with and without contrast
History: Moderate to severe head injury or repeated concussions **Exam:** May have focal neurological signs from contusions, hemorrhage, or ischemia; may have anosmia or other cranial nerve dysfunction (see Chapter 5)	Traumatic brain injury	Brain MRI without contrast
History: Timing of substance or drug use precipitates apathy **Exam:** Vital sign abnormalities, abnormal pupil size, stigmata of injections, associated signs and symptoms depending on substance	Substance-induced apathy (e.g., opioid, benzodiazepine, barbiturate; withdrawal from cocaine/stimulant; chronic marijuana use; antidopaminergic side effect)	Toxicology screen and confirmation

CTE = chronic traumatic encephalopathy; MRI = magnetic resonance imaging.

swings are a lifelong pattern and are triggered by rejection sensitivity, a diagnosis of a personality disorder is more likely. On the other hand, new affective lability that does not match the internal feeling state hints at an underlying neurological disorder causing pseudobulbar affect (PBA). PBA is also known by other names: pathological laughing and crying, involuntary emotional expression disorder, and emotional incontinence. The typical history and examination findings for PBA, seizures, and movement disorders are listed in Table 3.5.

Aggressive Behavior

Aggressive behavior, although a frequent reason for consultation, lacks an accepted standardized approach to diagnosis and treatment. Aggressive behavior can occur in the context of almost any psychiatric or neurological disorder. Unfortunately, pharmacological interventions are often used without first determining a specific cause of the behavior. As with epilepsy, which requires a description of semiology to determine the most effective treatment, the semiology of aggressive behavior can aid in treatment selection. An important first step is the so-called 4-P approach: obtaining a detailed description that includes the prodrome, if present; the precipitant; the purpose of the behavior if it can be discerned; and the pattern (Benjamin 1999, 2016). Prodromal behaviors may include sleep deprivation, hyperphagia, polydipsia, psychotic symptoms, anxiety or panic, sadness or depression, psychomotor excitement, euphoria, irritability, increased rituals, delirium, or signs of intoxication and withdrawal. Common precipitants include environmental changes (including caregiver changes), increased or decreased stimulation, internal conflict, psychosocial stressors, trivial provocation, or planned attack, or there may be no obvious precipitant.

Remorse or amnesia for the aggression are generally not helpful in determining whether the aggressive behavior is of psychiatric or neurological origin. A person with temporolimbic epilepsy or autism spectrum disorder may recall an incident and feel remorseful, whereas a person with intermittent explosive disorder or narcissistic personality disorder may claim amnesia for an incident.

Episode duration may offer a clue as to etiology. Focal seizures tend to last 20 seconds to 3 minutes. Migraine may last several hours. Panic attacks come on quickly and dissipate slowly over minutes to hours. Aggressive behavior in clouded consciousness or with a clear onset and conclusion suggests neurological etiology. Carefully planned or

Table 3.5 Evaluation of affective lability

Findings on evaluation	Diagnosis	Investigations
History: Affect and mood often congruent but with exceptions; DSM-5 criteria are referenced for associated symptoms; episodic in mood disorders, chronic lifelong in personality disorders **Exam:** Notable features may be present on the mental status exam (e.g., fast rate of speech, psychomotor agitation in mania) but neurological exam is normal	Primary psychiatric disorders (e.g., crying in MDD, laughing in bipolar mania, emotional lability in personality disorder)	Refer to DSM-5 (American Psychiatric Association 2022)
History: Affect and mood are incongruent and appear inappropriate to situation; mirthless laughter and "crocodile tears" are involuntary; patient may report anxiety or somatic symptoms during, usually <1 minute; stereotyped **Exam:** During seizure, the laughing and crying may appear forced or with grunting noises; there may be automatisms (e.g., lip smacking, swallowing) and staring; normal neurologic exam in between spells	Focal seizure (e.g., gelastic/laughing or dacrystic/crying seizures)	EEG

Table 3.5 Evaluation of affective lability (*continued*)

Findings on evaluation	Diagnosis	Investigations
History: Mood and affect are usually incongruent; possible anxiety precipitating movements; feels involuntary; premonitory urge and relief with movement in tics **Exam:** Forced muscle contraction in facial dystonia; quick movement in tics or production of noises that may sound like laughing and crying; irregular continuous movements in dyskinesia	Movement disorders (e.g., facial dystonia, focal or vocal tics, facial dyskinesia)	Clinical diagnosis
History: Sudden laughing or crying that is not consistent with or commensurate to internal mood; may be precipitated by innocuous personal questions such as inquiry about family; involuntary; duration seconds to minutes **Exam:** May be able to elicit with prompts (e.g., recall the moment your child graduated); abnormal neurological examination depending on underlying etiology, may also occur as part of pseudobulbar palsy (dysarthria, dysphagia, increased jaw jerk, hyperactive gag)	Pseudobulbar affect (e.g., due to TBI, MS, ALS, stroke, dementia)	Brain MRI (with or without contrast)

ALS = amyotrophic lateral sclerosis; EEG = electroencephalogram; MDD = major depressive disorder; MRI = magnetic resonance imaging; MS = multiple sclerosis; TBI = traumatic brain injury.

directed attacks, or those with claimed amnesia for the attack, are less likely to be of neurological origin. Interventions may be pharmacological, behavioral, or environmental, depending on the data obtained. Rather than listing differential diagnoses and diagnostic evaluations as in other sections, Table 3.6 lists the common patterns of aggressive behavior that can lead to different treatment approaches and some of their causes.

Pain Syndromes

Pain is a very common complaint with a long differential and often requires a multidisciplinary team that may include neurology, psychiatry, psychology, physiatry, physical therapy, anesthesiology, primary care, and sometimes surgery or complementary/alternative medicine. Pain is more than simply an unpleasant sensation from actual or potential tissue damage. It also includes the associated emotional experience (Raja et al. 2020), placing the subjective experience of pain in the borderland of neurology and psychiatry.

It is important to first categorize pain as acute or chronic. *Acute pain* is of shorter duration, dissipates when the underlying cause is addressed (e.g., healing after traumatic fracture), and generally serves an adaptive and protective role. *Chronic pain* can persist beyond the initial injury or usual course, which may lead to psychological and functional disability.

Pain can also be divided on the basis of mechanism: nociceptive, neuropathic, and nociplastic. *Nociceptive pain* arises from damage to tissue that activates nociceptors and can be further divided into somatic and visceral. In somatic pain, damage to skin, muscles, joints, and/or connective tissue results in sharp, throbbing, or pressure-like pain. In visceral pain, damage to internal organs classically results in cramping or aching pain. *Neuropathic pain* results from injury to the somatosensory nervous system (e.g., diabetic neuropathy) and is often described as burning, sharp, or shooting. Finally, in *nociplastic pain* (e.g., fibromyalgia), the patient may experience a sensation of widespread pain despite no evidence of tissue damage. One mechanism may be central sensitization that enhances the perception of pain after minor or even no peripheral stimulation.

Useful elements of the history include the following:

- Onset
- Duration
- Precipitant

Table 3.6 Evaluation of aggression

Description	Pattern	Causes
Aggression may correlate with exacerbation of psychiatric symptoms or reflect a co-occurring psychiatric disorder; recent substance use or abstinence after heavy use; onset of aggressive behavior in childhood; remorse for behavior may or may not occur	Aggression related to symptoms of psychiatric disorder	ADHD, autism spectrum disorder, conduct disorder, cluster B personality disorders, intermittent explosive disorder, oppositional defiant disorder, personality disorders, psychotic, mood, and anxiety disorders, substance-induced disorders
Non-neurotypical patient (especially if nonverbal) may bite, scratch, head bang, or strike self with closed fists, increasing with unstructured time or with positive or negative emotions; borderline personality disorder is associated with self-injury to relieve tension, self-punish, or gain attention	Self-injurious behavior	Nonverbal autism spectrum disorder or intellectual developmental disorder, borderline personality disorder, developmental syndromes such as Lesch-Nyhan, Smith-Magenis, or MECP2 (Rett) syndrome
Nonverbal neurodevelopmentally atypical individual; no prior history of aggressive behavior; approximate date of onset of aggressive behavior can be established; medical symptoms may or may not be present	New-onset aggressive behavior in a nonverbal individual	Headache, otitis media, dental pain, constipation, gastrointestinal distress, dysmenorrhea, visual problems (including presbyopia in midlife), urinary tract infection, occult infection, unseen traumatic brain injury, metabolic abnormality, akathisia, medication side effects

Table 3.6 Evaluation of aggression (*continued*)

Description	Pattern	Causes
Enduring pattern of irritability; onset may be temporally related to a change in medications or symptoms of a medical or neurological disorder	Chronic or enduring pattern of irritability	Medication or illicit drugs, substance withdrawal, posttraumatic brain injury, postictal state, seizure prodrome, hyperthyroidism, akathisia, premenstrual dysphoric disorder, PTSD, neurocognitive disorders, anxiety disorders, mood disorders, psychotic disorders, personality disorders or traits
History of or neuroimaging evidence of stroke, tumor, traumatic brain injury, focal encephalomalacia, or hemorrhage; unilateral or bilateral lesions on MRI; frontal-dysexecutive or right-hemisphere cognitive features on bedside exam; brief emotional outbursts out of proportion to stimulus	Focal neurobehavioral syndrome	Orbitofrontal syndrome, dorsolateral frontal syndrome, right-hemisphere syndrome, diencephalic syndrome, pseudobulbar palsy (including involuntary emotional expression disorder)
History of noticeable behavior change before or after seizures; irritability in the hours before a cluster of seizures; aggressive behavior during seizures is unusual and during postictal period is disorganized and untargeted (except in postictal psychosis) other than to reflexively strike out when touched; interictal aggressive behavior may follow perceived violation of rules in which the patient strongly believes	Limbic seizure-related behavior	Prodromal state, ictal state, postictal state, interictal personality or symptoms

- Whether the pain is intermittent or continuous
- Time of day the pain tends to occur
- Length of episodes (if episodic)
- Factors or positions that worsen or improve the pain
- Biological, therapeutic, and complementary treatments that have been tried, and what their effect was

It is helpful to understand whether the pain has interfered with the patient's occupation, education, relationships, activities of daily living (ADLs), instrumental ADL skills, or mobility. Because co-occurring depression and anxiety are common and may both result from but also influence the perception of pain, concurrent psychiatric diagnoses should be evaluated.

Common pain presentations are reviewed in Table 3.7. For a discussion of pain due to traumatic brain injury, see Chapter 5; for toxins, see Chapter 6, "Toxins, Substances, and Nutrition"; for headache and trigeminal neuralgia, see Chapter 11; for herpes zoster, see Chapter 12, "Neuroinfectious Diseases"; for multiple sclerosis, see Chapter 14, "Neuroimmunology."

Central neuropathic pain syndrome is characterized by pain due to disease or damage to central somatosensory tracts. It may be described as burning, freezing, squeezing, pricking, or shock-like electrical sensations. The affected area may be hypersensitive to touch or cold. The pain may be paroxysmal or continuous, and the somatosensory loss may spread beyond the area affected by the pain. Pain is manifested contralaterally from supraspinal lesions such as in thalamic pain syndrome. The patient may also have nonpainful dysesthesia or paresthesia. Patients with brainstem lesions may present with a "crossed" pain pattern with ipsilateral facial pain (with trigeminal nucleus damage) and contralateral hemi-body pain from involvement of the ascending spinothalamic tract.

In *complex regional pain syndrome,* the patient experiences severe burning or pain in the hand, foot, arm, or leg that typically develops following a fracture or other injury. The pain is out of proportion to the inciting trauma, and nerve damage may or may not be present. Symptoms may be sensory, vasomotor (skin temperature or color), sudomotor (sweating), or motor (weakness, tremor, dystonia). The patient experiences swelling, skin color and/or temperature change, and touch or cold sensitivity. Abnormal hair or nail growth may also occur. This syndrome occurs more frequently in women than men.

Table 3.7 Common pain syndromes

Syndrome	Characteristics of the pain	Associated symptoms
Central neuropathic pain syndrome	Burning, freezing, squeezing, pricking, or shock-like electrical sensations Paroxysmal or continuous Somatosensory loss may spread beyond the area affected by the pain	Nonpainful dysesthesia or paresthesia
Complex regional pain syndrome	Severe burning or pain in hand, foot, arm, or leg following a fracture or other injury Pain is out of proportion to the inciting trauma	Abnormal sweating, abnormal hair or nail growth
Diabetic neuropathy	Peripheral sensorimotor neuropathy: lancinating, burning, or sharp bilateral pain Sensory neuropathy: "stocking and glove" sensory loss Proximal neuropathy: radicular pain in the buttocks or thigh	Sexual dysfunction, orthostatic hypotension, bowel and bladder dysfunction, heart rate and blood pressure abnormalities, sweating abnormalities, problems with digestion
Fibromyalgia	Diffuse musculoskeletal pain, stiffness, and fatigue with tender points on examination; unrelated to physical trauma or neurological damage	Cognitive symptoms, sleep disturbance, gastrointestinal symptoms

Table 3.7 Common pain syndromes (*continued*)

Syndrome	Characteristics of the pain	Associated symptoms
Guillain-Barré syndrome	Muscular or radicular pain most intense in the legs and back; can be severe	Fatigue, blood pressure and heart rate variability, bowel and bladder dysfunction, deep vein thrombosis, pressure ulcers, respiratory insufficiency
Phantom limb and residual limb (stump) pain	Phantom limb pain: aching, burning, stinging or piercing pain that feels as if it originates in the missing extremity Residual limb pain: felt in the stump of an amputated extremity (typically caused by an ill-fitting prosthesis or postoperative inflammation)	Skin irritation (residual limb pain)
Radiculopathy and plexopathy	Radiculopathic pain: sharp and radiating; provoked with specific movements Plexopathy: deep, aching pain	Numbness, paresthesia, weakness, decreased reflexes
Spinal cord injury	Aching, burning, or lancinating pain in the extremities or other locations; myelopathic pain may be similar to radicular pain in character	Bowel and bladder symptoms, weakness

Source. Chang and Yang 2023; Ferraro et al. 2024; Rosner et al. 2023.

Diabetic neuropathy can take several forms. Peripheral sensorimotor mononeuropathy or polyneuropathy may result in muscle weakness or wasting, paresthesia, numbness, hyperesthesia to touch, and/or pain of the extremities beginning distally. The pain is typically bilateral, often is worse at night, and may be described as lancinating, burning, or sharp. Sensory polyneuropathy results in "stocking and glove" sensory loss (in a pattern involving bilateral feet/calves and hands), may cause problems with balance or coordination, and predisposes to skin ulcers, bone or joint damage, and infection, which can then lead to amputation. Diabetes may also result in autonomic neuropathy. Autonomic neuropathy seldom causes pain but is associated with sexual dysfunction, orthostatic hypotension, bowel and bladder dysfunction, heart rate and blood pressure abnormalities, sweating abnormalities, and problems with digestion.

Fibromyalgia is experienced as diffuse musculoskeletal pain, stiffness, and fatigue with tender points on examination. The pain is not related to physical trauma or neurological damage. Fibromyalgia is also associated with cognitive symptoms, sleep disturbances, and gastrointestinal symptoms. Onset commonly occurs in perimenopausal women.

In *Guillain-Barré syndrome*, muscular or radicular pain can occur at any point in the evolution of the condition and can be severe. Pain is typically most intense in the legs and back. Fatigue occurs both during the acute syndrome and during recovery. Blood pressure and heart rate variability, bowel and bladder dysfunction, deep vein thrombosis, and pressure ulcers can occur. Respiratory insufficiency often leads to transient intubation.

Amputees often experience phantom limb pain and residual limb (stump) pain. *Phantom limb pain* develops in the majority of amputees in the first 6 months after amputation. It then may gradually decrease. The pain can be aching, burning, stinging, or piercing and feels as if it originates in the missing extremity. *Residual limb pain (stump pain)* is felt in the stump of an amputated extremity and is typically caused by an ill-fitting prosthesis or by postoperative inflammation. It may be associated with skin irritation on the stump.

Radiculopathic pain is caused by compression of specific nerve roots exiting the spinal column. It more commonly originates in the lumbosacral region than in the cervical region and least commonly occurs in the thoracic region. The pain can be sharp and radiating and is provoked by specific movements. Pain from *plexopathy* is more likely to be deep and aching. Both radiculopathy and plexopathy may be associated with numbness, paresthesia, weakness, and decreased reflexes. Distribution depends on which nerves are affected.

Spinal cord injury pain may be associated with radicular pain due to damage to sensory nerve roots. This pain can be aching, burning, or lancinating in the extremities or other locations. It can also cause hemibody pain from involvement of the spinothalamic tract. Myelopathic pain may be felt in the arms, legs, or back and may be similar to radicular pain in character. Spinal cord injury may also be associated with bowel and bladder symptoms and weakness.

Review Questions

1. A 78-year-old man who wears glasses for correction of severe myopia develops sudden-onset hallucinations of flashing lights and describes multiple tiny black dots like pepper in his vision in the left eye. Which of the following is the most likely etiology of his symptoms?

   A. Charles Bonnet syndrome.
   B. Retinal tear.
   C. Seizure.
   D. Migraine.
   E. Peduncular hallucinosis.

2. A 35-year-old woman has been admitted to the hospital three times in the past 6 months with heightened anxiety, paranoia, nausea, and abdominal cramps. Six months ago, she began ketamine infusions for refractory depression. Which of the following tests will most likely lead to a correct diagnosis?

   A. Urine arylsulfatase A.
   B. Very-long-chain fatty acids.
   C. Cranial MRI.
   D. Serum and urine porphyrins.
   E. Heavy metal screen.

3. An 18-year-old woman develops chronic burning pain in her hand 1 month after recovering from an uncomplicated wrist fracture. Her hand is cold, swollen, and sensitive to the touch,

and the skin has a bluish tinge. Which of the following is the most likely cause?

A. Thalamic pain syndrome.
B. Mononeuropathy.
C. Complex regional pain syndrome.
D. Fibromyalgia.
E. Functional pain disorder.

Answers

Question 1: B. People with myopia are prone to spontaneous separation of the vitreous humor from the retina, which leads to retinal tears, especially in older age groups. The other conditions listed are less likely to cause monocular hallucinations.

Question 2: D. Acute intermittent porphyria attacks can be precipitated by ketamine and may include a combination of psychiatric and gastrointestinal symptoms. Porphyria attacks can be precipitated by a number of drugs, including ketamine.

Question 3: C. Complex regional pain syndrome is typically triggered by injury to an extremity. The symptoms are out of proportion to the injury, and no nerve damage needs to occur. The cause is unknown, but it occurs more frequently in women than men.

References

American Psychiatric Association: Diagnostic and Statistical Manual of Mental Disorders, 5th Edition, Text Revision. Washington, DC, American Psychiatric Association, 2022

Benjamin S: A Neuropsychiatric approach to aggressive behavior, in Neuropsychiatry and Mental Health Services. Edited by Ovsiew F. Washington DC, American Psychiatric Press, 1999, pp 149–196

Benjamin S: Treatment of Aggressive Behavior in Brain Damage. Focus Am Psychiatr Publ 14(4):473–476, 2016 31975827

Benjamin S, Lauterbach MD, Stanislawski AL: Congenital and acquired disorders presenting as psychosis in children and young adults. Child Adolesc Psychiatr Clin N Am 22(4):581–608, 2013 24012075

Chang MC, Yang S: Diabetic peripheral neuropathy essentials: a narrative review. Ann Palliat Med 12(2):390–398, 2023 36786097

Ferraro MC, O'Connell NE, Sommer C, et al: Complex regional pain syndrome: advances in epidemiology, pathophysiology, diagnosis, and treatment. Lancet Neurol 23(5):522–533, 2024 38631768

Miller A, Pratt H, Schiffer RB: Pseudobulbar affect: the spectrum of clinical presentations, etiologies and treatments. Expert Rev Neurother 11(7):1077–1088, 2011 21539437

O'Brien J, Taylor JP, Ballard C, et al: Visual hallucinations in neurological and ophthalmological disease: pathophysiology and management. J Neurol Neurosurg Psychiatry 91(5):512–519, 2020 32213570

Raja SN, Carr DB, Cohen M, et al: The revised International Association for the Study of Pain definition of pain: concepts, challenges, and compromises. Pain 161(9):1976–1982 2020 32694387

Rogers JP, Oldham MA, Fricchione G, et al: Evidence-based consensus guidelines for the management of catatonia: recommendations from the British Association for Psychopharmacology. J Psychopharmacol 37(4):327–369, 2023 37039129

Rosner J, de Andrade DC, Davis KD, et al: Central neuropathic pain. Nat Rev Dis Primers 9(1):73, 2023 38129427

Steffens DC, Fahed M, Manning KJ, Wang L: The neurobiology of apathy in depression and neurocognitive impairment in older adults: a review of epidemiological, clinical, neuropsychological and biological research. Transl Psychiatry 12(1):525 2022 36572691

4

Dementia

Mark Eldaief, M.D., M.M.Sc.
Bradford Dickerson, M.D., M.M.Sc.

Case Example

A 60-year-old man presents with a 4-year history of gradual cognitive decline, particularly involving difficulties with organization and planning. Recently, he has also been repeating questions and rapidly forgetting recently learned information. His wife had to assume his financial duties, despite his having had a successful career in finance. Otherwise, he is fully independent with chores and basic activities of daily living (ADLs). He has recently become very irritable, but his behavior remains appropriate in social situations, and he remains caring toward his family.

The evaluation and management of dementia are among the most common responsibilities facing psychiatrists, neurologists, and primary care physicians. In this chapter, I first build a framework for characterizing dementia, mild cognitive impairment (MCI), and normal aging. Then I review the epidemiology, diagnostic criteria, pathophysiology, imaging and biomarkers, genetics, psychiatric aspects, management, and treatment for the most common neurodegenerative conditions: Alzheimer disease, frontotemporal lobar degeneration (FTLD), Lewy body dementia (LBD), and vascular cognitive impairment (VCI)/vascular dementia. I briefly review Creutzfeldt-Jakob disease (CJD) and HIV-associated neurocognitive disorder (HAND), followed by normal-pressure hydrocephalus (NPH), cognitive impairment due to depression, and dementias presenting in young adulthood.

Approach to Patients With Cognitive Decline

The primary goal of the evaluation is to determine whether a patient has cognitive impairment or dementia and, if they do, to develop a tripartite diagnostic formulation: 1) cognitive functional status, 2) cognitive-behavioral syndrome, and 3) neurodegenerative brain disease (Wong et al. 2019) (Figure 4.1). *Cognitive functional status* refers to an individual's functional independence, classified as cognitively normal, subjective cognitive concern, MCI, or dementia. *Cognitive-behavioral syndrome* is a term used to capture the constellation of symptoms and signs of a patient's illness. In some cases, this is a descriptive term such as a *dysexecutive* or *amnestic syndrome*. In other cases, this term has a proper name such as *primary progressive aphasia* (PPA) or *posterior cortical atrophy* (PCA). *Neurodegenerative brain disease* refers to the underlying histopathology driving a patient's symptoms.

Cognitive deficits may occur in normal aging and most commonly involve domains of complex attention, processing speed, working memory, mental flexibility, abstract reasoning, response inhibition, episodic memory encoding and retrieval, verbal fluency, and visual construction (Harada et al. 2013). However, significant declines or significantly poor performance (e.g., 2 standard deviations below normative scores for age and education level) in these domains on objective testing should prompt further investigation into an incipient neurodegenerative disorder. A related issue is the growing number of individuals with subjective cognitive decline (SCD) who do not exhibit cognitive impairment on objective testing (Jessen et al. 2020). It is incumbent on clinicians to identify which patients presenting with SCD are most likely to progress to objective cognitive impairment.

MCI is synonymous with *mild neurocognitive disorder* in DSM-5 (American Psychiatric Association 2022). MCI indicates that a person has symptoms of cognitive dysfunction in daily life (ideally corroborated by an informant) but with relative preservation of functional independence (Petersen 2011). MCI is classified as being *amnestic, amnestic multidomain, non-amnestic single domain,* or *non-amnestic multi-*

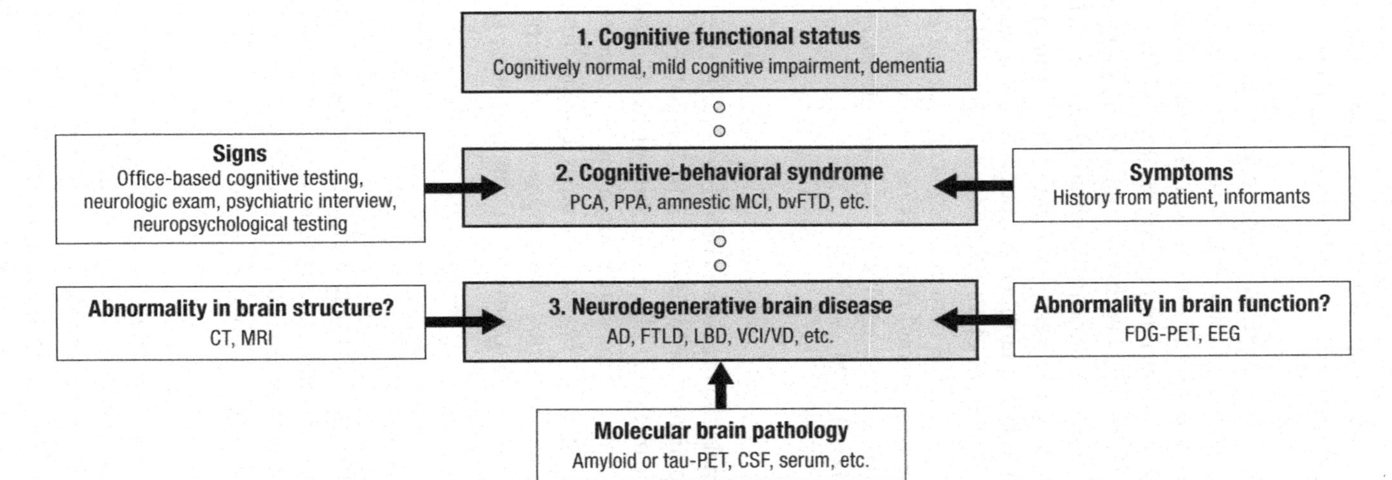

Figure 4.1 Formulation for cognitive impairment.

AD = Alzheimer disease; bvFTD = behavioral variant frontotemporal dementia; CSF = cerebrospinal fluid; CT = computed tomography; EEG = electroencephalography; FDG = ^{18}Fluorodeoxyglucose; FTLD = frontotemporal lobar degeneration; LBD = Lewy body dementia; MCI = mild cognitive impairment; MRI = magnetic resonance imaging; PCA = posterior cortical atrophy; PET = positron emission tomography; PPA = primary progressive aphasia; VCI = vascular cognitive impairment; VD = vascular dementia.

domain (Petersen et al. 1999). Some patients who are still functionally independent may present with a primarily behavioral syndrome and may or may not have MCI; such patients may fall under the functional construct of *mild behavioral impairment*.

Dementia is a descriptive, umbrella term referring to progressive impairment in cognition or behavior that 1) interferes with work or daily functioning, 2) represents a decline from previous abilities, and 3) is not explained by delirium or a concurrent primary psychiatric disorder (McKhann et al. 2011). In DSM-5, dementia falls under the category of major neurocognitive disorders (American Psychiatric Association 2022). Dementia is typically staged as very mild, mild, moderate, or severe. Functional status is often quantified through the Clinical Dementia Rating Scale (CDR) (Hughes et al. 1982; Morris 1993) (Table 4.1). Patients can be characterized by the sum of all six scores, reported as the "CDR sum of boxes." Supplemental domains for language and behavior have been added to the CDR; the full scale is often referred to as the FTLD CDR (Miyagawa et al. 2020).

History

Because many patients are unable to provide a comprehensive history, owing to either cognitive impairment or limited insight, it is helpful to also obtain a history from a caregiver. Salient elements of the history are listed in Table 4.2. Note that in some situations, a family member may describe a patient as having a problem with memory, but the clinician may determine through the elicitation of examples that the problem better reflects impairment in language, executive function, or other domains.

Examination

When examining patients with suspected dementia, a cognitive screening test such as the Mini-Mental State Examination or the Montreal Cognitive Assessment is a useful adjunct to the usual neurological evaluation. Considering which cognitive domains are affected may help localize the pathology.

- Speech/language: speech initiation, phrase length, prosody, repetition, articulation, multisyllabic word pronunciation, word-finding, reading, writing, comprehension
- Ideomotor praxis: transitive (e.g., pantomiming the use of a tool) and intransitive (e.g., waving goodbye) praxis

Table 4.1 Clinical Dementia Rating Scale

	Impairment level				
Factor	**None 0**	**Questionable 0.5**	**Mild 1.0**	**Moderate 2.0**	**Severe 3.0**
Memory	No memory loss or inconsistent slight forgetfulness	Consistent slight forgetfulness; partial recollection of events; "benign" forgetfulness	Moderate memory loss, more marked for recent events; defect interferes with everyday activities	Severe memory loss; only highly learned material retained; new material rapidly lost	Severe memory loss; only fragments remain
Orientation	Fully oriented	Fully oriented except for slight difficulty with time relationships	Moderate difficulty with time relationships; oriented to place of examination; may have geographic disorientation elsewhere	Severe difficulty with time relationships; usually disoriented to time, often to place	Oriented to person only

Table 4.1 Clinical Dementia Rating Scale (*continued*)

	Impairment level				
Factor	**None 0**	**Questionable 0.5**	**Mild 1.0**	**Moderate 2.0**	**Severe 3.0**
Judgment and problem solving	Solves everyday problems and handles business and financial affairs well; judgment good in relation to past performance	Slight impairment in solving problems and similarities and differences	Moderate difficulty in handling problems and similarities and differences; social judgment usually maintained	Severely impaired in handling problems and similarities and differences; social judgment usually impaired	Unable to make judgments or solve problems
Community affairs	Independent function at usual level in job, shopping, volunteer and social groups	Slight impairment in these activities	Unable to function independently at these activities although may still be engaged in some; appears normal to casual inspection	No pretense of independent function outside the home; appears well enough to be taken to functions outside a family home	No pretense of independent function outside the home; appears too ill to be taken to functions outside a family home

Table 4.1 Clinical Dementia Rating Scale (*continued*)

	Impairment level				
Factor	**None 0**	**Questionable 0.5**	**Mild 1.0**	**Moderate 2.0**	**Severe 3.0**
Home and hobbies	Life at home, hobbies, and intellectual interests well maintained	Life at home, hobbies, and intellectual interests slightly impaired	Mild but definite impairment of function at home; more difficult tasks abandoned	Only simple chores preserved; very restricted interests, poorly maintained	No significant function at home
Personal care	Fully capable of self-care	Fully capable of self-care	Needs prompting	Requires assistance in dressing, hygiene, keeping of personal effects	Requires much help with personal care; frequent incontinence

Source. Morris 1993. Used with permission.

Table 4.2 Salient elements of the history for cognitive impairment

Memory	• Rapidly losing learned information • Repeating questions • Forgetting details of conversations • Temporal disorientation • Forgetting names • Misplacing objects
Executive function	• Organizational deficits • Planning deficits • Mental inflexibility • Issues with problem solving • Poor reasoning
Attention	• Difficulties with sustained attention
Speech and language	• Word-finding difficulty • Grammatical errors • Single-word comprehension problems • Motor speech deficits (e.g., mispronunciation of multisyllabic words, oral-buccal apraxia, dysarthria)
Visuospatial function	• Spatial disorientation • Visual agnosia • Impaired visually guided reach • Depth perception issues • Prosopagnosia
Mood/behavior	• Disinhibited or inappropriate behavior • Decreased empathy • Increased irritability, agitation, verbal, or physical aggression • Changes in food preferences • New rituals or compulsions • Apathy • Depression • Psychosis
Functional status	• Perform vocation (if not retired) • Manage household finances • Perform household chores • Dress, bathe, groom, and toilet independently

- Cortical sensation: graphesthesia, stereognosis, two-point discrimination, and double simultaneous visual and tactile stimulation
- Dominant inferior parietal functions: calculation, writing, right-left orientation, and finger gnosis; collectively, deficits in these functions constitute Gerstmann syndrome
- Higher visual functions: oculomotor praxis (the ability to direct the eyes to a desired location), visually guided reaching (to detect optic ataxia), and the ability to simultaneously perceive multiple objects (the deficit is called simultanagnosia); the triad of oculomotor apraxia, optic ataxia, and simultanagnosia is referred to as Balint syndrome

The general neurological examination helps identify dementia subtypes. The cranial nerve exam should include a detailed examination of eye movements (e.g., speed and amplitude of saccadic eye movements). The tongue should be examined for the presence of fasciculations (spontaneous contractions of individual muscle groups under the tongue surface). The motor examination should also assess for muscle atrophy and fasciculations throughout the body; atrophy and fasciculations can indicate the presence of motor neuron disease. Signs of parkinsonism should be elicited, including masked facies, decreased blink rate, cogwheel rigidity, bradykinesia on rapid alternating movements, and resting tremor. The gait examination should assess for shuffling, asymmetric arm swing, slow turning, or freezing. A pull test should be performed to assess postural reflexes. In cases in which parkinsonism is detected, the full Unified Parkinson's Disease Rating Scale can be performed.

Neuropsychological Testing

Neuropsychological testing includes comprehensive assessments of memory, language, executive function, attention, and visuospatial function, with the specific battery tailored to the patient's clinical presentation. Scores are compared to age- and education-matched population means.

Structural Neuroimaging

Structural imaging should be considered in all patients who present with cognitive symptoms. MRI is preferable to CT, as it provides higher-resolution estimates of neuroanatomy. The main purpose of structural neuroimaging is to assess patterns of cortical and subcortical atrophy. Imaging also provides an index of subcortical/periventricular white matter disease. Other relevant vascular findings include detection of microhemorrhages on gradient echo/T2* or susceptibility weighted imaging (SWI) images, which may suggest the presence of cerebral amyloid angiopathy (CAA). Finally, structural neuroimaging can rule out other causes of cognitive impairment such as NPH, intracranial masses, strokes, or demyelinating diseases.

Positron Emission Tomography

^{18}Fluorodeoxyglucose positron emission tomography (FDG-PET) assesses cortical glucose uptake and, therefore, metabolism. Neurodegenerative diseases can be disambiguated by the patterns of hypometabolism observed (Mosconi et al. 2008). Amyloid PET imaging can detect amyloid 42 (A) in vivo (Ossenkoppele et al. 2015). There are three approved A agents (ligands): florbetapir, florbetaben, and flutemetamol (Scheltens et al. 2016). ^{18}F-Flortaucipir (aka T807 or AV1451) (Sander et al. 2016) is a fluorinated ligand that binds to paired helical filament tau protein in vivo. Tau binding in Alzheimer disease correlates better to regions of neurodegeneration and hypometabolism than does amyloid binding (Scheltens et al. 2016).

Cerebrospinal Fluid Studies

Cerebrospinal fluid (CSF) studies detect whether underlying Alzheimer disease pathology is present or, in rare cases, can rule out a nondegenerative explanation for a patient's cognitive symptoms. CSF is assessed for levels of Aβ, total tau protein (t-tau), and phosphorylated tau (p-tau). Generally, A levels of ≤500 pg/mL and p-tau levels of ≥61 pg/mL are highly suggestive of underlying Alzheimer disease, and together, these have diagnostic sensitivity and specificity of 85%–90% (Scheltens et al. 2016).

Serum Studies

Four plasma biomarkers have high sensitivity and specificity in Alzheimer disease: A42/A40, neurofilament light chain (NfL), p-tau 181, and p-tau 217 (de Wolf et al. 2020; Palmqvist et al. 2020).

Neurodegenerative Diseases

Alzheimer Disease

Epidemiology

Alzheimer disease is by far the most common cause of dementia worldwide. Age is the single greatest risk factor for Alzheimer disease. Prevalence rates increase exponentially with advanced age, doubling every 5 years past the age of 65 (Lane et al. 2018). Other risk factors include years of education, history of traumatic brain injury, and associated cardiovascular and cerebrovascular risk factors (Rujeedawa et al. 2021).

Diagnostic Criteria

Alzheimer disease typically presents with insidious memory decline. It is not uncommon for executive dysfunction and word-finding difficulty to also occur early on. Over time, these and other cognitive domains (e.g., visuospatial function) are affected to various degrees. Prodromal Alzheimer disease often presents as amnestic MCI, either single domain (memory) or multidomain (e.g., memory and executive function).

Pathophysiology

Alzheimer disease is pathophysiologically characterized by amyloid plaques and neurofibrillary tangles. Extracellular neuritic amyloid (A) plaques are typically distributed throughout the cerebral cortex. Neurofibrillary tangles are composed of hyperphosphorylated tau and are located within neuronal cell bodies and dendrites. Neurofibrillary tangle burden correlates more with cognitive deficits than amyloid does. Amyloid and tau may have complementary effects in the pathogenic cascade leading to Alzheimer disease (Gallardo and Holtzman 2019).

Imaging and Biomarkers

Alzheimer disease is the neurodegenerative disease for which the most biomarkers are currently available. Structural imaging in Alzheimer disease often reveals hippocampal atrophy or biparietal atrophy at levels beyond those expected for a patient's age (Dickerson et al. 2009). Patients with early-onset Alzheimer disease (EOAD) often present with frontal and parietal atrophy, reflecting the clinical observation that many of these patients have executive dysfunction. FDG-PET shows a characteristic pattern of temporoparietal hypometabolism (Mosconi et al. 2008). Furthermore, hypometabolism in the posterior cingulate is a sensitive marker of Alzheimer disease. Amyloid-PET imaging is often read as positive or negative for amyloid, depending on whether a certain threshold is reached. These scans are highly sensitive for Alzheimer disease pathology in patients with cognitive impairment. However, amyloid PET scans are positive in 10%–44% of cognitively normal individuals between the ages of 50 and 90 years (Chételat et al. 2020). Thus, amyloid-PET imaging is not particularly specific for Alzheimer disease in older individuals as a whole.

Genetics

Rarely, Alzheimer disease can be inherited in an autosomal-dominant form. Dominantly inherited mutations include mutations in the A precursor gene (*APP*), the presenilin 1 gene (*PSEN1*), or the presenilin 2 gene (*PSEN2*) (Rujeedawa et al. 2021). Individuals with pathogenic mutations of these genes typically present younger (under the age of 65). In addition, there is variability in the age at onset among different mutations, with *PSEN1* mutations presenting younger (mean 43.6 years) than those with *APP* mutations (mean 50.4 years) (Ryan et al. 2016). With respect to late-onset Alzheimer disease, the highest genetic risk is conferred by the apolipoprotein E gene (*APOE*), which is involved in cholesterol metabolism. Individuals can carry either the ε3 allele (which is protective) or the ε4 allele (which is pathogenic) of *APOE*. ε3/ε4 heterozygotes are 3–4 times more likely, and ε4/ε4 homozygotes are 12–15 times more likely, to develop Alzheimer disease than ε3/ε3 homozygotes (Lane et al. 2018).

Atypical Presentations of Alzheimer Disease

Logopenic variant primary progressive aphasia

Alzheimer disease patients can present with significant language symptoms, such as word-finding difficulty and speech hesitancy, even in the absence of significant memory loss. *Logopenic variant primary progressive aphasia* (lvPPA) is characterized by impaired single-word retrieval in spontaneous speech and during confrontation naming, and by impaired lengthy repetition (Gorno-Tempini et al. 2011). In addition, three of the following four criteria must be met: 1) phonologic errors in spontaneous speech and naming, 2) spared single-word comprehension and object knowledge, 3) spared motor speech, and 4) the absence of frank agrammatism (Gorno-Tempini et al. 2011).

Posterior cortical atrophy

Posterior cortical atrophy (PCA) is characterized by early, predominant visuospatial dysfunction (Benson et al. 1988). Diagnostic criteria were put forth by Crutch et al. (2017). Per these guidelines, PCA requires visuospatial or other parietal symptoms, with at least three of the following present: 1) space perception deficit, 2) simultanagnosia, 3) object perception deficit, 4) constructional dyspraxia, 5) environmental agnosia, 6) oculomotor apraxia, 7) dressing apraxia, 8) optic ataxia, 9) alexia, 10) left/right disorientation, 11) acalculia, 12) limb apraxia, 13) apperceptive prosopagnosia (inability to recognize that an object is actually a face), 14) homonymous visual field defect, or 15) finger agnosia (Crutch et al. 2017).

Behavioral or dysexecutive variant Alzheimer disease

Alzheimer disease patients, particularly EOAD patients, can present with a predominant behavioral or dysexecutive form of Alzheimer disease (Ossenkoppele et al. 2015). Such patients present more commonly with executive dysfunction than behavioral symptoms. Apathy is the most common behavioral symptom in these patients (Ossenkoppele et al. 2015).

Psychiatric Aspects of Alzheimer Disease

Psychiatric symptoms in Alzheimer disease often peak in the moderate stages of the disease (Radue et al. 2019). Common psychiatric symptoms in Alzheimer disease include irritability/agitation, psychosis (including delusions and hallucinations), apathy, and delirium (Radue et al. 2019). Nonpharmacological interventions for these symptoms include caregiver education, redirection, and structured approaches. If imminent risk of harm is present, the patient is referred to the emergency department. If symptoms are more chronic but nevertheless disruptive, selective serotonin reuptake inhibitors (SSRIs) are tried as a first-line agent (because of the black box warning for neuroleptics in elderly demented patients). In the presence of marked irritability or aggression, however, an atypical neuroleptic (e.g., quetiapine, aripiprazole, or risperidone) is recommended after discussion of risks and benefits (Radue et al. 2019).

Management and Treatment

Cholinesterase inhibitors (donepezil, rivastigmine, and galantamine) are approved for all stages of Alzheimer disease dementia. The noncompetitive *N*-methyl-D-aspartate (NMDA) receptor antagonist memantine is approved for moderate to severe stages of Alzheimer disease. Both medication classes are symptomatic treatments and not disease modifying. Several clinical trials have examined disease-modifying approaches. These have included several anti-amyloid strategies (e.g., secretase inhibitors and monoclonal antibodies directed at A) and, to a lesser extent, anti-tau strategies. There are now FDA-approved anti-amyloid treatments such as lecanemab, a humanized monoclonal antibody, has been shown to slow cognitive decline (van Dyck et al. 2023).

Frontotemporal Lobar Degeneration

Frontotemporal lobar degeneration (FTLD) is a clinically, histologically, and genetically heterogeneous group of diseases. It includes a behavioral and dysexecutive presentation—behavioral variant frontotemporal dementia (bvFTD)—as well as predominant language presentations—semantic variant primary progressive aphasia (svPPA)/semantic dementia and nonfluent variant primary progressive aphasia (nfvPPA). Associated FTLD syndromes can also present with significant motor symptoms, e.g., progressive supranuclear palsy (PSP), corticobasal degeneration (CBD), and FTD with motor neuron disease (FTD-MND) (FTD-amyotrophic lateral sclerosis [ALS]).

Epidemiology

FTLD has an average age of onset of 45–65 years and is the second most common neurodegenerative dementia, after Alzheimer disease, in individuals younger than 65 (Olney et al. 2017). It is important to recognize that some patients have an extremely young (20s) or old (80s) age of onset. Approximately 60% of FTLD are bvFTD presentations; language presentations constitute the remaining 40% (Onyike and Diehl-Schmid 2013).

Diagnostic Criteria

Patients with bvFTD typically present with significant behavioral symptoms hallmarked by apathy, disinhibition, or loss of empathy. Diagnostic criteria for bvFTD have been put forth by Rascovsky et al.

(2011). Per these criteria, three of the following six symptoms must be present for *possible* bvFTD: 1) early behavioral disinhibition; 2) early apathy or inertia; 3) early loss of empathy or sympathy; 4) early perseverative, stereotyped, or compulsive/ritualistic behavior; 5) hyperorality and dietary changes; and 6) a neuropsychological profile of executive deficits with relatively early sparing of memory and visuospatial function. *Probable* bvFTD is defined by the additional presence of biomarker evidence, such as prefrontal or anterior temporal atrophy on structural neuroimaging or hypometabolism on FDG-PET.

Clinical criteria for svPPA include impaired confrontation naming and impaired single-word comprehension, as well as three of the following: 1) impaired object knowledge (especially for low-frequency objects), 2) surface dyslexia or dysgraphia, 3) spared repetition, and 4) spared grammatical and motor speech production (Gorno-Tempini et al. 2011). Patients with svPPA can also present with socioemotional dysfunction (Eldaief et al. 2020).

Clinical criteria for nfvPPA include agrammatism in language production and effortful, halting speech with inconsistent speech sound errors and distortions (apraxia of speech). In addition, two of the following three criteria are required: 1) impaired comprehension of syntactically complex sentences, 2) spared single-word comprehension, and 3) spared object knowledge (Gorno-Tempini et al. 2011). Importantly, nfvPPA patients, particularly those with motor speech deficits such as PPA of speech, can develop motor symptoms that can be associated with phenotypic presentations of PSP or CBD (Grossman 2012).

Pathophysiology

The proteinopathies of FTLD are generally divisible into tauopathies and TAR DNA binding protein-43 proteinopathies. Tauopathies include 3R (Pick disease) and 4R (CBD and PSP) isoforms, along with multiple rarer tauopathies.

Imaging and Biomarkers

Structural MRI often reveals atrophy in the prefrontal and anterior temporal cortex. These regions also demonstrate hypometabolism on FDG-PET imaging. Depending on the FTD subtype and a patient's specific symptoms, atrophy or hypometabolism may be more temporally or frontally predominant. For example, svPPA typically affects the left anterior temporal lobe/temporal pole (Collins et al. 2017), whereas nfvPPA affects the left inferior frontal/frontal opercular region (Grossman 2012).

In cases of PSP, atrophy is observed in the dorsal midbrain, and hypometabolism can be seen in the superior frontal gyrus. In CBD, perirolandic atrophy and hypometabolism, as well as basal ganglia hypometabolism, are often observed. In addition, temporal variants of bvFTD have long been recognized (Edwards-Lee et al. 1997). Although many cases of FTLD are tauopathies, Tau-PET imaging is not very useful in FTLD (Lowe et al. 2016; Marquié et al. 2017). Unfortunately, nonimaging biomarkers are lacking in FTLD.

Genetics

Approximately 70% of FTLD cases are sporadic (Grossman 2012). Heritability in FTLD is conferred by three known autosomal dominant genes: progranulin (*GRN*), C9orf72-SMCR8 complex subunit (formerly chromosome 9 open reading frame 72) (*C9orf72*), and microtubule-associated protein tau (*MAPT*) (Baizabal-Carvallo and Jankovic 2016). Of these, *C9orf72* mutations are the most common genetic cause of FTD (Greaves and Rohrer 2019). Patients with *C9orf72* mutations can present with psychotic symptoms, including delusions and hallucinations (Devenney et al. 2019). In addition, *C9orf72* mutations can cause ALS in isolation or can cause a combined FTD-ALS syndrome. *MAPT* mutations can give rise to bvFTD, CBD, or PSP phenotypes, and more rarely to nfvPPA. *GRN* mutations are often associated with bvFTD or PPA or CBD syndrome, with asymmetric atrophy and parietal involvement on structural MRI. Moreover, patients with *GRN* mutations are more likely to exhibit white matter hyperintensities on T2-weighted MRI (Caroppo et al. 2014). The three major genetic forms of FTLD have typical associated clinical phenotypes, age of onset, and age at death (Moore et al. 2020).

Psychiatric Aspects of Frontotemporal Lobar Degeneration

Psychiatric symptoms are the hallmark of many forms of FTLD, resulting in FTLD being initially misdiagnosed as a primary psychiatric disorder (Olney et al. 2017). bvFTD can be clinically distinguished from primary psychiatric disorders by assessing clinical features of a patient's presentation (Ducharme and Dickerson 2015). Generally, patients who present with psychiatric symptoms are more likely to have a prior psychiatric history. The apathy in bvFTD can be differentiated from depression by a lack of dysphoria, feelings of self-reproach, or suicidal thoughts. Similarly, disinhibition in bvFTD can often be distinguished from that seen in mania by a lack of grandiosity. Also, whereas patients with OCD and bvFTD can both have restricted patterns of thinking, compulsions, and rituals, bvFTD patients are less likely to experience associated anxiety and obsessive, ego-dystonic thoughts (Ducharme and Dickerson 2015) and typically present later in life.

Management and Treatment

Unfortunately, there are currently no FDA-approved treatments for FTLD. Management of psychiatric symptoms involves the use of SSRIs and neuroleptics where appropriate (Khoury et al. 2021). It is also critical to address psychosocial and caregiver issues in bvFTD, as behavioral issues can be significantly disruptive. Speech therapy is often useful in language presentations of FTLD.

Lewy Body Dementia

Epidemiology

LBD is the second most common neurodegenerative disease after Alzheimer disease, affecting approximately 1.4 million Americans. Patients are predominantly male, with a typical age at onset in the 70s and early 80s (Sanford 2018). Lewy body pathology is found in 20%–25% of patients with dementia postmortem (Galasko 2017) and in 10%–15% of all samples from individuals older than 60 (Sanford 2018).

Diagnostic Criteria

LBD is a term subsuming the entities of dementia with Lewy bodies (DLB) and Parkinson disease dementia (PDD). These two are differentiated from one another by the temporal onset of symptoms: DLB is the term used when dementia occurs before, concurrently with, or within 1 year of the onset of motor symptoms. PDD is applied when parkinsonism precedes cognitive symptoms by more than 1 year (Sanford 2018). A diagnosis of LBD involves the presence of two or more of the following core criteria: 1) cognitive fluctuations, 2) visual hallucinations, 3) parkinsonism, and 4) rapid eye movement sleep behavior disorder (RBD). Visual hallucinations are typically well-formed and often involve animate objects (e.g., people or animals). Cognitive fluctuations can be severe, with some patients appearing transiently lethargic or encephalopathic. Parkinsonism in LBD patients exhibits overlap with idiopathic Parkinson disease: rigidity, bradykinesia, and postural instability. However, LBD patients often present with more bilateral symptoms, and rest tremor is less common. RBD is characterized by acting out dreams and can manifest several years before the diagnosis of LBD is made (see Chapter 15, "Sleep Disorders"). In addition, LBD patients have characteristic cognitive deficits, most notably in the domains of visuospatial and executive function.

Pathophysiology

The pathophysiological hallmark of LBD is the Lewy body: aggregated oligomers of misfolded α-synuclein protein found in neuronal cytoplasm. This process may begin in the enteric nervous system and then spread to the CNS. The vagus nerve is often implicated as a point of entry into the CNS, from which pathology is thought to spread rostrally (Sanford 2018).

Imaging and Biomarkers

Structural MRI may reveal posterior cortical volume loss, including the medial occipital cortex. FDG-PET shows hypometabolism in parietal and occipital cortices (Gomperts 2016), with a characteristic sparing of the posterior cingulate (unlike in Alzheimer disease, in which the posterior cingulate is almost invariably affected). This is referred to as the *cingulate island sign*. Dopamine transporter single-photon emission computed tomography scans, referred to as "DAT scans," reveal a reduction in striatal dopamine transporter binding (Sanford 2018) and have high sensitivity for predicting autopsy-confirmed LBD even at the MCI stage (Chen et al. 2021). Myocardial scintigraphy using ^{123}I-metaiodobenzylguanidine (MIBG), a molecular biomarker of cardiac sympathetic innervation, has become increasingly heavily weighted as part of the diagnostic criteria for DLB, as has polysomnographic evidence of RBD.

Genetics

Most LBD cases occur sporadically. When present, mutations causing LBD are observed in the leucine-rich repeat kinase-2 (*LRRK-2*), synuclein alpha (*SNCA*), and glucocerebrosidase A beta 1 (*GBA1*) genes (Sanford 2018).

Psychiatric Aspects of Lewy Body Dementia

Hallucinations are the most common psychiatric manifestation of LBD, although patients may also have delusions. Treatment of these symptoms can be challenging because LBD patients exhibit marked neuroleptic sensitivity. Neuroleptics, especially typical neuroleptics, can worsen parkinsonism (sometimes irreversibly) (Gomperts 2016). As such, neuroleptic use in LBD should be avoided unless psychotic symptoms are highly disruptive and other medications have failed. When neuroleptics are indicated, quetiapine, clozapine, or pimavanserin should be used (Gomperts 2016).

Management and Treatment

As in Alzheimer disease, acetylcholinesterase inhibitors are the mainstay of treatment for LBD because there is significant Lewy body deposition in the cholinergic nucleus basalis of Meynert. Patients can exhibit improvements in attention and cognition in response to this class of medications (Gomperts 2016; Sanford 2018). Dopamine agonists and other PD medications can be used in LBD, but they are typically less effective than they are in idiopathic PD.

Vascular Cognitive Impairment/ Vascular Dementia

Epidemiology

VCI and vascular dementia are differentiated from one another based on the presence of functional impairment in vascular dementia that affects activities of daily living. VCI and vascular dementia are rarely the sole cause of a patient's cognitive deficits (van der Flier et al. 2018). In contrast, VCI/vascular dementia may be invoked as a contributing factor in most dementias. For example, up to 75% of patients with dementia have evidence of vascular pathology at autopsy (van der Flier et al. 2018). Risk factors for VCI/vascular dementia include hypertension, diabetes, hyperlipidemia, smoking, and atrial fibrillation.

Diagnostic Criteria

Patients with VCI/vascular dementia classically present with executive dysfunction due to disruption in frontal-subcortical white matter (van der Flier et al. 2018). Accordingly, memory deficits tend to be characterized by impairments in encoding and retrieval, as opposed to storage deficits. Patients can also have accompanying focal neurological signs such as parkinsonism, weakness, sensory symptoms, or dysarthria (van der Flier et al. 2018). Formal criteria for vascular dementia call for a temporal relationship between a vascular event (e.g., a clinical stroke) and cognitive impairment, a clear relationship between the burden of vascular insults and the degree of cognitive impairment, and a lack of insidious progressive cognitive decline before the vascular insult.

Pathophysiology

VCI and vascular dementia can be broadly divided into two categories: strokes and subcortical white matter ischemic disease. White matter ischemic changes are often caused by microinfarcts and are seen as T2 hyperintensities on MRI. Both macro- and microinfarcts can be caused by vessel wall abnormalities, such as atherosclerosis, arteriosclerosis, or CAA (van der Flier et al. 2018).

Imaging and Biomarkers

Determination of VCI/vascular dementia is usually dependent on MRI. Diffusion-weighted MRI can detect infarcts in the acute stage; older strokes are detectable on T1- and T2-weighted sequences. T2 FLAIR is ideally suited to detect periventricular/subcortical white matter hyperintensities. GRE/T2* or SWI sequences can be used to detect susceptibility foci consistent with the microhemorrhages observed in CAA or strokes.

Genetics

Rarely, VCI/vascular dementia can result from a dominant mutation in the *NOTCH3* gene on chromosome 19. This results in the syndrome of cerebral autosomal dominant arteriopathy with subcortical infarcts and leukoencephalopathy, characterized by recurrent strokes and migraine headaches with aura progressing to dementia (Bersano et al. 2017).

Psychiatric Aspects of Vascular Cognitive Impairment/Vascular Dementia

Disruption of frontal-subcortical circuits can give rise to depression, psychosis, or apathy. As such, a vascular etiology for these symptoms is sometimes invoked when they occur later in life and when they are attended by significant frontal subcortical white matter hyperintensities. Depression in VCI/vascular dementia may respond less readily to SSRIs than uncomplicated depression does.

Management and Treatment

Management of VCI/vascular dementia is primarily directed at secondary prevention of further vascular insults, e.g., with strict blood pressure control (see Chapter 16, "Neurovascular Disorders").

Infectious Diseases

Creutzfeldt-Jakob Disease

A history of a rapidly progressive cognitive and functional decline (e.g., less than 1 year from symptom onset) should prompt consideration of a prion disease such as CJD. Caregivers can sometimes underestimate the duration of a patient's cognitive decline, so clinicians should verify that patients were truly cognitively normal just months before their clinical presentation. CJD can sometimes be distinguished from other dementias by certain motor manifestations such as ataxia, pyramidal symptoms, extrapyramidal symptoms, and most prominently, myoclonus (Watson et al. 2021). Workup for CJD should include brain MRI, electroencephalography (EEG), and lumbar puncture. Imaging abnormalities include diffusion and FLAIR hyperintensities such as cortical ribboning and basal ganglia hyperintensities (Watson et al. 2021). EEG abnormalities include periodic sharp wave complexes. The CSF of patients with sporadic CJD has elevated levels of 14-3-3 protein and PrP^{SC} protein as assessed with the real-time quaking-induced conversion (RT-QuIC) aggregation assay (Watson et al. 2021). Unfortunately, there is no treatment for CJD, and the condition is universally fatal.

HIV-Associated Neurocognitive Disorder

HAND includes HIV-associated dementia as well as milder neurocognitive symptoms. Fortunately, the refinement and widespread use of antiretroviral therapies have made HIV dementia rare (Winston and Spudich 2020). However, HIV continues to be associated with cognitive disorders as the result of HIV going untreated for a long duration before the start of antiretroviral treatment (Winston and Spudich 2020). In rare cases, a phenomenon called HIV RNA escape occurs, where antiretrovirals do not fully suppress HIV RNA in the CSF (Winston and Spudich 2020). Although antiretroviral treatment has markedly lessened cognitive issues at the population level, selected agents may cause cognitive impairment in individuals (Winston and Spudich 2020). Cognitive disorders can also be appreciated in HIV patients because of comorbid conditions such as mood disorders and substance use (Winston and Spudich 2020). Prescribing antiretrovirals and addressing HIV-associated comorbidities are the mainstays of treatment.

Other Dementias

Normal-Pressure Hydrocephalus

NPH is clinically characterized by the classic triad of gait disturbance, cognitive impairment, and urinary incontinence, often manifesting in that order. Cognitive deficits in NPH are subcortical, with cognitive slowing, executive dysfunction, and apathy (Damasceno 2009). Gait is characterized as difficult to initiate, broad-based, short-stepped, and "magnetic," with frequent falls (Damasceno 2009). Diagnosis is based on radiographic evidence of ventricular enlargement out of proportion to the degree of cortical atrophy. Specific diagnostic radiographic features have been proposed (Oliveira et al. 2019). The pathophysiology of NPH remains unresolved, but it can be secondary to processes that impair CSF absorption (e.g., prior subarachnoid hemorrhage). It can be difficult to disentangle NPH from other dementing etiologies such as Alzheimer disease. In fact, in one study, up to 20% of NPH patients undergoing shunt treatment had neuropathologically confirmed Alzheimer disease (Oliveira et al. 2019). In addition to neuroimaging, diagnosis is often supported by assessing for improvements following the removal of a large volume (e.g., 30–50 mL) of CSF via lumbar puncture. Assessments before and after this procedure can include formal neuropsychological testing, gait assessments by physical therapists, and caregiver reports. If improvements are convincingly shown, the standard treatment for NPH is the insertion of a ventriculoperitoneal shunt.

Cognitive Impairment Due to Depression

Historically referred to as *pseudodementia* and sometimes referred to as the *dementia syndrome of depression,* patients with depression can present with cognitive complaints. This can usually be differentiated from a neurodegenerative disorder by the nature and severity of the cognitive deficits, as assessed by formal neuropsychological testing. Executive deficits are the hallmark of cognitive impairment due to depression. Memory impairment is frontally based, with intact memory storage, and usually less severe than in cortical dementias.

Dementias Presenting in Young Adulthood

Very rarely, genetic, metabolic, and mitochondrial disorders can present with acquired and progressive cognitive dysfunction early or sometimes later in life. Many of these conditions are accompanied by other neurological symptoms such as movement disorders (e.g., pantothenate kinase-associated neurodegeneration, Huntington disease, and Wilson disease), epilepsy, neurocutaneous changes, and psychiatric symptoms.

Case Example, Continued

Elemental neurological examination is normal. Cranial MRI shows mild to moderate hippocampal, biparietal, and mild dorsolateral prefrontal atrophy. FDG-PET shows bilateral temporoparietal hypometabolism, which involves the posterior cingulate, as well as very mild frontal hypometabolism. CSF examination revealed an A42 level of 315.6 pg/mL (reference >500) and p-tau level of 89.1 pg/mL (reference <61).

The combination of the patient's age (60), prominent executive dysfunction, and behavioral symptoms might lead this patient to be misdiagnosed as having bvFTD. However, behavioral symptoms do *not* include disinhibition, loss of empathy, compulsions, nor a predilection for sweets. Although he does exhibit irritability and paranoia, these behavioral symptoms are less common in bvFTD and are more often seen in Alzheimer disease. Furthermore, it is not uncommon for patients with EOAD to initially present with a dysexecutive profile.

This patient's cognitive-behavioral syndrome is best classified as amnestic multidomain. Basic ADLs remain intact, but the patient is no longer able to work and struggles with managing household finances. Therefore, cognitive-functional status is best classified as mild dementia. Underlying histopathology is likely to be Alzheimer disease, as his CSF and neuroimaging results are consistent with Alzheimer disease. Thus, the final diagnosis is dysexecutive variant Alzheimer disease. The patient is started on a cholinesterase inhibitor and will likely be placed on combination therapy with memantine when the dementia becomes moderate.

Key Clinical Points

- Cognitive functional status can be characterized as cognitively normal, subjective cognitive concern, mild cognitive impairment, very mild dementia, or dementia.
- Dementias can be classified based on cognitive-behavioral syndromes and underlying neurodegenerative brain diseases, not necessarily with a 1:1 correspondence.
- Psychiatric symptoms are common across dementia diagnoses. The impact of these symptoms on patients' and caregivers' quality of life often surpasses the impact of cognitive symptoms.
- Atypical presentations of Alzheimer disease include language (logopenic variant primary progressive aphasia), visuospatial (posterior cortical atrophy), and frontal (behavioral/dysexecutive) presentations.
- Frontotemporal lobar degeneration typically presents with some combination of behavioral symptoms, executive dysfunction, and language deficits.

Review Questions

1. Which of the following genes is most likely to be abnormal in a person who develops clinical signs of Alzheimer disease at age 40?

   A. *APOE*
   B. *APP*
   C. *C9orf72*
   D. *PSEN1*
   E. *PSEN2*

2. A 50-year-old man has experienced a functional decline, associated with gradually diminishing speech, for at least 3 years. He has aphasia characterized by fluent anomic language with impaired comprehension of single words, impaired confrontation naming, and preserved repetition. He also has object agnosia. Which of the following dementia types is most likely?

   A. Vascular dementia
   B. Frontal variant Alzheimer disease

C. Behavioral variant FTD (bvFTD)
D. Nonfluent variant primary progressive aphasia (nfvPPA)
E. Semantic variant primary progressive aphasia (svPPA)

3. A 40-year-old woman who has been treated for psychosis for 5 years has been suffering functional decline characterized by increasing apathy, decreasing executive function, and socially inappropriate behavior. On examination, her grip strength is mildly reduced in both hands. Which of the following causes is most likely?

    A. *GRN* mutation
    B. *MAPT* mutation
    C. Lewy bodies
    D. *C9orf72* mutation
    E. 4R-tauopathy

Answers

Question 1: D. The *APP, PSEN1*, and *PSEN2* genes are all associated with EAOD (early-onset Alzheimer disease), but *PSEN1* is associated with the earliest age of onset. *C9orf72* is associated with FTD, and *APOE* is a risk factor gene for late-onset Alzheimer disease.

Question 2: E. Although fluent anomia can occur with the progression of Alzheimer disease, the pattern of fluent aphasia with impaired confrontation naming, single-word comprehension, and preserved repetition in combination with object agnosia is most consistent with svPPA.

Question 3: D. *C9orf72* mutations are associated with delusions and hallucinations, behavioral variant FTD, and elements of amyotrophic lateral sclerosis (ALS). *GRN* and *MAPT* mutations are seen in other forms of FTLD. Dementia with Lewy bodies may include psychotic symptoms but is not as likely to resemble bvFTD and is not associated with ALS. Corticobasal degeneration and progressive supranuclear palsy are 4R tauopathies and can include an FTD-like picture but are not ordinarily preceded by psychosis.

References

American Psychiatric Association: Diagnostic and Statistical Manual of Mental Disorders, 5th Edition, Text Revision. Washington, DC, American Psychiatric Association, 2022

Baizabal-Carvallo JF, Jankovic J: Parkinsonism, movement disorders and genetics in frontotemporal dementia. Nat Rev Neurol 12(3):175–185, 2016 26891767

Benson DF, Davis RJ, Snyder BD: Posterior cortical atrophy. Arch Neurol 45(7):789–793, 1988 3390033

Bersano A, Bedini G, Oskam J, et al: CADASIL: treatment and management options. Curr Treat Options Neurol 19(9):31, 2017 28741120

Caroppo P, Le Ber I, Camuzat A, et al: Extensive white matter involvement in patients with frontotemporal lobar degeneration: think progranulin. JAMA Neurol 71(12):1562–1566, 2014 25317628

Chen Q, Lowe VJ, Boeve BF, et al: β-Amyloid PET and 123I-FP-CIT SPECT in mild cognitive impairment at risk for Lewy body dementia. Neurology 96(8):e1180–e1189, 2021 33408148

Chételat G, Arbizu J, Barthel H, et al: Amyloid-PET and 18F-FDG-PET in the diagnostic investigation of Alzheimer's disease and other dementias. Lancet Neurol 19(11):951–962, 2020 33098804

Collins JA, Montal V, Hochberg D, et al: Focal temporal pole atrophy and network degeneration in semantic variant primary progressive aphasia. Brain 140(2):457–471, 2017 28040670

Crutch SJ, Schott JM, Rabinovici GD, et al: Consensus classification of posterior cortical atrophy. Alzheimers Dement 13(8):870–884, 2017 28259709

Damasceno BP: Normal pressure hydrocephalus: diagnostic and predictive evaluationon. Dement Neuropsychol 3(1):8–15, 2009 29213603

de Wolf F, Ghanbari M, Licher S, et al: Plasma tau, neurofilament light chain and amyloid-β levels and risk of dementia; a population-based cohort study. Brain 143(4):1220–1232, 2020 32206776

Devenney EM, Ahmed RM, Hodges JR: Frontotemporal dementia. Handb Clin Neurol 167:279–299, 2019 31753137

Dickerson BC, Bakkour A, Salat DH, et al: The cortical signature of Alzheimer's disease: regionally specific cortical thinning relates to symptom severity in very mild to mild AD dementia and is detectable in asymptomatic amyloid-positive individuals. Cereb Cortex 19(3):497–510, 2009 18632739

Ducharme S, Dickerson BC: The neuropsychiatric examination of the young-onset dementias. Psychiatr Clin North Am 38(2):249–264, 2015 25998114

Edwards-Lee T, Miller BL, Benson DF, et al: The temporal variant of frontotemporal dementia. Brain 120(Pt 6):1027–1040, 1997 9217686

Eldaief MC, Perez DL, Quimby M, et al: Atrophy in distinct corticolimbic networks subserving socioaffective behavior in semantic variant primary progressive aphasia. Dement Geriatr Cogn Disord 49(6):589–597, 2020 33691310

Galasko D: Lewy body disorders. Neurol Clin 35(2):325–338, 2017 28410662

Gallardo G, Holtzman DM: Amyloid-β and tau at the crossroads of Alzheimer's disease. Adv Exp Med Biol 1184:187–203, 2019 32096039

Gomperts SN: Lewy body dementias: dementia with Lewy bodies and Parkinson disease dementia. Continuum (Minneap Minn) 22(2 Dementia):435–463, 2016 27042903

Gorno-Tempini ML, Hillis AE, Weintraub S, et al: Classification of primary progressive aphasia and its variants. Neurology 76(11):1006–1014, 2011 21325651

Greaves CV, Rohrer JD: An update on genetic frontotemporal dementia. J Neurol 266(8):2075–2086, 2019 31119452

Grossman M: The non-fluent/agrammatic variant of primary progressive aphasia. Lancet Neurol 11(6):545–555, 2012 22608668

Harada CN, Natelson Love MC, Triebel KL: Normal cognitive aging. Clin Geriatr Med 29(4):737–752, 2013 24094294

Hughes CP, Berg L, Danziger WL, et al: A new clinical scale for the staging of dementia. Br J Psychiatry 140:566–572, 1982 7104545

Jessen F, Amariglio RE, Buckley RF, et al: The characterisation of subjective cognitive decline. Lancet Neurol 19(3):271–278, 2020 31958406

Khoury R, Liu Y, Sheheryar Q, et al: Pharmacotherapy for frontotemporal dementia. CNS Drugs 35(4):425–438, 2021 33840052

Lane CA, Hardy J, Schott JM: Alzheimer's disease. Eur J Neurol 25(1):59–70, 2018 28872215

Lowe VJ, Curran G, Fang P, et al: An autoradiographic evaluation of AV-1451 Tau PET in dementia. Acta Neuropathol Commun 4(1):58, 2016 27296779

Marquié M, Normandin MD, Meltzer AC, et al: Pathological correlations of [F-18]-AV-1451 imaging in non-Alzheimer tauopathies. Ann Neurol 81(1):117–128, 2017 27997036

McKhann GM, Knopman DS, Chertkow H, et al: The diagnosis of dementia due to Alzheimer's disease: recommendations from the National Institute on Aging-Alzheimer's Association workgroups on diagnostic guidelines for Alzheimer's disease. Alzheimers Dement 7(3):263–269, 2011 21514250

Miyagawa T, Brushaber D, Syrjanen J, et al: Use of the CDR® plus NACC FTLD in mild FTLD: data from the ARTFL/LEFFTDS consortium. Alzheimers Dement 16(1):79–90, 2020 31477517

Moore KM, Nicholas J, Grossman M, et al: Age at symptom onset and death and disease duration in genetic frontotemporal dementia: an international retrospective cohort study. Lancet Neurol 19(2):145–156, 2020 31810826

Morris JC: The Clinical Dementia Rating (CDR): current version and scoring rules. Neurology 43(11):2412–2414, 1993 8232972

Mosconi L, Tsui WH, Herholz K, et al: Multicenter standardized 18F-FDG PET diagnosis of mild cognitive impairment, Alzheimer's disease, and other dementias. J Nucl Med 49(3):390–398, 2008 18287270

Oliveira LM, Nitrini R, Román GC: Normal-pressure hydrocephalus: a critical review. Dement Neuropsychol 13(2):133–143, 2019 31285787

Olney NT, Spina S, Miller BL: Frontotemporal dementia. Neurol Clin 35(2):339–374, 2017 28410663

Onyike CU, Diehl-Schmid J: The epidemiology of frontotemporal dementia. Int Rev Psychiatry 25(2):130–137, 2013 23611343

Ossenkoppele R, Jansen WJ, Rabinovici GD, et al: Prevalence of amyloid PET positivity in dementia syndromes: a meta-analysis. JAMA 313(19):1939–1949, 2015 25988463

Palmqvist S, Janelidze S, Quiroz YT, et al: Discriminative accuracy of plasma phospho-tau217 for Alzheimer disease vs other neurodegenerative disorders. JAMA 324(8):772–781, 2020 32722745

Petersen RC: Clinical practice: mild cognitive impairment. N Engl J Med 364(23):2227–2234, 2011 21651394

Petersen RC, Smith GE, Waring SC, et al: Mild cognitive impairment: clinical characterization and outcome. Arch Neurol 56(3):303–308, 1999 10190820

Radue R, Walaszek A, Asthana S: Neuropsychiatric symptoms in dementia. Handb Clin Neurol 167:437–454, 2019 31753148

Rascovsky K, Hodges JR, Knopman D, et al: Sensitivity of revised diagnostic criteria for the behavioural variant of frontotemporal dementia. Brain 134(Pt 9):2456–2477, 2011 21810890

Rujeedawa T, Carrillo Félez E, Clare ICH, et al: The clinical and neuropathological features of sporadic (late-onset) and genetic forms of Alzheimer's disease. J Clin Med 10(19):4582, 2021 34640600

Ryan NS, Nicholas JM, Weston PSJ, et al: Clinical phenotype and genetic associations in autosomal dominant familial Alzheimer's disease: a case series. Lancet Neurol 15(13):1326–1335, 2016 27777022

Sander K, Lashley T, Gami P, et al: Characterization of tau positron emission tomography tracer [18F]AV-1451 binding to postmortem tissue in Alzheimer's disease, primary tauopathies, and other dementias. Alzheimers Dement 12(11):1116–1124, 2016 26892233

Sanford AM: Lewy body dementia. Clin Geriatr Med 34(4):603–615, 2018 30336990

Scheltens P, Blennow K, Breteler MM, et al: Alzheimer's disease. Lancet 388(10043):505–517, 2016 26921134

van der Flier WM, Skoog I, Schneider JA, et al: Vascular cognitive impairment. Nat Rev Dis Primers 4:18003, 2018 29446769

van Dyck CH, Swanson CJ, Aisen P, et al: Lecanemab in early Alzheimer's disease. N Engl J Med 388(1):9–21, 2023 36449413

Watson N, Brandel JP, Green A, et al: The importance of ongoing international surveillance for Creutzfeldt-Jakob disease. Nat Rev Neurol 17(6):362–379, 2021 33972773

Winston A, Spudich S: Cognitive disorders in people living with HIV. Lancet HIV 7(7):e504–e513, 2020 32621876

Wong B, Lucente DE, MacLean J, et al: Diagnostic evaluation and monitoring of patients with posterior cortical atrophy. Neurodegener Dis Manag 9(4):217–239, 2019 31392920

5

Traumatic Brain Injury

Brigid C. Dwyer, M.D.
Alexandra M. Stillman, M.D.
Douglas I. Katz, M.D.

Case Example: Mild Traumatic Brain Injury

A 55-year-old woman is rear-ended while stopped at a traffic light. She is wearing her seatbelt. She recalls driving her car a few minutes before the crash and subsequently sitting in her vehicle, confused as to what had just transpired. Her airbag deployed, but she does not recall this happening. Bystanders report that she lost consciousness for approximately 1 minute. She is transported by ambulance to an emergency department, where she is fully oriented but complains of a headache and disequilibrium. She repeatedly asks staff, "Why is it so bright in here?" She complains of nausea and vomits once. Head CT shows no evidence of trauma-induced abnormalities. She returns home that evening and rests for 2 days but has difficulty returning to her normal activities. Nausea and a constant headache persist for a week; light sensitivity, sound sensitivity, and disequilibrium improve but recur when she spends more than a few minutes on her smartphone or when she attempts to do household chores. She frequently misplaces her keys, wallet, and phone. Her sleep is restless, and she wakes up frequently. She has difficulty concentrating and easily becomes frustrated, tearful, and irritable.

Case Example: Severe Traumatic Brain Injury

A 29-year-old man is discovered on the roadside by a bystander next to the motorcycle he had been riding. He has a head injury, as well as multiple orthopedic injuries. He does not track objects, does not move spontaneously, and demonstrates only reflex posturing movements in response to pain. He is intubated and brought urgently to the nearest level I trauma center, where he is stabilized and admitted to the neurocritical care unit. A head CT and angiogram performed on arrival show acute subdural and subarachnoid hemorrhages involving the frontal, temporal, and parietal lobes as well as the brain parenchyma. An MRI reveals severe diffuse axonal injury with petechial hemorrhages involving the subcortical white matter and corpus callosum. He requires monitoring and management of his intracranial pressure for several days. He begins tracking and withdrawing his right side to pain after 10 days, and after 3 weeks, he begins following simple commands. A percutaneous endoscopic gastrostomy is placed for nutrition. He is discharged to an acute rehabilitation facility. As his physical and cognitive abilities improve, he exhibits disinhibited and agitated behaviors.

Traumatic brain injury (TBI) is among the most common neurological disorders and is a leading cause of death and disability. TBI can have devastating consequences and is considered a chronic disorder that can lead to long-standing and lifelong problems, including cognitive impairment, behavioral dysregulation, mood disorders, somatic problems, and other chronic symptoms. In this chapter, we review the epidemiology, pathophysiology, and severity rating of TBIs and discuss the clinical manifestation and treatment of mild, moderate, and severe TBIs.

Epidemiology

The estimated global incidence of TBI ranges from 27 million to more than 50 million new cases yearly (GBD 2016 Traumatic Brain Injury and Spinal Cord Injury Collaborators 2019). The global disability rate is among the highest of all neurological disorders, at 111 per 100,000 population. In the United States, an estimated 3.17 million people live with permanent sequelae of TBI (Zaloshnja et al. 2008). TBI incidence is highest in the youngest and oldest age groups of the population. Falls, which are especially common in young children and the elderly, have become the leading cause of TBIs. Traffic-related injuries have decreased in recent years but remain a leading cause in late adolescence and early adulthood. Rates of TBI are significantly higher in males than females, at an almost 2-to-1 ratio (Haarbauer-Krupa et al. 2021).

The Centers for Disease Control and Prevention estimated the total cost of TBI in the United States at 40.6 billion dollars in 2016 (Miller et al. 2021). TBI can cause major life disruptions, including loss of productivity, strain on relationships, social isolation, risks of substance misuse, and other challenges. TBI has been associated with an increased risk for degenerative neurological disorders such as Parkinson disease, chronic traumatic encephalopathy, and other dementias (Haarbauer-Krupa et al. 2021).

Pathophysiology

The pathophysiology of TBI is highly complex, with varying combinations of pathological damage across a range of severities. It is useful, although somewhat oversimplified, to consider TBI pathology in terms of primary and secondary neuropathological consequences, divided further into focal and diffuse categories of pathology. The *primary injury* is the damage that occurs at the time of injury, and the *secondary injury* is the damage occurring because of the delayed effects of the primary injury, such as brain swelling, loss of vasoregulation, excitotoxicity, metabolic disturbance, and immunological reactions. Clinical manifestations are largely determined by the type, distribution, severity, and location of the combined neuropathological events after brain injury. Focal and diffuse pathological processes are often combined, but for clinical diagnosis, it is helpful to evaluate their potential effects separately. Structural neuroimaging is useful for diagnosing focal and diffuse pathology. Precise clinical pathophysiological diagnosis is sometimes challenging, with diffuse and secondary injuries for which diagnostic biomarkers are limited.

The most common type of diffuse injury is *diffuse axonal injury,* whereby shear strain injury to axons leads to widespread axonal disruption throughout different parts of the brain. The most common type of focal injury is *contusion,* essentially a bruise to the brain, typically located in the frontal and temporal cortices and extending to varying depths in the adjacent white matter. Other forms of focal injury are larger deep brain hemorrhages and extra-axial hemorrhages in the form of epidural and subdural hematomas. Focal lesions and brain swelling that can occur with both focal and diffuse injury can cause secondary damage by restricting circulation along with rising intracranial pressures and by shifting the brain within and between cerebral compartments.

Following acute and subacute pathophysiological events, residual brain damage can be associated with long-standing loss of brain function related to localized damage and diffuse disconnections within and between multiple brain networks. Neurotransmitter systems are widely affected during the acute period of injury, with sudden surges of glutamate, L-aspartate, dopamine, norepinephrine, serotonin, γ-aminobutyric acid, and other neurotransmitters. This is followed by normalization of neurotransmitter activity, which may take weeks, but some neurotransmitter systems, particularly acetylcholine, may remain depleted (Arciniegas et al. 2021). These neurotransmitter systems are potential targets of neuroprotection early after injury and targets of pharmacological treatment for cognitive, behavioral, and emotional symptoms later after injury.

Severity of Injury

The conventional clinical parameters used to define TBI severity include depth of unconsciousness during the acute period, usually defined by the Glasgow Coma Scale; duration of unconsciousness; and duration of posttraumatic confusion or amnesia (Table 5.1). Mild TBI, largely synonymous with concussion, is by far the most common form of TBI. Mild TBI is often considered separately from moderate to severe TBI because of differences in neuropathology, clinical features, course, and outcome.

The most consistent clinical consequences of TBI involve cognitive, emotional, and behavioral dysfunction. Other neurological functions that can be affected include motor control, balance, oculomotor function, and perceptual capacities. The natural history of recovery after TBI can typically be defined by three phases: loss of consciousness, followed by a posttraumatic confusional state (PTCS) closely linked to posttraumatic amnesia (PTA), followed by a postconfusional phase of improving higher-level cognitive functioning and social awareness. Depending on the severity, TBI results in variable degrees of altered consciousness and loss of consciousness (see Table 5.1).

Patients with very severe injuries may stall within one phase or another in the course of recovery and have persistent neurocognitive or neurobehavioral symptoms. As patients progress through the natural history of recovery after TBI, the defining cognitive limitations

Table 5.1 Nonpenetrating traumatic brain injury severity classification

Criterion	Mild	Moderate	Severe
Loss of consciousness	0–30 minutes	30 minutes to 24 hours	>24 hours
Glasgow Coma Scale score	13–15	9–12	3–8
Posttraumatic amnesia	0–24 hours	1–7 days	>7 days

typically progress from deficits in arousal and consciousness to basic attention and anterograde amnesia, and then to higher-level attention, memory retrieval, executive functioning, processing speed, self-awareness, and social awareness.

Focal injury disrupts functional brain networks, which may result in recognizable syndromes associated with particular locations of focal damage. Damage to areas of the frontal, temporal-limbic, and neocortical networks largely determines the usual clinical effects of focal TBI, disturbing cognitive and behavioral functioning. The residual syndromes of prefrontal lesions include alterations in affect and behavior (e.g., disinhibition, apathy), impairment in attention, working memory, memory retrieval, and executive functioning. Lesions in anterior and inferior temporal areas may also contribute to behavioral disturbances. Larger lesions extending to medial temporal areas may produce specific impairments in memory encoding, consolidation, and retrieval (amnesia). Other localizing temporal syndromes include anomia or aphasia with dominant hemisphere involvement.

Approach to Patients With Traumatic Brain Injury

Obtaining an accurate, detailed history is essential to making a diagnosis of TBI. The clinical effects of brain injury must be interpreted within the larger context of preinjury personal factors (e.g., age, education, occupation, preexisting problems, psychosocial issues, personality types) and postinjury strengths and liabilities (e.g., family support, social network, financial stability, comorbidities, pain syndromes, psychiatric disorders, addictions). The approach to the patient varies with the severity and pathophysiologies of the TBI.

Mild Traumatic Brain Injury

The diagnosis of mild TBI can be challenging if the injury is not associated with loss of consciousness or PTA or is completely reliant on retrospective, subjective accounts. Clearly established accounts of post-injury unconsciousness, PTA, and confusional signs within the time thresholds noted in Table 5.1 or acute neurological signs, support a more definitive diagnosis of mild TBI. Small hemorrhages on neuroimaging also definitively support a diagnosis of TBI that has been termed *complicated mild TBI.* The diagnosis of mild TBI is often made on the basis of a variety of symptoms that typically occur with mild TBI as part of the postconcussion syndrome, such as headache, dizziness, light sensitivity, noise sensitivity, imbalance, fatigue, irritability, mood swings, difficulty concentrating, and memory problems. Many of these symptoms are nonspecific and may occur without concussion or with other trauma (Meehan and Bachur 2009). Therefore, a definitive diagnosis of mild TBI (concussion) cannot be made on the basis of symptoms alone but should be considered in the overall context of detailed history, physical examination, and other clinical assessments. Recently updated consensus diagnostic criteria for mild TBI require 1) a biomechanically plausible mechanism of injury and a combination of clinical signs, 2) two acute symptoms with at least one clinical or laboratory finding attributable to brain injury, or 3) CT or MRI neuroimaging evidence supporting TBI. Furthermore, these findings cannot be better accounted for by another diagnosis (Silverberg et al. 2023).

Initial management after a concussion includes recommendations for rest to aid recovery. However, rest may have adverse effects, such as fatigue, diurnal sleep disruption, reactive depression, anxiety, and physiological deconditioning, particularly if rest is prolonged (DiFazio et al. 2016; Willer and Leddy 2006). As recovery progresses, the somatic symptoms of concussion should improve, although emotional symptoms can worsen, especially if the patient undergoes a prolonged period of rest (Thomas et al. 2015). Consensus currently favors a period of rest lasting no more than 3–5 days after injury, followed by a gradual resumption of both physical and cognitive activities as tolerated, remaining below the level at which symptoms are exacerbated. Mild aerobic exercise may speed recovery from postconcussion syndrome, even in patients who did not exercise before the injury (Leddy et al. 2010). It is reasonable to have patients return to work or school gradually rather than attempt to immediately return at full capacity. With these interventions, most patients have full resolution of their symptoms and successful return to preinjury levels of performance.

Somatic Symptoms

Posttraumatic headache is the most common sequela of concussion (Packard 1999). Surprisingly, it is more common after mild traumatic brain injury or concussion than after moderate or severe traumatic brain injury (Couch and Bearss 2001). A prior history of headache, particularly migraine, is a known risk factor for the development of posttraumatic headache (Lucas et al. 2014). Posttraumatic headache disorders may be driven by multiple traumatic etiologies, including direct brain injury and musculoskeletal head or neck injury. Migraine, followed by tension and cervicogenic headache, is the most common type of posttraumatic headache (Dwyer and Zasler 2020). Care should be taken to avoid headaches from medication overuse. See Chapter 11, "Headache."

Dizziness is common after concussion. Dizziness is typically a subjective sense of poor coordination, gait instability, or disequilibrium. Patients may also complain of nausea and motion sensitivity. Dizziness may be secondary to pathological mechanisms in the brain or in the middle or inner ear, or it may be a result of cervical injury.

One cause of inner-ear posttraumatic vertigo is benign paroxysmal positional vertigo, which can be diagnosed with a Dix-Hallpike maneuver and is usually successfully treated in the office with the Epley maneuver (Valovich et al. 2015). Management involves encouraging patients to move gradually and safely to help the vestibular system accommodate. Dizziness usually resolves spontaneously, and medications are of little help. Vestibular rehabilitation involving habituation exercises can often can accelerate improvement and decrease symptoms (Valovich et al. 2015). Eye motility problems are a common contributor to dizziness and disequilibrium. Examples include convergence spasm, which is typically of functional origin, or convergence insufficiency, as well as problems with tracking and saccadic movements (Master et al. 2016).

Sleep disturbance, manifesting as fatigue, daytime somnolence, and alteration of the sleep-wake cycle, is common after concussion and can influence recovery (Mahmood et al. 2004). Sleep hygiene education should be the first intervention, including maintaining regular sleep-wake times; avoiding late-day naps; eliminating caffeine, nicotine, and alcohol use; and minimizing screen time at least an hour before bedtime (Figueiro et al. 2011; Lewy et al. 1980). See Chapter 15, "Sleep Disorders."

Cognitive Symptoms

Cognitive complaints are common after concussion. Patients report forgetfulness, distractibility, loss of concentration, and mental fatigue. With a program of gradual increase in mental activity, parallel to recovery of physical capacity, most patients make a gradual recovery within a few weeks (Dikmen et al. 1986). When cognitive difficulties persist, clinicians should consider injury-related problems, such as headache, pain, disequilibrium, sleep disturbance, and anxiety, which may contribute to subjective cognitive symptoms and impaired cognitive functioning. Subjective dysexecutive symptoms are highly correlated with measures of emotional and mental health, and depression is most strongly predictive of executive functioning complaints (Stillman et al. 2020). Emotional and psychological factors are major determinants in recovery (Iverson et al. 2015; Massey et al. 2015).

Psychiatric Symptoms

Acute-onset anxiety or depression often occurs after concussion (Dikmen et al. 2004; O'Donnell et al. 2004). A preinjury history of anxiety is likely a prognostic factor (Iverson et al. 2015). Patients with a preinjury history of anxiety, depression, or PTSD are more likely to develop emotional symptoms after a concussion, although emotional problems may develop in any patient after a concussion (Meares et al. 2011). The circumstances under which an injury is sustained may be psychologically traumatic (e.g., car accident, assault), leading to an acute stress reaction or disorder. If untreated, this may result in PTSD, especially in persons who may be more vulnerable to this condition. Injury and persisting symptoms may have repercussions in many aspects of the patient's life (e.g., loss of wages; the inability to handle normal work, school, and family responsibilities), leading to further psychological stress. Referral to a therapist trained in skills-based psychotherapies such as cognitive-behavioral therapy or exposure therapy is often helpful. Pharmacological treatment can be a useful adjunct.

Prolonged Symptoms

Most patients with concussion have resolution of symptoms and can return to preinjury levels of performance, but some have prolonged symptoms and sequelae. Patients who have persistent symptoms that appear inconsistent with the severity of their injury may have developed a functional neurological disorder (see Chapter 10) or may be exaggerating their symptoms intentionally. On neuropsychological testing, this can take the form of failed effort testing or failed validity testing (e.g., less than chance responses). Studies show that complex, multifactorial reasons underlie symptom exaggeration, and this is often incorrectly interpreted as a conscious process (Silver 2012).

Patients who have persistent postconcussive symptoms generally fall into four categories: 1) patients who sustained a high-force mechanism of injury; 2) those with a history of multiple concussions, particularly occurring close in time; 3) patients with other neurological conditions; and 4) those with other injury or non-injury factors prolonging recovery, including age-related factors. It has been proposed that pre-existing personality factors (pre-injury neuroticism, pessimism, and low resilience) and psychosocial conditions also play a role in the persistence of symptoms (Fordal et al. 2022; Rogers and Read 2007).

Moderate and Severe Traumatic Brain Injury

Moderate to severe TBI requires more urgent diagnostic assessment and management of problems that may occur acutely, such as subdural or epidural hematomas, high intracranial pressures, hypoxia, ischemia, hydrocephalus, seizures, autonomic disturbances, and other secondary complications. The 30-day mortality rate of moderate to severe TBI is relatively high, approximately 29% (Brown et al. 2004).

As described previously, the natural history of more severe injuries is more prolonged, with lingering problems in cognition affecting attention, memory, and executive functioning. After moderate to severe TBI, 60% of patients report long-lasting issues with attention (Ponsford et al. 2014). Judgment, decision-making, and social interaction are often affected. Patients commonly exhibit reduced self-awareness and insight into their deficits, in contrast to patients with mild TBI, who are usually aware of, often discouraged about, and even hypervigilant with regard to impairments.

The mood and behavioral changes associated with moderate to severe TBI are also of great clinical importance and consequence. Decreased ability to regulate emotions and behavior may lead to agitation and aggression after moderate to severe TBI, especially during the PTCS, and may persist after resolution of the PTCS. Impulsivity and disinhibited behavior can compromise safety. Mood lability is also a hallmark of moderate to severe TBI.

Depression, anxiety, decreased motivation, and apathy are common after moderate to severe TBI, and depression is 5.25 times more likely to occur with a preexisting history (Gould et al. 2011). Anxiety disorders may be among the earliest clinical developments (Gould et al. 2011). Psychosis and mania have an approximately 2%–3% incidence in populations with severe TBI, with or without axonal injury (Diaz et al. 2012; Gould et al. 2011). Many patients have a pre-injury history of psychosis, and the risk of a new psychiatric diagnosis is highest in the first year (Alway et al. 2016).

Treatment

Rehabilitation

Patients with moderate to severe TBI often require ongoing medical care after acute hospital management and benefit from rehabilitation in an inpatient rehabilitation facility (IRF). IRF care includes at least 3 hours a day of therapies by physical, occupational, and speech therapists aimed at treating problems in mobility, activities of daily living (ADLs), and cognitive/behavioral functioning. Postacute rehabilitation of patients with moderate to severe TBI often involves management of cognitive and behavioral regulation problems, including agitation and aggression, that are characteristic of the PTCS. Patients often have balance and other motor problems that affect mobility and safety, especially in the setting of decreased insight and awareness. Cognitive, behavioral, and motor impairments may affect the patient's ability to safely and independently carry out ADLs. As recovery evolves, therapists may use restorative and compensatory rehabilitation strategies to improve function and reduce dependency and supervision requirements to facilitate transition to home care (Katz and Dwyer 2021).

Patients with severe TBI usually have impairments in cognitive functioning that affect their capacity to make decisions independently. Psychiatric consultants may be called on to assess decisional capacity. In most cases, maintaining necessary levels of supervision and substituted decision-making until a patient's cognitive capacity improves is sufficient to maintain safety and protect a patient's well-being. In some cases, the health care proxy should be initiated for medical decision-making. Assigning a power of attorney may be sufficient to temporarily protect financial or legal interests. In more difficult cases, probate court may become involved to assign a guardian or conservator to protect a patient's interests, at least temporarily.

Pharmacotherapy

Pharmacological treatments for behavioral dysregulation, mood disorder, anxiety, and cognitive impairment are often part of management in TBI. Pharmacotherapy for depression in TBI appears to be effective (Salter et al. 2016). Selective serotonin reuptake inhibitors (SSRIs) or serotonin-norepinephrine reuptake inhibitors (SNRIs) are typically used instead of tricyclic antidepressants (TCAs) because they are likely to be more effective and have fewer side effects, including less reduction in seizure threshold (Fann et al. 2009). However, TCAs may be preferred if concurrently targeting headaches, pain, or insomnia. TCA dosages for depression are higher than those used to treat headache and pain. Additionally, stimulants may be useful to treat depression after TBI and have been shown to be beneficial for cognition, particularly aspects of attention and processing speed post-TBI (Lee et al. 2005)

The incidence of generalized anxiety disorder post-TBI is estimated to be up to 24%, much higher than in the general population. Typically, SSRIs or SNRIs are considered first-line treatment. Benzodiazepines should be avoided if possible. They can cause cognitive impairment and behavioral disinhibition, and there is concern that they may slow recovery post-TBI (Schallert et al. 1986).

Antipsychotics and benzodiazepines are the most commonly used medications in the treatment of acute aggressive, agitated, and self-injurious behaviors in patients with neuropsychiatric disorders (Pabis and Stanislav 1996). However, these medications should be minimized if possible in TBI, especially first-generation, typical antipsychotics and those with greater dopamine D_2 receptor–blocking activity. In addition to adverse and paradoxical effects, there is some evidence that benzodiazepines and typical antipsychotics can impair neuroplasticity after TBI (Hoffman et al. 2008). Atypical antipsychotics, particularly those with less dopamine-blocking activity, such as quetiapine and clozapine, probably have the least adverse potential for recovery and cognition and may be effective in managing behavioral dyscontrol. Of course, in an emergency situation, if a patient is a danger to themselves or others, typical antipsychotics and/or benzodiazepines may be a reasonable choice. Other sedating medications such as trazodone may also be effective. There is evidence that beta-blockers such as propranolol are effective in reducing aggressive behavior after TBI. Antiepileptic agents that also act as mood stabilizers such as valproic acid and lamotrigine can be effective and are usually well tolerated (Chatham Showalter and Kimmel 2000). There is some evidence that dopamine agonists, such as amantadine, can also improve behavioral regulation after TBI (Hammond et al. 2017).

Manic behavior after TBI is less common than depression or anxiety, and it can be treated with mood stabilizers such as valproate when it does occur. Pseudobulbar affect occurs in more than 10% of people with TBI (Tateno et al. 2004). SSRIs are considered first-line treatment (Wortzel et al. 2008), but combination treatment with dextromethorphan and quinidine can also be effective. Apathy is common post-TBI. Some studies suggest that methylphenidate or amantadine may be effective (Gualtieri and Evans 1988; Van Reekum et al. 1995).

For cognitive consequences of TBI, first-line treatment should be nonpharmacological, including modification of environmental factors, psychoeducation, and cognitive rehabilitation. Management should include eliminating any medications that may be contributing to cognitive impairment, especially if they are not medically necessary. Attentional issues are common. Stimulants are the gold standard of treatment for attentional and processing-speed deficits post-TBI, but they must be used cautiously in people with cardiovascular issues and those with psychotic symptoms. Memory issues are common after TBI and are typically treated with stimulants or cholinesterase inhibitors (Kim et al. 2006).

Case Example: Mild Traumatic Brain Injury, continued

The patient's neurological examination is normal, and a brain MRI without contrast is also unremarkable. Physical therapy and occupational therapy are ordered to address her ongoing symptoms. She explores in detail what level of physical or mental activity would exacerbate her symptoms at any given time and begins to feel reassured by her growing capabilities as well as her ability to use workarounds such as cell phone reminders, Post-It notes, and a pill box for medications. She begins taking amitriptyline for posttraumatic tension headache prophylaxis and insomnia. After 3 months, she begins collaborating with human resources at her workplace to return to work, where her work hours are gradually increased from 4- to 8-hour shifts. She uses a screen dimmer and secures a dark, quiet break room in case of unexpected symptom flares. After 6 months, she gradually discontinues the use of memory aids and returns to her normal level of physical activity.

Case Example: Severe Traumatic Brain Injury, continued

For his mood and behavioral management, the patient is prescribed divalproex sodium, propranolol, and trazodone. He begins an aggressive course of physical, occupational, and speech therapies at an acute rehabilitation center specializing in TBI. After 5 weeks, he begins to speak in simple phrases, but he has significant anomia and remains disoriented for nearly 3 months. With further improvement in orientation, instances of agitation and resistance to nursing care decrease. However, he occasionally tries to stand from his wheelchair, stating that he is ready to go home, and requires redirection. He is eventually able to retain the primary reason for his hospitalization, but he still has difficulty with initiation and sequencing. He is moderately apathetic and requires strict scheduling of medications to regulate his sleep cycle. He is discharged home to the care of his parents with a full-time patient care assistant, visiting nurse, and ongoing home therapies.

Key Clinical Points

- Traumatic brain injury (TBI) is among the most common neurological disorders and is a leading cause of death and disability.
- The pathophysiology of TBI is highly complex, with varying combinations of pathological damage across a range of severities: mild, moderate, and severe. It is useful to consider TBI pathology in terms of primary and secondary neuropathologic consequences, divided into focal and diffuse pathologies.
- The natural history of TBI typically follows 3 phases: loss of consciousness, followed by a posttraumatic confusional state (PTCS) closely linked to posttraumatic amnesia (PTA), followed by a postconfusional phase of improving higher-level cognitive functioning and social awareness.
- Peak symptoms are expected within hours to days of TBI, with gradual improvement of somatic and neurological symptoms thereafter. Psychiatric symptom recovery may be more variable.
- Patients with TBI may suffer from symptoms of depression, anxiety, apathy, and sometimes mania or other psychotic symptoms.
- When prescribing medications for chronic TBI-induced headaches, care should be taken to avoid medication overuse headache.
- Substantial behavioral dyscontrol may be treated with mood stabilizers, sedating antidepressants, beta-blockers, and atypical antipsychotics.

Review Questions

1. Which of the following diagnoses is most predictive of executive dysfunction following traumatic brain injury?

   A. Dorsolateral prefrontal damage.
   B. Basal ganglia damage.
   C. Depression.
   D. PTSD.
   E. Medial temporal damage.

2. On the basis of duration of loss of consciousness (LOC), Glasgow Coma Scale (GCS) on arrival, and duration of posttraumatic amnesia (PTA), which of the following descriptions of nonpenetrating TBI is most consistent with mild traumatic brain injury?

   A. LOC 15 minutes, GCS 14, PTA 2 weeks.
   B. LOC 8 hours, GCS 13, PTA 1 week.
   C. LOC 24 hours, GCS 12, PTA 24 hours.
   D. LOC 15 minutes, GCS 13, PTA 12 hours.
   E. LOC 8 hours, GCS 12, PTA 4 days.

3. Which of the following is the most common posttraumatic sequela of mild TBI?

   A. Ocular motility abnormalities.
   B. Gait instability.
   C. Dizziness.
   D. Vertigo.
   E. Headache.

Answers

Question 1: C. Psychological symptoms are common after TBI, and the presence of depression has been shown to be the most predictive of executive dysfunction. Executive dysfunction does occur following dorsolateral frontal damage, but depression is more common.

Question 2: D. TBI severity for nonpenetrating trauma is determined by the depth of coma (GCS) and duration of coma and posttraumatic amnesia (LOC, PTA), as shown in Table 5.1. Mild TBI is defined as LOC ≤30 minutes, GCS 13–15, and PTA <24 hours.

Question 3: E. Posttraumatic headache is typically migrainous and occurs more often in mild than in moderate or severe TBI. All of the other symptoms occur, but with less frequency than headache.

References

Alway Y, Gould KR, Johnston L, et al: A prospective examination of Axis I psychiatric disorders in the first 5 years following moderate to severe traumatic brain injury. Psychol Med 46(6):1331–1341, 2016 26867715

Arciniegas DB, Quinn DK, Silver JM: Pharmacotherapy of cognitive impairment, in Brain Injury Medicine, 3rd Edition. Edited by Zasler ND, Katz DI, Zafonte RD. New York, Demos Medical Publishing, 2021, pp 1137–1149

Brown AW, Leibson CL, Malec JF, et al: Long-term survival after traumatic brain injury: a population-based analysis. NeuroRehabilitation 19(1):37–43, 2004 14988586

Chatham Showalter PE, Kimmel DN: Agitated symptom response to divalproex following acute brain injury. J Neuropsychiatry Clin Neurosci 12(3):395–397, 2000 10956575

Couch JR, Bearss C: Chronic daily headache in the posttrauma syndrome: relation to extent of head injury. Headache 41(6):559–564, 2001 11437891

Diaz AP, Schwarzbold ML, Thais ME, et al: Psychiatric disorders and health-related quality of life after severe traumatic brain injury: a prospective study. J Neurotrauma 29(6):1029–1037, 2012 22111890

DiFazio M, Silverberg ND, Kirkwood MW, et al: Prolonged activity restriction after concussion: are we worsening outcomes? Clin Pediatr (Phila) 55(5):443–451, 2016 26130391

Dikmen S, McLean A, Temkin N: Neuropsychological and psychosocial consequences of minor head injury. J Neurol Neurosurg Psychiatry 49(11):1227–1232, 1986 3794728

Dikmen SS, Bombardier CH, Machamer JE, et al: Natural history of depression in traumatic brain injury. Arch Phys Med Rehabil 85(9):1457–1464, 2004 15375816

Dwyer B, Zasler N: Post-traumatic cephalalgia. NeuroRehabilitation 47(3):327–342, 2020 32986623

Fann JR, Hart T, Schomer KG: Treatment for depression after traumatic brain injury: a systematic review. J Neurotrauma 26(12):2383–2402, 2009 19698070

Figueiro MG, Wood B, Plitnick B, et al: The impact of light from computer monitors on melatonin levels in college students. Neuroendocrinol Lett 32(2):158–163, 2011 21552190

Fordal L, Stenberg J, Iverson GL, et al: Trajectories of persistent postconcussion symptoms and factors associated with symptom reporting after mild traumatic brain injury. Arch Phys Med Rehabil 103(2):313–322, 2022 34695386

GBD 2016 Traumatic Brain Injury and Spinal Cord Injury Collaborators: Global, regional, and national burden of traumatic brain injury and spinal cord injury, 1990–2016: a systematic analysis for the Global Burden of Disease Study 2016. Lancet Neurol 18(1):56–87, 2019 30497965

Gould KR, Ponsford JL, Johnston L, et al: The nature, frequency and course of psychiatric disorders in the first year after traumatic brain injury: a prospective study. Psychol Med 41(10):2099–2109, 2011 21477420

Gualtieri C, Evans R: Stimulant treatment for the neurobehavioral sequelae of traumatic brain injury. Brain Inj 2(4):273–290, 1988 3060211

Haarbauer-Krupa J, Pugh MJ, Prager EM, et al: Epidemiology of chronic effects of traumatic brain injury. J Neurotrauma 38(23):3235–3247, 2021 33947273

Hammond FM, Malec JF, Zafonte RD, et al: Potential impact of amantadine on aggression in chronic traumatic brain injury. J Head Trauma Rehabil 32(5):308–318, 2017 28891908

Hoffman AN, Cheng JP, Zafonte RD, et al: Administration of haloperidol and risperidone after neurobehavioral testing hinders the recovery of traumatic brain injury-induced deficits. Life Sci 83(17–18):602–607, 2008 18801378

Iverson GL, Silverberg ND, Mannix R, et al: Factors associated with concussion-like symptom reporting in high school athletes. JAMA Pediatr 169(12):1132–1140, 2015 26457403

Katz DI, Dwyer B: Clinical neurorehabilitation: using principles of neurological diagnosis, prognosis, and neuroplasticity in assessment and treatment planning. Semin Neurol 41(2):111–123, 2021 33663002

Kim YH, Ko MH, Na SY, et al: Effects of single-dose methylphenidate on cognitive performance in patients with traumatic brain injury: a double-blind placebo-controlled study. Clin Rehabil 20(1):24–30, 2006 16502746

Leddy JJ, Kozlowski K, Donnelly JP, et al: A preliminary study of subsymptom threshold exercise training for refractory post-concussion syndrome. Clin J Sport Med 20(1):21–27, 2010 20051730

Lee H, Kim S-W, Kim J-M, et al: Comparing effects of methylphenidate, sertraline and placebo on neuropsychiatric sequelae in patients with traumatic brain injury. Hum Psychopharmacol 20(2):97–104, 2005 15641125

Lewy AJ, Wehr TA, Goodwin FK, et al: Light suppresses melatonin secretion in humans. Science 210(4475):1267–1269, 1980 7434030

Lucas S, Hoffman JM, Bell KR, Dikmen S: A prospective study of prevalence and characterization of headache following mild traumatic brain injury. Cephalalgia 34(2):93–102, 2014 23921798

Mahmood O, Rapport LJ, Hanks RA, et al: Neuropsychological performance and sleep disturbance following traumatic brain injury. J Head Trauma Rehabil 19(5):378–390, 2004 15597029

Massey JS, Meares S, Batchelor J, et al: An exploratory study of the association of acute posttraumatic stress, depression, and pain to cognitive functioning in mild traumatic brain injury. Neuropsychology 29(4):530–542, 2015 25822464

Master CL, Scheiman M, Gallaway M, et al: Vision diagnoses are common after concussion in adolescents. Clin Pediatr (Phila) 55(3):260–267, 2016 26156977

Meares S, Shores EA, Taylor AJ, et al: The prospective course of postconcussion syndrome: the role of mild traumatic brain injury. Neuropsychology 25(4):454–465, 2011 21574719

Meehan WP 3rd, Bachur RG: Sport-related concussion. Pediatrics 123(1):114–123, 2009 19117869

Miller GF, DePadilla L, Xu L: Costs of nonfatal traumatic brain injury in the United States, 2016. Med Care 59(5):451–455, 2021 33528230

O'Donnell ML, Creamer M, Pattison P, et al: Psychiatric morbidity following injury. Am J Psychiatry 161(3):507–514, 2004 14992977

Pabis DJ, Stanislav SW: Pharmacotherapy of aggressive behavior. Ann Pharmacother 30(3):278–287, 1996 8833564

Packard RC: Epidemiology and pathogenesis of posttraumatic headache. J Head Trauma Rehabil 14(1):9–21, 1999 9949243

Ponsford J, Bayley M, Wiseman-Hakes C, et al: INCOG recommendations for management of cognition following traumatic brain injury, part II: attention and information processing speed. J Head Trauma Rehabil 29(4):321–337, 2014 24984095

Rogers JM, Read CA: Psychiatric comorbidity following traumatic brain injury. Brain Inj 21(13–14):1321–1333, 2007 18066935

Salter KL, McClure JA, Foley NC, et al: Pharmacotherapy for depression posttraumatic brain injury. J Head Trauma Rehabil 31(4):E21–E32, 2016 26479398

Schallert T, Hernandez TD, Barth TM: Recovery of function after brain damage: severe and chronic disruption by diazepam. Brain Res 379(1):104–111, 1986 3742206

Silver JM: Effort, exaggeration and malingering after concussion. J Neurol Neurosurg Psychiatry 83(8):836–841, 2012 22696584

Silverberg ND, Iverson GL; ACRM Brain Injury Special Interest Group Mild TBI Task Force Members: The American Congress of Rehabilitation Medicine diagnostic criteria for mild traumatic brain injury. Arch Phys Med Rehabil 104(8):1343–1355, 2023 37211140

Stillman AM, Madigan N, Torres K, et al: Subjective cognitive complaints in concussion. J Neurotrauma 37(2):305–311, 2020 31407632

Tateno A, Jorge RE, Robinson RG: Pathological laughing and crying following traumatic brain injury. J Neuropsychiatry Clin Neurosci 16(4):426–434, 2004 15616168

Thomas DG, Apps JN, Hoffmann RG, et al: Benefits of strict rest after acute concussion: a randomized controlled trial. Pediatrics 135(2):213–223, 2015 25560444

Valovich McLeod TC, Hale TD: Vestibular and balance issues following sport-related concussion. Brain Inj 29(2):175–184, 2015 25291297

Van Reekum R, Bayley M, Garner S, et al: N of 1 study: amantadine for the amotivational syndrome in a patient with traumatic brain injury. Brain Inj 9(1):49–53, 1995 7874096

Willer B, Leddy JJ: Management of concussion and post-concussion syndrome. Curr Treat Options Neurol 8(5):415–426, 2006 16901381

Wortzel HS, Oster TJ, Anderson CA, et al: Pathological laughing and crying : epidemiology, pathophysiology and treatment. CNS Drugs 22(7):531–545, 2008 18547124

Zaloshnja E, Miller T, Langlois JA, et al: Prevalence of long-term disability from traumatic brain injury in the civilian population of the United States, 2005. J Head Trauma Rehabil 23(6):394–400, 2008 19033832

6

Toxins, Substances, and Nutrition

Taylor Young, M.D., M.A.
Elizabeth DeGrush, D.O.

Case Example

A 47-year-old woman is referred to the clinic for treatment of depression and alcohol use disorder. She arrives late in the day, 2 days before her scheduled appointment. Staff report concerns about alcohol intoxication. The woman states that she thinks there is something wrong with her eyes because she has been dropping things and bumping into things in her apartment. She adamantly denies using alcohol recently. Her boyfriend states that she has been isolating herself and losing weight. She has a long history of alcohol use, and her last drink was 2 days ago. Recently, she started smoking heroin and fentanyl but denies intravenous drug use.

In this chapter, we cover the interrelated topics of substances of abuse, toxicity due to heavy metals or homeopathic remedies, and nutritional deficiency syndromes, focusing on the more common neurological signs, symptoms, and syndromes within each category. The number of substances that can cause neurological sequelae is vast, so we focus on the more common causes.

Approach to Patients With Disorders Due to Toxins, Substances, and Nutrition

History

Substance use, toxic exposures, and nutrition should be addressed routinely in all patient encounters, particularly for new patients and those with neurological symptoms. The history should include legal and illicit substances, prescribed medications, over-the-counter medications, herbal remedies, nutritional supplements, nutritional status, and environmental exposures. Because some patients may not be forthcoming or may be unaware, the clinician must attend to clues such as prior substance use disorders, laboratory abnormalities, known constellations of symptoms, findings on neurological examination, and collateral information to further guide the evaluation.

Examination

When there is clinical suspicion for substance abuse, toxic exposure, or nutritional deficiency, a complete neurological examination, including cognition and mental status, should be performed. Examination of vital signs, pupils, and the motor system for evidence of tremor or myoclonus, as well as gait, the neuromuscular system, and cerebellar signs, is of special interest. The examination for sequelae of traumatic brain injury, which frequently co-occurs with substance abuse, is also important (see Chapter 5, "Traumatic Brain Injury").

Recreational and Illicit Drugs

Common symptoms of acute intoxication and withdrawal for frequently encountered recreational and illicit drugs are listed in Table 6.1.

Alcohol

Alcohol can have both acute and chronic effects on the central and peripheral nervous systems. The complications of chronic alcohol use and withdrawal can be life-threatening. Alcohol withdrawal delirium (delirium tremens or DTs) is a medical emergency. Generalized con-

Table 6.1 Signs and symptoms of acute intoxication and withdrawal from commonly used substances

Substance	Intoxication	Withdrawal
Caffeine	Increased alertness, sense of well-being, rapid thoughts and speech, psychomotor agitation, dizziness, tinnitus, headache, nausea, vomiting, psychosis, rigidity, tremor, hypertension/hypotension, cardiac arrhythmia, seizures, coma, death	Fatigue, headache, flu-like symptoms, dysphoric mood, irritability, impaired concentration
Alcohol	Signs as found in order of increasing blood alcohol concentration: increased talkativeness, relaxation, mild euphoria, mild motor impairment, ataxia, nystagmus, hyperreflexia, mood lability, agitation, delayed reaction times, impaired recall, marked dysarthria, amnestic episodes (blackouts and brownouts), diplopia, nausea, vomiting, hypoventilation, hypothermia, cardiac arrhythmia, coma, death	2–48 hours: Autonomic hyperactivity (diaphoresis, tachycardia, hypertension, fever, flushing), tremor, insomnia, nausea and vomiting, transient hallucinations or illusions (typically visual or tactile), anxiety, psychomotor agitation, seizures >48 hours: Delirium tremens, autonomic instability Additional reported complications: Parkinsonism, chorea, dystonia, myoclonus, catatonia (Brust 2014)

Table 6.1 Signs and symptoms of acute intoxication and withdrawal from commonly used substances (*continued*)

Substance	Intoxication	Withdrawal
Cannabis	Impaired coordination, euphoria, anxiety, slowed perception of time, impaired judgment, impaired short-term memory, social withdrawal, injected conjunctiva, increased appetite, dry mouth, tachycardia, illusions, hallucinations	1–2 days: Insomnia, shakiness, decreased appetite, sweating, chills 6–8 days: Irritability, anxiety, restlessness, depressed mood 8–20 days: Anger, aggression (Connor et al. 2021)
Stimulants	Increased alertness, euphoria, agitation, hyperactivity, hypervigilance, anxiety, anger, tremor, stereotyped behaviors, ataxia, increased sociability, mydriasis, tachycardia, hypertension, hyperthermia, hallucinations, illusions, delirium, seizures, dyskinesias, dystonia, coma	Fatigue, insomnia or hypersomnia, vivid dreams, increased appetite, psychomotor agitation or retardation
Opioids	Miosis, somnolence, apathy, slurred speech, inattention, impaired memory, hypotension, hypothermia, respiratory depression	Dysphoria, nausea, vomiting, diarrhea, mydriasis, lacrimation, rhinorrhea, salivation, abdominal pain, piloerection, fever, diaphoresis, myalgias, yawning, insomnia
Hallucinogens	Alterations in consciousness, cognition, emotion, and perception; psychosis	
Nitrous oxide	Anxiolytic, dissociative, and hallucinogenic effects (Garakani et al. 2016)	

Table 6.1 Signs and symptoms of acute intoxication and withdrawal from commonly used substances (*continued*)

Substance	Intoxication	Withdrawal
Toluene	Headaches, fatigue, slowed cognitive function, ataxia, nystagmus, confusion, dizziness, euphoria	
Kratom	Stimulant and analgesic properties (Eggleston et al. 2019)	
Dextromethorphan	Euphoria, hallucination, ataxia, mydriasis, dissociative sedation, respiratory depression, tachycardia, hypertension, psychosis, agitation, dysregulation (Ritter et al. 2020)	
Anticholinergics	Anhidrosis, mydriasis, flushing, hyperthermia, urinary retention, hallucinations, encephalopathy	

vulsive seizures can occur during alcohol withdrawal. These may be treated with benzodiazepines and do not necessarily indicate a diagnosis of epilepsy. Focal seizures in this context require additional evaluation. Antiseizure medications do not prevent alcohol withdrawal seizures. Amnestic episodes from impaired memory consolidation, known as *alcoholic blackouts,* can occur in the setting of acute intoxication. They are an indicator of the severity of alcohol use but are not seizures or events predictive of a chronic cognitive disorder. The many neurological complications of alcohol use are summarized in Table 6.2.

Cannabis

Cannabis is the most widely used illicit substance worldwide, and it has wide-ranging effects on the central nervous, cardiovascular, and pulmonary systems. Cannabis has been decriminalized in many areas of the United States, and there is growing interest in potential therapeutic uses within the medical community.

In addition to increasing the risk of developing other substance use disorders, cannabis use has been associated with neuropsychiatric outcomes, including a dose-dependent relationship between cannabis use and the risk of schizophrenia or other psychotic disorders, an association between long-term cannabis use and the risk of violence or aggression, and several cases of catatonia (Dellazizzo et al. 2020; Marconi et al. 2016; Sheikh et al. 2021).

Cognitive changes related to cannabis are common and vary with use pattern. Intoxication with cannabis impairs attention, motor inhibition, and possibly emotion recognition (Wittemann et al. 2021). In the acute phase of regular use, cannabis impairs working and episodic memory (Curran et al. 2016). Heavy cannabis use is associated with deficits in verbal learning and verbal working memory (Wittemann et al. 2021). Chronic cannabis use affects working and episodic memory, attention, motor control, and motivation. Cognitive changes are largely mediated by tetrahydrocannabinol (THC), and cannabidiol (CBD) may ameliorate these effects when used with THC (Curran et al. 2016). The risk of cognitive deficits increases with earlier onset of use, and there is some evidence for improvement in cognitive deficits with abstinence (Harvey 2019; Kroon et al. 2021).

Cannabis hyperemesis syndrome is an emerging form of cyclic vomiting associated with chronic and heavy cannabis use. Typically, individuals with this syndrome have used cannabis weekly to daily for more than 1 year, experience episodes of severe nausea and vomiting

Table 6.2 Neurological complications of alcohol use

Syndrome	Setting	Features
Alcoholic hallucinosis	During or after a period of heavy alcohol use superimposed on chronic alcohol use	**Presentation:** hallucinations (auditory > visual), delusions (e.g., persecutory/referential), mood disturbance due to hallucinations, clear consciousness, duration <7 days **Other:** increase in suicidal ideation; some cases are related to an independent psychotic disorder (Narasimha et al. 2019) **Management:** benzodiazepines ± antipsychotics
Delirium tremens	Severe alcohol withdrawal	**Presentation:** encephalopathy, symptoms of alcohol withdrawal, onset 48–72 hours after alcohol cessation, duration 3–4 days, often followed by prolonged somnolence; potentially fatal (Grover and Ghosh 2018) **Management:** ICU, benzodiazepines, supportive care, thiamine (Grover and Ghosh 2018)
Syndrome of subacute encephalopathy with seizures in alcoholics	Alcohol withdrawal, chronic alcohol use, acute alcohol intoxication	**Presentation:** seizures (focal motor, focal impaired awareness, focal status epilepticus, nonconvulsive status epilepticus), encephalopathy, abnormal EEG (focal slowing, lateralized periodic discharges, electrographic seizures), transient neurological deficits (hemiparesis, aphasia, neglect, hemianopsia, cortical blindness) **Management:** antiepileptic drugs may prevent seizure recurrence (Fernández-Torre and Kaplan 2019)

Table 6.2 Neurological complications of alcohol use (*continued*)

Syndrome	Setting	Features
Cognitive changes (not meeting requirements for mild cognitive impairment or dementia)	Chronic alcohol use	**Affected domains:** general intelligence, memory, executive function, working and short-term memory, inhibition and impulsivity, emotion and psychosocial skills, visuospatial and psychomotor activity **Pathophysiology:** alterations to gray and/or white matter predominantly affecting the frontocerebellar and mesocorticolimbic networks **Management:** thiamine, alcohol cessation (Oscar-Berman et al. 2014)
Mild cognitive impairment and dementia	Chronic alcohol use	**Affected domains:** visuospatial skills, memory, executive function **Pathophysiology:** toxic effects on cortex, cortical-limbic circuits, and white matter **Management:** cessation, thiamine; possible benefit from memantine, rivastigmine, and cognitive rehabilitation (Sachdeva et al. 2016)
Cerebellar degeneration	Chronic alcohol use	**Presentation:** cerebellar signs (ataxic gait > dysmetria, dysdiadochokinesis, nystagmus) **Pathophysiology:** Toxic effects of alcohol and its metabolites, thiamine and other nutritional deficiencies, hepatic dysfunction (Fitzpatrick et al. 2008)
Marchiafava-Bignami disease	Chronic alcohol use	**Presentation:** encephalopathy or unconsciousness, gait ataxia, dysarthria, diplopia, mutism, signs of cerebral disconnection, pyramidal signs, rigidity, primitive reflexes, seizures **Pathophysiology:** progressive demyelination and necrosis of corpus callosum **Management:** thiamine, some evidence for steroids (Hillbom et al. 2014)

Table 6.2 Neurological complications of alcohol use (*continued*)

Syndrome	Setting	Features
Myelopathy	Chronic alcohol use	**Presentation:** paresthesias in lower extremities progressing to spastic paraparesis **Pathophysiology:** toxic effects of alcohol and its metabolites, portosystemic shunting of blood secondary to cirrhosis, nutritional deficiencies of B_{12} and folate (Sage et al. 1984)
Peripheral neuropathy	Chronic alcohol use	**Presentation:** slow progression of paresthesias, pain (dull aching, burning, hyperesthesia, allodynia), numbness and sensory deficits (vibration/proprioception), diminished reflexes, weakness beginning in distal lower extremities **Management:** alcohol cessation, thiamine/other B vitamins (Julian et al. 2019)
Myopathy	Acute alcohol intoxication or chronic use	**Presentation:** acute-onset weakness, pain, swelling with intoxication *or* gradual onset weakness with rare reports of pain in chronic alcohol use **Pathophysiology:** nutritional deficiency, decreased anabolism, increased catabolism **Management:** alcohol cessation (Simon et al. 2017)

EEG = electroencephalogram.

precipitated by cannabis use, and may compulsively take hot showers to alleviate symptoms. Symptoms typically resolve with cessation of cannabis use. The pathology is thought to involve a paradoxical effect of chronic cannabis use on the brainstem and hypothalamic-pituitary-adrenal axis (Perisetti et al. 2020).

Cannabis use has also been associated with reversible cerebral vasoconstriction syndrome (RCVS), which is a neurological emergency because of the associated risk of stroke, seizure, or hemorrhage. RCVS is described further in Table 6.3.

Stimulants

Stimulants are used to increase alertness and focus, and their effects are mediated largely by dopaminergic and noradrenergic systems. Commonly abused stimulants include cocaine, amphetamines, and prescription medications such as methylphenidate. Symptoms of intoxication and withdrawal are listed in Table 6.1.

Stimulants have been associated with ischemic and hemorrhagic stroke, seizures, cognitive impairment, parkinsonism, and psychosis (Lappin and Sara 2019). Chronic stimulant abuse has been associated with deficits in learning, memory, attention, executive function, cognitive flexibility, and screening stimuli for salience. Excess dopamine and serotonin, leading to downregulation of dopamine receptors and decreased dopamine release in the caudate, striatum, and midbrain, are thought to be the mechanisms of the cognitive deficits (Lappin and Sara 2019). Chronic stimulant use can increase existing choreiform dyskinesias or tics and can occasionally result in a syndrome of repetitive compulsive stereotypies known as *punding*. Stimulants (cocaine in particular) have been associated with RCVS and, less frequently, posterior reversible encephalopathy syndrome (PRES). PRES is further described in Table 6.3.

In the case of cocaine, the toxic effects are not from the substance itself but from agents used to "cut" and thus adulterate it. For example, levamisole, an anthelmintic agent, has been linked to neutropenia, agranulocytosis, vasculitis, vasculopathy, and leukoencephalopathy (Brunt et al. 2017).

Opioids

Opioids, widely prescribed for analgesia and widely abused for their calming, euphoric effect (see Table 6.1), are a leading cause of sub-

Table 6.3 Neurological syndromes associated with medication and substance abuse

Syndrome	Precipitants	Features
Reversible cerebral vasoconstriction syndrome	Cannabis, cocaine, LSD, SSRIs/SNRIs, triptans, sympathomimetics, oral contraceptives, vascular dissection, stress, exertion, sex; can also occur spontaneously	**Presentation:** "Thunderclap" headache (neurological emergency, may be reoccurring), focal neurological deficits, seizures **Pathophysiology:** Segmental intracerebral vascular stenosis that resolves within 3 months **Complications:** Stroke, subarachnoid hemorrhage, intracerebral hemorrhage **Treatment:** Verapamil (Burton and Bushnell 2019)
Posterior reversible encephalopathy syndrome	BP >180/140 mmHg, wide fluctuation in BP, renal disease, cocaine, chemotherapy and immunosuppressive agents (tacrolimus, bevacizumab, sunitinib, sorafenib), preeclampsia, eclampsia, sepsis, autoimmune disorders	**Presentation:** Encephalopathy, depressed consciousness, headache, seizures (focal, generalized tonic-clonic, status epilepticus), visual disturbance (blurriness, hemianopsia, cortical blindness), focal neurological deficits, vasogenic edema predominantly affecting the posterior brain regions on MRI **Pathophysiology:** Dysregulated cerebral blood flow, disruption of the blood-brain barrier **Treatment:** BP control, symptomatic management (Fischer and Schmutzhard 2017)

Table 6.3 Neurological syndromes associated with medication and substance abuse (*continued*)

Syndrome	Precipitants	Features
Toxic leukoencephalopathy	Heroin (particularly inhaled), morphine, fentanyl, chemotherapy, immunosuppression, antimicrobials, toluene, alcohol, tobacco, benzodiazepines, cocaine, amphetamines, MDMA, psilocybin, cannabis, arsenic, lead, carbon monoxide, pesticides, radiation	**Presentation:** Three stages over weeks to months: 1) gait and limb ataxia; soft/slurred speech, apathy, akathisia, 2) increased ataxia, spastic paraparesis, choreoathetosis, myoclonus, primitive reflexes; 3) fever, hypotonic paresis, stretching spasms, and akinetic mutism; confluent symmetric T2/FLAIR hyperintensities restricted to white matter; may involve corpus callosum **Treatment:** Some evidence for amantadine and antioxidants (Burke et al. 2021; Filley et al. 2017)

BP = blood pressure; FLAIR = fluid-attenuated inversion recovery; LSD = lysergic acid diethylamide; MDMA = 3,4-methylenedioxymethamphetamine; SNRIs = serotonin-norepinephrine reuptake inhibitors; SSRIs = selective serotonin reuptake inhibitors.

stance-related morbidity and mortality. Nonfatal opioid overdoses are an increasing cause of anoxic brain injury.

Oral, intravenous, and intrathecal use of opioids has been associated with myoclonus and hyperalgesia (Woodward et al. 2017). Opioids, including tramadol, tapentadol, meperidine, methadone, oxycodone, and fentanyl, have been associated with serotonin syndrome (see Chapter 9, "Movement Disorders"). Tramadol can also lower the seizure threshold. Heroin and other opioids have been linked to toxic leukoencephalopathy, sometimes referred to as *chasing the dragon* syndrome because of its association with inhaling heroin smoke. See Table 6.3 for further details on toxic leukoencephalopathy.

Hallucinogens

The term *hallucinogens* refers to a group of psychoactive substances that generally cause transient perceptual disturbances (see Table 6.1). These substances include lysergic acid diethylamide (LSD), phenylcyclohexyl piperidine (PCP), mescaline, psilocybin, 3,4-methylenedioxymethamphetamine (MDMA), ketamine, and *N,N*-dimethyltryptamine. Recently, there has been renewed interest in the use of hallucinogens in the treatment of psychiatric disorders, chronic pain syndromes, and headaches. The neurological sequelae of hallucinogen use are not well described; they include psychosis and hallucinogen persisting perception disorder (HPPD). HPPD, which is not well understood, is a condition in which individuals reexperience perceptual disturbances associated with prior hallucinogen use. HPPD has most frequently been associated with LSD; however, it has been reported with PCP, MDMA, cannabis, synthetic cannabinoids, and risperidone (Martinotti et al. 2018).

Nitrous Oxide

When used for recreational purposes, nitrous oxide may be referred to as whippets, poppers, or laughing gas. Accidental exposure or intentional abuse can lead to B_{12} deficiency and neuropsychiatric symptoms, including myelopathy, myeloneuropathy, and subacute combined degeneration, which are described in greater detail later in this chapter ("Cyanocobalamin"). No practical laboratory tool is available for diagnosis of nitrous oxide abuse or toxicity; as a result, diagnoses are often missed (Garakani et al. 2016).

Toluene

Toluene is a solvent commonly used in paint, spray paint, airplane glue, and cleaning products that is abused by "sniffing from a bag," a practice also known as huffing. It is easily obtained because of the low cost of the products that contain it, and individuals may also be exposed occupationally. Chronic exposure has been linked to a form of toxic leukoencephalopathy associated with dementia, ataxia, cranial nerve abnormalities, and corticospinal abnormalities (Filley et al. 2017).

Kratom

Kratom is a traditional Southeast Asian herbal remedy made from the *Mitragyna speciosa* plant. Although it is illegal in several U.S. states and cities, kratom is unregulated and has been explored for use in opioid dependence because of its activity at the μ opioid receptor. Kratom exposure has been linked to seizures, hallucinations, respiratory depression, delirium, dizziness, vertigo, slurred speech, tremors, and death (Eggleston et al. 2019).

Synthetic Cannabinoids

Synthetic cannabinoids are intended to mimic the effects of cannabis and are commonly sold as Spice or K2. They have been linked to agitated behavior, seizures, and toxic leukoencephalopathy (Breivogel et al. 2020).

Over-the-Counter Medications

Dextromethorphan

Dextromethorphan (DXM) is a readily available over-the-counter antitussive that is commonly abused for its hallucinogenic, euphoric, and dissociative properties. It is also available in novel therapeutics for the treatment of pseudobulbar affect and depression. DXM acts primarily as a noncompetitive *N*-methyl-D-aspartate receptor antagonist. Symptoms of intoxication are dose dependent and range from mild perceptual disturbances, mild motor impairment, and mild cognitive impairment to intense hallucinations and persistent psychosis with agitated and dysregulated behavior (Ritter et al. 2020). In high doses, DXM can also precipitate seizures (Majlesi et al. 2011).

Anticholinergics

Medications with anticholinergic effects are readily available over the counter. The anticholinergic toxidrome is classically taught as "dry as a bone, blind as a bat, red as a beet, hot as a hare, full as a flask, and mad as a hatter," referring to dry skin, blurred vision, skin flushing, hyperthermia, urinary retention, and confusion or agitation, respectively. Neurological signs of anticholinergic toxicity include mydriasis, blurred vision, ataxia, hyperreflexia, tremor, seizures, and worsening of cognitive impairments (Mintzer and Burns 2000).

Vitamins

Thiamine

Thiamine (B_1) is a water-soluble vitamin that is essential in carbohydrate metabolism. Thiamine deficiency is also called beriberi; it includes wet beriberi, which is seen in nutritional deficiency in children in impoverished countries, and dry beriberi, which is seen in adults with thiamine deficiency due to chronic alcoholism, severe chronic systemic illness, or malnutrition. (Smith et al. 2021). Thiamine deficiency can lead to two neuropsychiatric disorders—Wernicke encephalopathy and Korsakoff syndrome—that exist on a continuum. Wernicke encephalopathy can occur after about 4 weeks of regular alcohol use and malnourishment and is classically described as a triad of acute ataxia or gait abnormality, ophthalmoplegia or eye movement abnormality, and confusion. If untreated for an extended period, Wernicke encephalopathy can progress to the more permanent and debilitating Korsakoff syndrome. Korsakoff syndrome is characterized by profound recent and anterograde amnesia and a tendency to confabulate. Although the two syndromes are well known, thiamine deficiency is often missed and can be confused with alcoholic hallucinosis, hepatic encephalopathy, and delirium. Thiamine levels can be suggestive, but there is no clear symptomatic cutoff. Neuroimaging, including brain MRI, is not diagnostic but can be useful in supporting the diagnosis. During the acute stage, the MRI may show T2 hyperintensity in the mammillary bodies, periaqueductal gray matter, and medial thalamus. More chronic findings on MRI include mammillary body atrophy, third ventricle enlargement, and damage to superior cerebellar regions, brainstem structures, and hypothalamus (Chandrakumar et al. 2018).

A high index of suspicion of thiamine deficiency and a low threshold for thiamine repletion are critical prior to or concurrent with the administration of any intravenous fluids containing glucose. Treatment for presumed Wernicke encephalopathy in alcoholics is not entirely agreed upon, but most sources recommend 500 mg of thiamine hydrochloride through intravenous infusion three times daily for 2–3 days, then transitioning to 250 mg/day of thiamine for 3–5 days, followed by oral supplementation of 100 mg/day. Gait and ocular symptoms may improve in a few days; however, delirium can persist for weeks, even with successful treatment (Chandrakumar et al. 2018). Thiamine repletion has no known side effects or toxicity, but failure to administer thiamine early enough or in sufficient dosages can have severe consequences (Smith et al. 2021).

Pyridoxine

Pyridoxine (B_6) is a vitamin that is easily obtained from a regular diet, and deficiency is extremely rare. On the other hand, pyridoxine is readily available in high, potentially toxic doses in energy drinks and nutritional supplements at most grocery stores. Toxicity due to chronic high-dose pyridoxine use can lead to a small fiber neuropathy progressing into a large fiber neuropathy over time. Risk factors for pyridoxine deficiency include chronic alcoholism, renal impairment, dialysis, or transplantation, some autoimmune diseases, and genetic defects. Pyridoxine deficiency due to a genetic disorder does not often lead to neuropathy, but it can be associated with neonatal epilepsy. Pyridoxine deficiency in the setting of neurotoxic medications such as chemotherapy can result in peripheral neuropathy, which responds to supplementation (Hadtstein and Vrolijk 2021). Pyridoxine deficiency in adults is typically associated with other B vitamin deficiencies.

Cyanocobalamin

Cyanocobalamin (B_{12}) deficiency can be caused by a lack of adequate absorption from the gut due to severe nutritional deficiency; intrinsic factor deficiency (which leads to pernicious anemia); severe dietary restrictions (including strict vegan diets); and, occasionally, certain medications, such as H_2 blockers and metformin (Kumar 2014; Shipton and Thachil 2015). Pernicious anemia accounts for a minority of cases compared with the dietary deficiencies found in individuals with chronic alcoholism and among the elderly.

B_{12} is stored in the liver, and years of deficiency may be required to deplete supplies and cause symptoms (Shipton and Thachil 2015). Neurological symptoms include paresthesias, hallucinations, personality changes, mood alteration, ataxia, memory loss, and generalized limb weakness. Physical examination findings can include loss of sensation (vibration, proprioception, pain, temperature), gait disturbance, and altered reflexes (increased or decreased depending on the level of involvement). Subacute combined degeneration refers to B_{12} deficiency–induced demyelination of the dorsal and lateral columns of the spinal cord. Diagnosis is based on examination and laboratory findings: a low (<200 pg/mL) or borderline low (200–300 pg/mL) B_{12} level paired with a high methylmalonic acid (MMA) or homocysteine level (Shipton and Thachil 2015). Subtle neurological symptoms with borderline B_{12} values and a normal complete blood count (CBC) are possible (Lindenbaum et al. 1988), so many authors suggest treatment for B_{12} levels <400 pg/mL. MRI may demonstrate hyperintensities in the posterior and lateral columns of the spinal cord and rarely in the white matter of the brain, which sometimes can be enhanced with contrast (Kumar 2014). Often, abnormal findings on imaging or diagnostic studies as well as physical examination findings linger even after treatment is started (Hemmer et al. 1998).

Patients with absorption issues such as intrinsic factor deficiency may require 1,000 μg cyanocobalamin IM daily for 5–7 days, followed by monthly injections of 500–1000 mcg. Sublingual formulations that can bypass the gut are available, but high-dose oral formulations are often sufficient (Kumar 2014). Treatment is continued until symptoms either resolve or plateau and levels normalize. Although it was thought that high levels of B_{12} were not toxic, some associations with liver disease, potential malignancy, blood disorders, and skin disorders have been noted in patients receiving very-high-dose repletion therapy or those with excessively high B_{12} levels (>950 pg/mL) (Morales-Gutierrez et al. 2020; Shipton and Thachil 2015).

Folate

Folate (B_9) and B_{12} are both involved in DNA synthesis and can cause neuropsychiatric as well as blood disorders, although folate's involvement in neurological disorders remains controversial. There are case reports of pure folate deficiency causing peripheral neuropathy, spinal cord degeneration, dementia, and mood symptoms. All of these conditions are much less common than in B_{12} deficiency, but B_9 should always be checked in concert with B_{12} and a confirmatory test such as MMA level (Reynolds 2014).

Niacin

Niacin (B_3) is obtained via a regular diet and is converted into nicotinic acid, which easily penetrates the blood-brain barrier. Severe dietary deficiency of B_3 or severe nutritional deficiency due to AIDS, anorexia, or other disorders is known as pellagra. In addition to the classic "3Ds" symptoms of diarrhea, dermatitis, and dementia, pellagra can cause atypical psychiatric symptoms such as paranoia, aggression, and suicidality.

Vitamin D

Vitamin D is a steroid hormone that is ingested from animal products or synthesized from sun exposure and requires two steps to become physiologically active (Feige et al. 2020). In addition to calcium homeostasis, cholecalciferol (vitamin D_3) may have a role in preventing or reducing progression in multiple sclerosis (Feige et al. 2020). Vitamin D toxicity is possible at levels above 150 ng/mL (which can occur with supplementation of 100,000 IU/day or more); symptoms are related to hypercalcemia and can mimic the progression of multiple sclerosis in some cases (Feige et al. 2020).

Carbon Monoxide

Carbon monoxide (CO) displaces oxygen in red blood cells and makes it harder for the oxygen that remains to be delivered to tissues (Bleecker 2015). CO poisoning is most common in the winter months because of the use of heaters that emit CO in poorly ventilated areas (Bleecker 2015). Headache is an early symptom, eventually progressing to loss of consciousness with prolonged exposure. Delayed neurological symptoms due to reversible CNS demyelination can arise as long as a month after a lucid and symptom-free period and can include fatigue, cognitive and behavioral changes, occasional parkinsonism, rarely cortical blindness, and white matter changes on MRI (Bleecker 2015). Treatment is 100% oxygen or hyperbaric oxygen in severe cases (Bleecker 2015).

Nontraditional Medications and Herbal Remedies

Interest is increasing in homeopathic and herbal remedies, many of which can have neurological sequelae. Specific inquiry is required because patients seldom volunteer the use of homeopathic remedies. Common agents, their effects, and interactions are listed in Table 6.4.

Metals

Copper and Zinc

Copper deficiency, although unusual, can cause neurological illness and can be caused by malabsorption from bariatric surgery, inflammatory bowel disease, Crohn disease, ulcerative colitis, celiac disease, or prolonged diarrheal illness. Other causes include hyperalimentation without supplementation, anorexia, malnutrition, or hereditary disorders of copper metabolism. The usual symptoms include paresthesias in the feet and legs and sensory ataxia, which mimic B_{12} deficiency (Poujois et al. 2018). Treatment is parenteral repletion, but symptoms may linger long after treatment (Poujois et al. 2018). Because of competition in the absorptive process, zinc toxicity can cause copper deficiency (Joshi et al. 2019); one source of excess zinc is denture creams or pastes.

Excess copper also causes neuropsychiatric illness, such as Wilson disease, which is caused by an autosomal recessive genetic abnormality in the *ATP7B* gene. Characteristic findings include liver and basal ganglia damage due to copper accumulation. Symptoms may include dystonia, tremor, parkinsonism, ataxia, and dysarthria. Kayser-Fleischer rings, brown rings around the cornea, can be detected by slit lamp examination. Personality changes, irritability, depression, and behavioral changes can occur in rare cases of copper toxicity. Chelation therapy and avoidance of foods high in copper are the mainstays of treatment (Lorincz 2010).

Lead

Exposure to high levels of lead causes long-lasting neurological effects, especially for children during brain development. High levels of lead

Table 6.4 Potential toxicities and interactions of commonly used alternative medicines

Supplement	Common uses	Toxicities or interactions
Ashwagandha	Relaxation, anxiety, depression	High doses in ethanol solutions could be toxic (Paul et al. 2021)
Valerian root	Relaxation, anxiety	Hypertension, throat burning, abdominal discomfort; potentiates other GABAergic/sedative medications (Freitas et al. 2021)
Gingko biloba	Proposed neuroprotective, cardioprotective, and anti-cancer properties	Vomiting and diarrhea; generalized convulsive seizures; interactions with aspirin, warfarin, trazodone, omeprazole, antihypertensive agents, and antihyperglycemics; bleeding due to platelet dysfunction (Mei et al. 2017)
St John's Wort (hypericum)	Depression	CYP system medication interactions; may cause serotonin syndrome if combined with SSRIs or SNRIs (Hammerness et al. 2003)
Ginseng	Memory, mood enhancement	Insomnia, nervousness, headache, tachycardia, arrhythmias when used with digoxin or steroids; risk of bleeding when used with anticoagulants (Mancuso and Santangelo 2017)

CYP = cytochrome P450; SSRIs = selective serotonin reuptake inhibitors; SNRIs = serotonin-norephinephrine reuptake inhibitors.

exposure cause cognitive decline, headaches, personality changes, intellectual changes, and, in severe cases, coma and death (Mason et al. 2014). Chronic findings on examination may include weakness (especially distally), tremors, and decreased hearing. Long-term exposure has been correlated with psychiatric syndromes such as schizophrenia, depression, and bipolar disorder (Vorvolakos et al. 2016). Chelation and removal of the exposure (e.g., lead paint or plumbing in older homes) is the treatment of choice.

Arsenic

Ingestion of large amounts of arsenic can result in death. Chronic ingestion of small amounts in drinking water can cause peripheral motor and sensory neuropathy (Mochizuki 2019).

Mercury

Prior to the advent of modern safety measures, exposure to mercury occurred in hat felting and in the production of thermometers or light bulbs. Signs of toxicity are varied but include tremors, neuropathy, confusion, and memory loss. The latter two symptoms may take a longer period of time to resolve with treatment (Calabrese et al. 2018).

Case Example, Continued

The patient's vital signs are within normal limits. She is appropriately dressed but underweight. She is drowsy but fully oriented. Attention is moderately impaired. Her stated mood is "mildly depressed," and her affect is somewhat flat and constricted in range. She denies hallucinations or delusions. Her speech is hypophonic and slow. Cranial nerve examination reveals full visual fields, pupils 3.5 mm and equally reactive, extraocular movements intact without diplopia or nystagmus, and no dysarthria. Motor examination is notable for slightly reduced bulk and pronator drift on the right without abnormal movements. Sensory examination is unremarkable. Reflexes are 3+ and symmetric throughout with bilateral crossed adductors and bilateral plantar flexion. There is right greater than left dysmetria on finger-nose-finger testing and rebound phenomena in all four extremities. Heel-to-shin testing is intact. Gait is unsteady, with a tendency to fall to the right. The patient is started on high-dose thiamine and placed on an alcohol withdrawal protocol.

Toxicology screen is positive for opioids and caffeine but negative for alcohol and other substances of abuse. Comprehensive metabolic panel, CBC, and urinalysis are within normal limits. B_{12} level is 410. CT scan of the head and CT angiogram of the head and neck are unremarkable. Routine electroencephalography shows generalized slowing. Brain MRI without contrast shows diffuse, bilateral, nearly symmetric T2/fluid-attenuated inversion recovery hyperintensities in the subcortical and periventricular white matter, most prominent in the splenium of the corpus callosum, bilateral thalami, posterior limbs of the internal capsules, brainstem, and bilateral cerebellar hemispheres.

Her examination, recent use of inhaled opioids, and MRI abnormalities are most consistent with a diagnosis of toxic leukoencephalopathy. Although these MRI findings may be consistent with PRES in the appropriate clinical setting, the absence of hypertension, stimulant use, or typical precipitating agents would argue against it. The absence of stroke, headaches, and stenotic vessels or occlusions on CT angiography argues against RCVS. There are no ophthalmoplegia, confabulation, or typical MRI findings to suggest Wernicke encephalopathy from thiamine deficiency.

Once a diagnosis of toxic leukoencephalopathy is made, treatment is primarily supportive. Physical and occupational therapy evaluations are ordered, and the patient is assessed for readiness for substance rehabilitation.

Key Clinical Points

- Clinicians should have a low threshold for considering high-dose thiamine (500 mg IV every 8 hours for 3 days) in any patient with altered mental status or encephalopathy.
- Subacute combined degeneration (due to B_{12} deficiency), posterior reversible encephalopathy syndrome (PRES), reversible cerebral vasoconstriction syndrome (RCVS), toxic leukoencephalopathy, and stroke can mimic symptoms of acute and chronic alcohol use.
- Numerous substances, including chemotherapeutics, antimicrobials, drugs of abuse, and environmental toxins, can cause toxic leukoencephalopathy.
- Serum levels of B_{12} in the low normal range can cause neuropsychiatric symptoms and should be supplemented to a target level greater than 400 pg/mL.
- Both deficiency and excess of vitamin B_6 can cause peripheral neuropathy.
- In cases of neurological symptoms with unclear etiology, clinicians should consider potentially toxic exposures and explore substance use, prescription medications, over-the-counter medication use, nutrition, and potential environmental exposures.
- Individuals commonly abuse multiple substances, which may confound the clinical picture.

Review Questions

1. A 50-year-old patient with alcohol use disorder presents with encephalopathy, ataxia, dysarthria, and seizures. MRI of the brain reveals necrosis and demyelination of the corpus callosum. Which of the following diagnoses is most consistent with this presentation?

   A. Wernicke encephalopathy.
   B. Delirium tremens.
   C. Syndrome of subacute encephalopathy with seizures in alcoholic patients.
   D. Marchiafava-Bignami disease.
   E. Dementia from alcohol use.

2. Which of the following is *not* a typical complication of chronic alcohol use?

   A. Cerebellar degeneration.
   B. Myelopathy.
   C. Peripheral neuropathy.
   D. Cognitive impairment.
   E. Posterior reversible encephalopathy syndrome.

3. A patient presents to the emergency department with sudden onset of the "worst headache of my life." Lumbar puncture and head CT do not show hemorrhage. CT angiography of the brain shows alternating stenosis and dilation of vessels, which gives the impression of beads. Use of which of the following is implicated in the diagnosis?

   A. Cocaine.
   B. Zinc.
   C. Pyridoxine.
   D. Nitrous oxide.
   E. Carbon monoxide.

Answers

Question 1: D. Although all choices are possible sequelae of alcohol use disorder, the MRI finding is more specific for the diagnosis of Marchiafava-Bignami disease.

Question 2: E. All choices are possible complications of chronic alcohol use except posterior reversible encephalopathy syndrome, which may be caused by high blood pressure, cocaine, autoimmune disorders, and certain medications.

Question 3: A. The vignette is consistent with reversible cerebral vasoconstriction syndrome. Precipitants of this syndrome include cocaine, cannabis, LSD, selective serotonin reuptake inhibitors, norepinephrine-serotonin reuptake inhibitors, triptans, sympathomimetics, oral contraceptives, vascular dissection, stress, exertion, and sex.

References

Bleecker ML: Carbon monoxide intoxication. Handb Clin Neurol 131:191–203, 2015 26563790

Breivogel CS, Wells JR, Jonas A, et al: Comparison of the neurotoxic and seizure-inducing effects of synthetic and endogenous cannabinoids with Δ9-tetrahydrocannabinol. Cannabis Cannabinoid Res 5(1):32–41, 2020 32322674

Brunt TM, van den Berg J, Pennings E, et al: Adverse effects of levamisole in cocaine users: a review and risk assessment. Arch Toxicol 91(6):2303–2313, 2017 28314885

Brust JCM: Acute withdrawal: diagnosis and treatment. Handb Clin Neurol 125:123–131, 2014 25307572

Burke H, Jiang S, Cohen-Oram A: Heroin-induced toxic leukoencephalopathy from "chasing the dragon" and the proposed synergistic effect of amantadine and antioxidants in its treatment. J Acad Consult Liaison Psychiatry 62(3):353–356, 2021 34102131

Burton TM, Bushnell CD: Reversible cerebral vasoconstriction syndrome. Stroke 50(8):2253–2258, 2019 31272323

Calabrese EJ, Iavicoli I, Calabrese V, et al: Elemental mercury neurotoxicity and clinical recovery of function: a review of findings, and implications for occupational health. Environ Res 163:134–148, 2018 29438899

Chandrakumar A, Bhardwaj A, 't Jong GW: Review of thiamine deficiency disorders: Wernicke encephalopathy and Korsakoff psychosis. J Basic Clin Physiol Pharmacol 30(2):153–162, 2018 30281514

Connor JP, Stjepanović D, Budney AJ, et al: Clinical management of cannabis withdrawal. Addiction 117(7):2075–2095, 2022 34791767

Curran HV, Freeman TP, Mokrysz C, et al: Keep off the grass? Cannabis, cognition and addiction. Nat Rev Neurosci 17(5):293–306, 2016 27052382

Dellazizzo L, Potvin S, Athanassiou M, et al: Violence and cannabis use: a focused review of a forgotten aspect in the era of liberalizing cannabis. Front Psychiatry 11:567887, 2020 33192691

Eggleston W, Stoppacher R, Suen K, et al: Kratom use and toxicities in the United States. Pharmacotherapy 39(7):775–777, 2019 31099038

Feige J, Moser T, Bieler L, et al: Vitamin D supplementation in multiple sclerosis: a critical analysis of potentials and threats. Nutrients 12(3):783, 2020 32188044

Fernández-Torre JL, Kaplan PW: Subacute encephalopathy with seizures in alcoholics syndrome: a subtype of nonconvulsive status epilepticus. Epilepsy Curr 19(2):77–82, 2019 30955427

Filley CM, McConnell BV, Anderson CA: The expanding prominence of toxic leukoencephalopathy. J Neuropsychiatry Clin Neurosci 29(4):308–318, 2017 28506192

Fischer M, Schmutzhard E: Posterior reversible encephalopathy syndrome. J Neurol 264(8):1608–1616, 2017 28054130

Fitzpatrick LE, Jackson M, Crowe SF: The relationship between alcoholic cerebellar degeneration and cognitive and emotional functioning. Neurosci Biobehav Rev 32(3):466–485, 2008 17919727

Freitas C, Khanal S, Landsberg D, et al: An alternative cause of encephalopathy: valerian root overdose. Cureus 13(9):e17759, 2021 34659971

Garakani A, Jaffe RJ, Savla D, et al: Neurologic, psychiatric, and other medical manifestations of nitrous oxide abuse: a systematic review of the case literature. Am J Addict 25(5):358–369, 2016 27037733

Grover S, Ghosh A: Delirium tremens: assessment and management. J Clin Exp Hepatol 8(4):460–470, 2018 30564004

Hadtstein F, Vrolijk M: Vitamin B-6-induced neuropathy: exploring the mechanisms of pyridoxine toxicity. Adv Nutr 12(5):1911–1929, 2021 33912895

Hammerness P, Basch E, Ulbricht C, et al: St John's wort: a systematic review of adverse effects and drug interactions for the consultation psychiatrist. Psychosomatics 44(4):271–282, 2003 12832592

Harvey PD: Smoking cannabis and acquired impairments in cognition: starting early seems like a really bad idea. Am J Psychiatry 176(2):90–91, 2019 30704281

Hemmer B, Glocker FX, Schumacher M, et al: Subacute combined degeneration: clinical, electrophysiological, and magnetic resonance imaging findings. J Neurol Neurosurg Psychiatry 65(6):822–827, 1998 9854956

Hillbom M, Saloheimo P, Fujioka S, et al: Diagnosis and management of Marchiafava-Bignami disease: a review of CT/MRI confirmed cases. J Neurol Neurosurg Psychiatry 85(2):168–173, 2014 23978380

Joshi S, McLarney M, Abramoff B: Copper deficiency related myelopathy 40 years following a jejunoileal bypass. Spinal Cord Ser Cases 5:104, 2019 31871769

Julian T, Glascow N, Syeed R, et al: Alcohol-related peripheral neuropathy: a systematic review and meta-analysis. J Neurol 266(12):2907–2919, 2019 30467601

Kroon E, Kuhns L, Cousijn J: The short-term and long-term effects of cannabis on cognition: recent advances in the field. Curr Opin Psychol 38:49–55, 2021 32823178

Kumar N: Neurologic aspects of cobalamin (B12) deficiency. Handb Clin Neurol 120:915–926, 2014 24365360

Lappin JM, Sara GE: Psychostimulant use and the brain. Addiction 114(11):2065–2077, 2019 31321819

Lindenbaum J, Healton EB, Savage DG, et al: Neuropsychiatric disorders caused by cobalamin deficiency in the absence of anemia or macrocytosis. N Engl J Med 318(26):1720–1728, 1988 3374544

Lorincz MT: Neurologic Wilson's disease. Ann N Y Acad Sci 1184:173–187, 2010 20146697

Majlesi N, Lee DC, Ali SS: Dextromethorphan abuse masquerading as a recurrent seizure disorder. Pediatr Emerg Care 27(3):210–211, 2011 21378523

Mancuso C, Santangelo R: Panax ginseng and Panax quinquefolius: from pharmacology to toxicology. Food Chem Toxicol 107(Pt A):362–372, 2017 28698154

Marconi A, Di Forti M, Lewis CM, et al: Meta-analysis of the association between the level of cannabis use and risk of psychosis. Schizophr Bull 42(5):1262–1269, 2016 26884547

Martinotti G, Santacroce R, Pettorruso M, et al: Hallucinogen persisting perception disorder: etiology, clinical features, and therapeutic perspectives. Brain Sci 8(3):47–65, 2018 29547576

Mason LH, Harp JP, Han DY: Pb neurotoxicity: neuropsychological effects of lead toxicity. BioMed Res Int 2014:840547, 2014 24516855

Mei N, Guo X, Ren Z, et al: Review of Ginkgo biloba-induced toxicity, from experimental studies to human case reports. J Environ Sci Health Part C Environ Carcinog Ecotoxicol Rev 35(1):1–28, 2017 28055331

Mintzer J, Burns A: Anticholinergic side-effects of drugs in elderly people. J R Soc Med 93(9):457–462, 2000 11089480

Mochizuki H: Arsenic neurotoxicity in humans. Int J Mol Sci 20(14):3418, 2019 31336801

Morales-Gutierrez J, Díaz-Cortés S, Montoya-Giraldo MA, et al: Toxicity induced by multiple high doses of vitamin B12 during pernicious anemia treatment: a case report. Clin Toxicol (Phila) 58(2):129–131, 2020 31018715

Narasimha VL, Patley R, Shukla L, et al: Phenomenology and course of alcoholic hallucinosis. J Dual Diagn 15(3):172–176, 2019 31161915

Oscar-Berman M, Valmas MM, Sawyer KS, et al: Profiles of impaired, spared, and recovered neuropsychologic processes in alcoholism. Handb Clin Neurol 125:183–210, 2014 25307576

Paul S, Chakraborty S, Anand U, et al: Withania somnifera (L.) Dunal (Ashwagandha): a comprehensive review on ethnopharmacology, pharmacotherapeutics, biomedicinal and toxicological aspects. Biomed Pharmacother 143:112175, 2021 34649336

Perisetti A, Gajendran M, Dasari CS, et al: Cannabis hyperemesis syndrome: an update on the pathophysiology and management. Ann Gastroenterol 33(6):571–578, 2020 33162734

Poujois A, Djebrani-Oussedik N, Ory-Magne F, et al: Neurological presentations revealing acquired copper deficiency: diagnosis features, aetiologies and evolution in seven patients. Intern Med J 48(5):535–540, 2018 29034989

Reynolds EH: The neurology of folic acid deficiency. Handb Clin Neurol 120:927–943, 2014 24365361

Ritter D, Ouellette L, Sheets JD, et al: "Robo-tripping": Dextromethorphan toxicity and abuse. Am J Emerg Med 38(4):839–841, 2020 31812232

Sachdeva A, Chandra M, Choudhary M, et al: Alcohol-related dementia and neurocognitive impairment: a review study. Int J High Risk Behav Addict 5(3):e27976, 2016 27818965

Sage JI, Van Uitert RL, Lepore FE: Alcoholic myelopathy without substantial liver disease: a syndrome of progressive dorsal and lateral column dysfunction. Arch Neurol 41(9):999–1001, 1984 6477238

Sheikh B, Hirachan T, Gandhi K, et al: Cannabis-induced malignant catatonia: a medical emergency and review of prior case series. Cureus 13(8):e17490, 2021 34548987

Shipton MJ, Thachil J: Vitamin B12 deficiency: A 21st century perspective. Clin Med (Lond) 15(2):145–150, 2015 25824066

Simon L, Jolley SE, Molina PE: Alcoholic myopathy: pathophysiologic mechanisms and clinical implications. Alcohol Res 38(2):207–217, 2017 28988574

Smith TJ, Johnson CR, Koshy R, et al: Thiamine deficiency disorders: a clinical perspective. Ann N Y Acad Sci 1498(1):9–28, 2021 33305487

Vorvolakos T, Arseniou S, Samakouri M: There is no safe threshold for lead exposure: a literature review. Psychiatriki 27(3):204–214, 2016 27837574

Wittemann M, Brielmaier J, Rubly M, et al: Cognition and cortical thickness in heavy cannabis users. Eur Addict Res 27(2):115–122, 2021 33080597

Woodward OB, Naraen S, Naraen A: Opioid-induced myoclonus and hyperalgesia following a short course of low-dose oral morphine. Br J Pain 11(1):32–35, 2017 28386402

7

Neurodevelopmental Disorders

Clay E. Smith, M.D.
Miya R. Asato, M.D.

Case Example

A 28-month-old boy presents with tantrums and difficulty with communication. He was recently placed into foster care because of concerns about neglect and maternal alcohol use. His foster mother notices that he seems anxious and that he wants to run out of the house repeatedly. He has frequent tantrums and struggles with behavior regulation. He enjoys walking around the house putting objects in a play shopping cart. He also likes watching a small repertoire of videos and will get upset if other children in the family want to watch something else. He will not speak other than scream and say "baba" when he wants milk. He eats soft starchy foods and refuses to eat meat or produce. He is starting to make eye contact and demonstrates a social smile.

Behavior concerns can be one of the first presenting symptoms of an underlying neurodevelopmental disorder. Neurodevelopmental disorders are conditions related to differences in brain structure and function with onset during childhood. These conditions are characterized by impairment in motor abilities, cognition, communication, or behavior and may have effects across the lifespan (Mullin et al. 2013). The DSM-5 (American Psychiatric Association 2022) diagnoses of autism spectrum disorder (ASD), intellectual developmental disorder (IDD) (intellectual disability), attention deficit/hyperactivity disorder (ADHD), and specific learning disorder are conceptually based on behavioral and social constructs and are not yet consistently classified as distinct neurobiological conditions. One neurodevelopmental disorder will often co-occur with one or more other disorders. For example, children with ADHD may have specific learning disabilities and a developmental coordination disorder. Early presentations of one type of distinctive behavior may evolve into more discrete diagnoses such as ADHD or anxiety with increasing age. The evaluation of adults with a history of neurodevelopmental disorders is informed by this chapter's discussion of the evaluation of children with these disorders.

Approach to Patients With Neurodevelopmental Disorders

When evaluating a child with atypical development for behavioral difficulties, several historical components should be explored. Initial behavior concerns during the toddler years may raise concern for global developmental delay or autism spectrum disorder based on developmental history, and presentations at older ages may be manifestations of underlying learning disabilities. In children younger than 5, delayed milestones in several areas constitute global developmental delay. If a child is brought into the office by a foster mother, clinicians should inquire about the biological mother's pregnancy, birth, and other postnatal factors such as infant illness. In light of concerns about developmental delay, it is relevant to discern whether the presentation is characterized by regression or lack of expected progression. Such ascertainment may be impossible owing to the social situation and limited knowledge of the caregiver. Asking about developmental progress and achievement in specific domains may help the clinician and caregiver assign a developmental age. Inquiring about the family structure, home, and neighborhood environment provides valuable insights into social determinants of health. Family history relative to physical, psychiatric, and developmental conditions can provide clues into potential hereditary factors. A history of maternal or caregiver depression may affect a child's emotional, language, and social development. Low academic achievement in family members may suggest undiagnosed developmental disorders.

For children who are already in childcare or school settings, feedback from teachers or childcare personnel provides valuable insight into the presenting problem, evolution of symptoms, response to environmental factors, and additional areas of concern not identified by family members. Evaluation and progress report forms from early intervention services are additional sources of professional assessment. Developmental assessments are particularly helpful if new caregivers are unable to provide longitudinal history.

Much of the neurodevelopmental examination can be conducted without the child appreciating that they are being evaluated. Mental status, language (receptive and expressive), affect, and social skills can easily be observed throughout the visit. Cranial nerves and much of the motor examination can be obtained from watching the child move around the examination room. Abnormal neurological findings traditionally correlate with discernible pathology in the nervous system, such as detection of limb weakness due to a contralateral stroke. In contrast, neurological "soft signs" do not have discrete corresponding pathology and may instead be more reflective of an immature nervous system (see Table 7.1). A constellation of multiple soft signs in conjunction with functional difficulties such as trouble manipulating clothing fasteners or mastering handwriting may indicate an underlying developmental coordination disorder, a common occurrence in children with and without other neurodevelopmental disorders. This is often missed in children with scholastic difficulty who struggle with written assignments; it may be misattributed to an attentional disorder.

In the general physical examination, it is important to identify dysmorphic features (see Table 7.2), congenital somatic differences (e.g., extremity deformities or asymmetry), neurocutaneous markings, or hepatosplenomegaly indicating a metabolic storage disorder. In addition to cutaneous findings, neurocutaneous syndromes may include intellectual or learning disabilities and seizures due to the common neuroepithelial origin of involved tissues (see Table 7.3). Growth patterns can reveal metabolic or genetic conditions that feature growth failure or gigantism as a systemic feature. When the clinician identifies possible dysmorphic features in the child, it can be helpful to ask a parent for family pictures to assess whether some of the traits may be hereditary. The discovery of unusual physical features should prompt consideration of evaluation by a geneticist or neurodevelopmental phy-

Table 7.1 Neurological soft signs versus potential signs of CNS disease

	Potential significance	
Neurological finding	**Localizing**	**Nonlocalizing**
Clumsiness—gross and fine motor	Cerebellar disease, cortical motor damage, cortical sensory damage	Developmental coordination disorder
Overflow and mirror movements	Elicited by motor effort, associated with cortical motor damage	Seen in typical development and persistent in NDDs
Inability to move eyes without head movement	Oculomotor or cortical motor weakness	Motor planning difficulties, can be seen in ADHD
Intermittent, gaze-evoked horizontal nystagmus	Cerebellar or brainstem disease	Can be congenital, associated with various CNS disorders, medication related
Hyperreflexia or few beats of clonus	Upper motor neuron damage	Can result from systemic disorders (e.g., thyroid), anxiety

ADHD = attention deficit/hyperactivity disorder; CNS = central nervous system; NDD = neurodevelopmental disorder.

Source. Adapted from Benjamin S. Lauterbach, M.D.: The neurological examination adapted for neuropsychiatry. CNS Spectrums 23(3):219–227, 2018. Copyright © 2018. Used with permission.

sician. Sensory deficits in vision and hearing are important to identify as part of the general examination and are often easily corrected.

Developmental assessment is key to determining whether intellectual or learning disability is suspected. Derivation of the developmental quotient (developmental age divided by chronological age, multiplied by 100) using standardized tools is useful for young children (as a proxy for IQ). As children reach school age, they are more reliably able to undergo formal IQ testing to identify intellectual disability in conjunction with clinical assessment. An informal approach is to ask parents what age they think their child is developmentally

Table 7.2 Key body areas to survey for dysmorphic features on physical examination

Stature	Mouth and lips
Hair growth pattern	Teeth
Ear structure, size, placement	Hand size
Nose size, structure	Fingers and thumbs
Face size, structure	Nails
Philtrum	Feet structure and size

Source. Reprinted from Benjamin S. Lauterbach, M.D.: The neurological examination adapted for neuropsychiatry. CNS Spectrums 23(3):219–227, 2018. Copyright © 2018. Used with permission.

Table 7.3 Dermatologic features in common neurocutaneous syndromes

Neurocutaneous syndrome	Dermatologic features
Neurofibromatosis type 1	Axillary and inguinal freckling, café-au-lait macules (six or more, >5–15 mm), cutaneous neurofibromas, plexiform neurofibromas, Lisch nodules
Tuberous sclerosis (some findings may be acquired)	Hypomelanotic macules (ash-leaf spots), shagreen patches, subungual fibromas, angiofibromas, adenoma sebaceum
Sturge-Weber syndrome	Port wine stain in trigeminal distribution
Ataxia-telangiectasia	Telangiectasias on ears, cheeks, trunk; premature graying of hair; progeric facies; hypopigmented macules; café-au-lait spots

Source. Adapted from Benjamin S. Lauterbach, M.D.: The neurological examination adapted for neuropsychiatry. CNS Spectrums 23(3):219–227, 2018. Copyright © 2018. Used with permission.

and divide that by chronological age to estimate the degree of delay or deviation. Children with a low developmental quotient (70% or less) should be referred for formalized developmental assessment and medical evaluation.

A low developmental quotient is an important clinical red flag to guide referrals, but it is not necessarily an indicator of prognosis, particularly for children in whom the cause and natural history is unknown and for children who have not yet received any intervention. Serial visits with repeated assessments and noting the timing of interventions will help clarify the direction and velocity of developmental progression. Developmental velocity (change in development over time) determines whether development is accelerating, decelerating, or remaining static in terms of milestone attainment and whether this trajectory reflects any known natural history of the underlying etiology. Medical workup and treatments for cognitive delay or limitations may differ depending on whether the process is static, episodic, or progressive in nature. For example, a child presenting with progressive behavioral changes and academic difficulties who is found to have metachromatic leukodystrophy, as diagnosed by MRI and measurement of aryl sulfatase A levels, may be eligible for hematopoietic stem cell transplantation, which could alter the progressive nature of the underlying disease. Although most children with behavioral changes and academic difficulties do not need imaging and biochemical assays, a thorough neurological examination could reveal unreported gait changes and signs of peripheral neuropathy, thus indicating the need for a thorough medical workup.

Autism Spectrum Disorder

Applying a neurodevelopmental approach is increasingly important given the increasing recognition of the complex interplay of neurobiological factors that underlie the spectrum of autism presentations. The diagnostic criteria for ASD, which include difficulties in social communication, reciprocal social interaction, and restrictive and repetitive behaviors, result in children coming to medical attention at relatively young ages.

Advanced genetic testing for ASD and other neurodevelopmental disorders (NDDs) is increasingly a routine part of the medical evaluation and includes microarray and fragile X screening for males (Hyman et al. 2020). Whole-exome sequencing as a first-tier test in children with neurodevelopmental disorders including ASD increases the diagnostic yield of genetic testing (Srivastava et al. 2019). Additional testing such as electroencephalography (EEG), MRI, and metabolic screening is guided by clinical presentation, medical history, and family history. Children with ASD and coexisting intellectual disability and characteristic physical or congenital anomalies are the most likely to benefit from genetic evaluation, which may change medical management or facilitate access to specialized treatments.

Genetic causes of ASD include fragile X, Rett syndrome, tuberous sclerosis complex, neurofibromatosis type 1, Angelman, Klinefelter, and macrocephaly-PTEN syndromes. Children with less recognizable features may also have genetically based ASD related to one of the many hundreds of reported genetic variants (Butler et al. 2015) that appear to affect synaptic plasticity and changes in neuronal connectivity. In sum, however, less than half of all individuals with ASD have clear genetic etiologies (Bourgeron 2015). Rapidly advancing genetic technology sometimes necessitates updated testing using new technologies, and families should be educated about the advantages of pursuing molecular testing. Comprehensive genetic reevaluation may reveal results that affect adult health outcomes. For example, systemic tumors occur in people with ASD and *PTEN* mutations or tuberous sclerosis, and cardiomyopathy occurs in some mitochondrial disorders. Some underlying variants (e.g., *POLG*-associated disorders) are associated with liver failure when exposed to valproic acid, which may be uncovered when a patient is treated with valproic acid for a psychiatric disorder. Genetic testing is also informative for family planning and for siblings who may be asymptomatic carriers. Working closely with medical specialists and genetic counselors to provide pre- and posttesting counseling is now standard of care.

Beyond etiology, children with ASD often have common coexisting neurodevelopmental conditions that affect daily functioning and health. Conditions such as ADHD, intellectual disability, learning disabilities, speech and language disorders, and developmental coordination disorders may share common genetic mechanisms affecting neurodevelopment. The bidirectional relationship between ASD and coexisting NDDs suggests a need to screen and treat detected conditions throughout the lifespan. Team-based evaluations including neurodevelopmental specialists, psychologists, allied health professionals, and education professionals may be helpful in identifying underrecognized conditions and formulating treatment plans. Children with ASD may have co-occurring and sometimes earlier-onset neurological conditions such as epilepsy, encephalopathy, sleep disorders, and movement disorders. Certain co-occurring conditions are recognized to be more common in specific ASD-associated mutations. For example, children with the *SCN2A* variant are prone to epileptic encephalopathy, which includes refractory seizures and cognitive/developmental decline, whereas children with a *SYNGAP1* mutation may have different types of seizures without an associated encephalopathy. Sleep disturbance in a patient with ASD may be due to a variety of causes including nocturnal epilepsy, periodic limb movements of sleep, and anatomical obstruction, as well as other systemic or behavioral causes. Medical evaluation should be offered to patients with sleep disturbance to diagnose and address these disorders in conjunction with behavioral training and judicious pharmacotherapy.

Intellectual Developmental Disorder

IDD is characterized by deficits in both intellectual and adaptive functions, with onset during the developmental period. Both DSM-5 and the American Association on Intellectual and Developmental Disabilities classify the level of intellectual disability based on the intensity of support needed to achieve a person's optimal level of functioning. The score on standardized IQ tests is no longer the guiding criterion for intellectual developmental disorder. Prior diagnostic criteria focused on impairment in general mental ability corresponding to an IQ measurement ≥2 standard deviations below the mean (i.e., ≤70) (American Psychiatric Association 2022), along with impairment in adaptive or daily function. Adaptive functioning can be assessed using standardized instruments such as the Adaptive Behavior Assessment System, which provides conceptual, social, and practical adaptive domain scores and a general composite score. The Vineland Adaptive Behavior Scale and the Diagnostic Adaptive Behavior Scale provide similar subscales and composite scores. About 1.4% of school-aged children in the United States have been diagnosed with IDD (Zablotsky et al. 2017).

Children with milder forms of IDD may not be recognized until school age, when academic skill deficits may become apparent. Genetic causes are identified in more than 50% of cases of IDD. Down syndrome is the most common genetic cause of intellectual disability. X-linked disorders, such as fragile X syndrome, account for 5%–10% of intellectual disability in males. The approach for genetic testing in IDD is similar to that in ASD. Treatable conditions such as lead intoxication, hypothyroidism, and other inborn errors of metabolism should be considered. Important physical examination findings include distinctive facial features seen in fetal alcohol spectrum syndrome and lysosomal storage disorders, liver enlargement seen in glycogen storage disorders, and failure to thrive seen in urea cycle defects. Family history may also be important to note in light of reported maternal pregnancy losses, unexplained childhood deaths, relatives with intellectual disability, advanced parental age, and parental consanguinity. Inquiries around maternal health, prenatal illness, trauma (pre- and postnatal), neonatal illness, and other environmental factors (e.g., lead exposure in the home) are important to assess when gathering the history.

Brain MRI may be indicated based on the severity of the intellectual disability or if the clinical examination yields findings such as ataxia with known anatomical correlates (such as the molar tooth sign in Joubert syndrome). EEG may be considered if there are concerns for active seizures or waxing and waning of mental status or cognitive skills.

Learning Disabilities

Learning disabilities can present in school-aged children with psychiatric concerns related to internalizing or externalizing behaviors, or they may co-occur with a number of psychological or medical conditions. Factors such as cognition, mood, anxiety, exposure, and sleep should always be considered in evaluating a possible learning disability. Learning difficulties may place individuals at risk for psychiatric disorders, and psychiatric disorders are often highly associated with learning disorders.

In 2019–2020, specific learning disability (SLD) was the most common disability category for students receiving special education services under the Individuals with Disabilities Education Act (IDEA). Nearly 2.4 million students were considered to have SLD as their qualifying diagnosis (National Center for Education Statistics 2021). Differences in qualifying criteria have contributed to apparent discrepancies in prevalence data.

SLDs represent a continuum of ability, with no sharp delineation by objective measure between their presence or absence. Variability in assessment measures and diagnosis, a continuum of severity, and comorbidity lead to phenotypic heterogeneity. Diagnosis is based on the synthesis of detailed history, school reports, and psychoeducational assessment. The difficulties in a child's learning and application of academic skills must persist despite targeted intervention. The child's performance should be found to be both significantly and quantifiably below expectations for chronological age and lead to functional impairment. The symptoms should have begun during school age, although they may not be apparent until the schoolwork exceeds the child's ability. Finally, the learning impairment is not better accounted for by intellectual disability, sensory or other neurodevelopmental issues, inadequate instruction, or lack of proficiency in the language of instruction. SLD subtypes include difficulties with word reading, reading comprehension, spelling, writing, numbers, and mathematical reasoning, with some further broken down into more specific impairments (DSM-5). Diagnoses may be made by a school psychologist, clinical psychologist, or physician trained in pediatric development but often rely on data acquired from multiple disciplines.

A child may present because of academic difficulty, problems such as disengagement with schooling or oppositional behavior, or indirect consequences of the SLD. Presentations of SLD vary by age. Young children at risk may be identified by difficulties with phonological awareness or an inability to play rhyming games or identify syllables in words. Later, they may have difficulties manipulating words, for instance, subtracting the "b" from *bat* to create *at*. In kindergarten, children may struggle with letter-sound correspondence or connecting numbers with values. Early elementary children may have difficulties with decoding words and show persistent difficulty in confusing sight words such as *saw* and *was*. Simple addition and subtraction concepts may be difficult. Older children who may have mastered decoding may still have inefficient and effortful reading with issues in comprehension or written expression. Schools will often offer intervention for struggling students before formally assessing children for SLDs.

A child's inability to keep up in class may cause significant distress. The child may avoid reading aloud in the classroom, develop somatic complaints about attending school, or become disruptive or oppositional. An evaluation for SLD should be considered for children who demonstrate academic underachievement. SLDs that are not adequately identified or addressed may be manifested by mood issues similar to an adjustment disorder. Parents may be unaware of the impact or extent of a child's academic struggles, so requesting that parents seek teachers' feedback may elucidate the cause of behavior or somatic symptoms.

The diagnostic criteria for SLDs stipulate that the learning difficulty is not better explained by other neurodevelopmental disorders such as IDD or ADHD. However, these conditions are not always mutually exclusive, as they may co-occur with SLD. A study of nearly 1,000 school-aged children in outpatient or inpatient psychiatry practices found the highest rates of SLDs in bipolar disorder (79%); ADHD, combined subtype (71%); ASD (67%); ADHD, inattentive subtype (66%); and spina bifida (60%). Elevated rates were seen in oppositional-defiant disorder, adjustment disorder, anxiety, and depression, to a lesser degree (18%–19%) (Mayes and Calhoun 2006). Rates of suicidal thoughts or behavior are increased in individuals with poor reading ability or SLD (Daniel et al. 2006; Fuller-Thomson et al. 2018). Student attrition and co-occurring depressive symptoms contribute to poor mental health outcomes, whereas high rates of social/emotional support are associated with better outcomes (Mugnaini et al. 2009).

The syndrome of nonverbal learning disability (NVLD), not included in DSM-5, is most often defined by visuospatial deficits and performance IQ significantly lower than verbal IQ on neuropsychological testing. Other deficits described with NVLD include social/emotional problems, impairment in math abilities, and impaired motor coordination (Fisher et al. 2022). Difficulty in distinguishing purely visuospatial deficits from attention and executive function deficits on formal testing makes it difficult to differentiate NVLD from other established neurodevelopmental disorders such as SLD in mathematics, ASD, and ADHD. However, there is currently no other defined SLD that specifically addresses core visuospatial deficits.

Genomewide association, sibling comparison, volumetric imaging, and functional MRI studies are being used to investigate the genetics and pathophysiology of SLDs. However, SLD research is complicated by differences in diagnostic criteria, severity, and the manner of accounting for other cognitive and environmental variables.

Management of SLDs can seem overwhelming to families, with a multitude of proprietary teaching methods, tutoring programs, or practices available in the community. Effective practices are systematic, sequential, and explicit in their instruction and should be reflected in the child's individualized education program (IEP).

Attention-Deficit/Hyperactivity Disorder

ADHD is characterized by hyperactive/impulsive and/or inattentive symptoms. These symptoms begin in youth and are pervasive, impairing, and excessive for the individual's developmental level. The estimated prevalence of ADHD varies, but based on data from the 2016 National Survey of Children's Health, 6.1 million (9.4%) U.S. children ages 2–17 years had received an ADHD diagnosis. The heritability of ADHD has been estimated as anywhere from 18% to 74% (Faraone and Larsson 2019; Sprich et al. 2000).

In parent-reported data collection, 63.8% of children had a co-occurring condition. Behavioral or conduct problems, anxiety problems, depression, ASD, and Tourette syndrome were the most common (DuPaul et al. 2013). The estimated comorbidity of SLD in ADHD is 31%–45% (Danielson et al. 2018). With such high rates, it can be difficult to discern the causes of behavioral challenges. Diagnosis requires a measured assessment so as not to misattribute symptoms of inattention and hyperactivity-impulsivity to the SLD. Diagnostic overshadowing, in which symptoms may be written off as owing to intellectual developmental disorder, is possible as well. IDD and ADHD are not mutually exclusive, and a clinician must determine whether the behavior is appropriate for an individual's developmental level. Additional referrals such as psychoeducational or neuropsychological assessment may be required.

Biomarkers for ADHD in imaging, neurophysiology, or genetics are an ongoing field of study, but the evidence is insufficient to necessitate their use in clinical settings. Electrophysiological measures in ADHD have been investigated for decades. EEG may be useful in the differential diagnostic workup, but on its own has limited specificity for diagnosing ADHD (Loo and Barkley 2005).

The pillars of treatment in ADHD are behavioral interventions and pharmacotherapy. Comorbidities must be considered in either approach. Behavioral or environmental changes may be informal adjustments to routine or more structured adjustments under the guidance of a professional, as in parent-child interaction therapy. In a preschool-aged child, behavioral interventions are a preferred first step. However, even children in preschool age may require pharmacotherapy if symptoms are refractory to parent training in behavior management or if services are inaccessible. Indicators of severity may include multiple injuries related to hyperactivity-impulsivity or multiple expulsions from daycare programs. Behavioral and environmental modifications should include appropriate accommodations in the public school system.

Key Genetic Conditions Seen in Practice

Several disorders that may be seen in a neurodevelopmentally oriented clinical practice are linked to psychiatric disorders. For example, 22q11 microdeletion disorders are increasingly recognized as a risk factor for childhood-onset schizophrenia (Sporn et al. 2004). In addition, patients with fragile X mutations or premutation states can present with a spectrum of symptoms such as anxiety, ADHD, and autism presenting in early childhood, before intellectual disability is fully appreciated. Given the potential hereditary implications of some of these disorders, searching for the underlying etiology of neuropsychiatric disorders is a priority. Tables 7.4 and 7.5 review common neurogenetic and neurodevelopmental disorders.

Common Approaches for the Management of Neurodevelopmental Disorders

Once a neurodevelopmental diagnosis is provided to a family, the family needs to understand the natural history of the condition and how the condition may affect daily functioning, school experiences, and developmental maturation in more general terms. Given that many conditions may be associated with primary medical disorders, information as to whether the neurodevelopmental condition is primary or secondary may be helpful to put the new diagnosis or subsequent diagnoses into context. Expectations about the role of therapies, specialized education, medical treatments, and the roles of the child and family in management should be outlined and modified with each visit. Outlining the roles of different specialists within the clinical, school, and community settings will clarify how each professional may help the child in different ways to attain goals for optimal functional outcomes, as well as convey to the family the importance of multidisciplinary collaboration.

For school-based interventions, the child's IEP can specify targeted interventions to improve longer-term functional and educational outcomes. For example, children with dyslexia benefit from evidence-based reading interventions, and children with speech apraxia benefit from intensive speech therapy and access to augmentative communication technology. Children with developmental coordination disorder may struggle to navigate homework requiring handwritten responses but are more successful when taught to type assignments or use dictation-to-text technology. Many of these services may be offered in the school setting, although families may need additional outpatient services through their medical insurance to access a full range of expe-

Table 7.4 Selected neurogenetic syndromes

Syndrome	Genetic etiology	Clinical features	Neuropsychiatric features
22q deletion syndromes	22q11.2 deletion	Congenital heart disease, palatal/pharyngeal anomalies, short stature, round ears, hypocalcemia/hypoparathyroidism	Autism, ADHD, anxiety, mood disorders, schizophrenia spectrum disorders, heterogeneous cognitive profile
Angelman syndrome[a]	15q11.2–13 deletion of maternal origin (uniparental disomy, imprinting, deletion)	Microcephaly, prognathism, deep-set eyes, macrostomia, widely spaced teeth, brachycephaly, hypopigmented skin and hair, strabismus, drooling, hand flapping	Epilepsy, ataxia, sleep disorders, hyperactivity, happy demeanor, paroxysms of laughter, intellectual disability
Down syndrome	Trisomy 21	Flat face, epicanthic folds, small ears, macroglossia, short stature, short neck and fingers, hearing and vision deficits, hyperextensible joints, transverse palmar crease, congenital heart disease, obstructive sleep apnea, thyroid dysfunction, autoimmunity	Anxiety and mood disorders; hypotonia; autism spectrum disorder; mild to moderate intellectual disability; Alzheimer disease, typically developing in 40s

Table 7.4 Selected neurogenetic syndromes (*continued*)

Syndrome	Genetic etiology	Clinical features	Neuropsychiatric features
Fragile X syndrome	*FMR1* trinucleotide repeat expansion >200 repeats	Long, narrow face; large ears; high forehead; prognathism; epicanthic folds; dental crowding; macro-orchidism; flat feet; speech and language problems	Mild to moderate intellectual disability, autistic-like behaviors, anxiety, attention difficulties
FXTAS	Premutation range (*FMR1*) 55–200 repeats Males >> females, age ≥50	Intention tremor, ataxia parkinsonian features, autonomic dysfunction, peripheral neuropathy	Dementia, anxiety, mood disorders, frontal-executive dysfunction
HPRT1 disorders (e.g., Lesch-Nyhan syndrome)	*HPRT1* variant X-linked recessive	Hyperuricemia, gouty arthritis, nephrolithiasis	Compulsive self-injury, finger and lip biting; moderate to severe intellectual disability; dystonia
Smith-Magenis syndrome	*RAI1* deletion or variant	Hypotonia, hyporeflexia, coarse facial features, progressive, dental anomalies, failure to thrive, childhood-onset obesity, short stature	Mild to moderate intellectual disability, chronic sleep disturbance, stereotypies, self-hugging, polyembolokoilamania, onychotillomania, self-injurious behaviors, anxiety disorders, ADHD, seizures, peripheral neuropathy

Table 7.4 Selected neurogenetic syndromes (*continued*)

Syndrome	Genetic etiology	Clinical features	Neuropsychiatric features
Prader-Willi syndrome	15q11-q13 (deletion, uniparental disomy, imprinting error)	Failure to thrive, short stature, small hands and feet, hypotonia, underdeveloped genitalia, cryptorchidism, hypothalamic hypogonadism, obesity	Hyperphagia, body-focused repetitive behaviors, anxiety disorders, ADHD, mild to moderate intellectual disability, sleep disorders
Williams syndrome	7q11.23 deletion	Elfin facies; small, widely spaced teeth; aortic root abnormalities; supravalvular aortic stenosis	Superficial sociability, anxiety/phobias, mild to moderate intellectual disability, ADHD, poor visuospatial skills, pragmatic language deficits, often musically talented, learn by memorization, outgoing, extreme interest in other people

ADHD = attention-deficit/hyperactivity disorder; FXTAS = fragile-X-associated tremor/ataxia syndrome.
[a]Williams 2010.

Table 7.5 Common neurodevelopmental diagnoses

Diagnosis	Etiologies	Clinical features	Neuropsychiatric features
Spastic diplegia (CP)[a]	Periventricular leukomalacia	Paraparesis and spasticity of the lower extremities	Epilepsy 10% Intellectual disability 25%–35%
Spastic hemiplegia (CP)[a]	Hemispheric injury (e.g., perinatal stroke)	Unilateral weakness and spasticity	Epilepsy 40% Intellectual disability 25%
Spastic quadriplegia (CP)[a]	Extensive cerebral injury (e.g., anoxia)	Feeding disorders, spasticity and movement disorders	Epilepsy 33%–50% Intellectual disability 85%
Extrapyramidal CP[a]	Associated with low birth weight, anoxia, kernicterus	Choreoathetosis, risk of hearing impairment	Epilepsy 10%–30% Intellectual disability 30%–60%
Mixed CP[1]	Extensive CNS injury	Spastic paraparesis and choreoathetosis	Epilepsy and intellectual disability ~95%
Fetal alcohol spectrum disorders	Exposure to maternal alcohol ingestion	Growth retardation, microcephaly, small palpebral fissures, thin upper lip	Mild to borderline intellectual disability, conduct disorder, oppositional defiant disorder, anxiety/adjustment disorders, depression, substance use
Epilepsy	Trauma, infection, genetics, inflammatory, autoimmune, vascular	Differs by seizure type and etiology	Some epilepsy may be associated with anxiety, mood disorder, ADHD, suicidal ideation, cognitive deficits depending on pathophysiology[b]

ADHD = attention-deficit/hyperactivity disorder; CNS = central nervous system; CP = cerebral palsy.
[a]Kaufman et al. 2023; Reid et al. 2018; Sellier et al. 2012; Ott et al. 2003.
[b]Ott et al. 2003.

rienced specialty services. For families who have challenges meeting their child's learning needs, referrals to parent advocacy groups and health law services may be helpful.

For medically complex children, information sharing and communication can be complicated when the child's team is large and located in different places. Parents may feel overwhelmed with the managerial role that is suddenly thrust on them. Engaging social workers, nurses, insurance case managers, and other community supports can provide guidance and organization as the parent adapts to their child's new diagnosis. Developing a portable record may be helpful for the parent to keep information, test results, and contact information of team members organized. Parents of children with complex needs may need clarification about whom to call for a particular need or emergency. Team-based approaches for educational and community support were reviewed earlier in "Learning Disabilities." Medical homes, a group of professionals who provide care coordination for a given population, are one solution (Kuo et al. 2016).

Addressing parent adaptation over time—by either individual support or support groups—is important, as parents may experience an array of feelings such as frustration for diagnostic delays, guilt, anger, and sorrow. Acknowledging feelings, validating worries, and identifying needs for social support may be a primary focus of medical visits after a diagnosis is made.

The predominant symptoms of NDDs may change over time. Primary features of hyperactivity and impulsivity may be predominant in ADHD at young ages, but as academic demands increase, challenges with sustained attention and executive function may emerge. Anxiety around performance or self-awareness of the disability may compound the clinical picture. Inquiries around functioning in multiple settings (e.g., home, school, community) help focus discussion around targets and approaches for treatment and choice of additional resources. For example, a child with ADHD with average intelligence but subtle learning disabilities may not meet their school's threshold for formal educational evaluation or allocation of learning support services, so referral to a neuropsychologist may be helpful to clarify areas of weakness, identify specific SLDs, and recommend interventions. Children with ADHD may also have language disorders such as social pragmatic communication and auditory processing disorders, which may be missed and left unaddressed. Social impairment in ADHD is common and qualitatively different from that seen in ASD. Individuals with ADHD may have issues with attending to social cues or show deficits in self-regulation that peers find aversive.

At early ages, terms such as "developmental delay" may provide misleading cues to the parent that their child will catch up to peers. School-based evaluation (which is accessible to all students through IDEA) can help distinguish learning disabilities from intellectual disabilities. Assessment of adaptive behavior is also relevant to determine the degree of functional impairment, whether to support the diagnosis of intellectual disabilities or to assess the impact of another neurodevelopmental diagnosis.

Case Example, Continued

ASD and global developmental delay are suspected based on the clinical history. Given the complexity of the case history, the child is referred for neurodevelopmental and neuropsychological evaluation. Physical examination is notable for anxious behavior, hypotonia, a high-arched palate, and hyperflexible joints. Hearing screening is normal. Metabolic screening and referral to a genetic counselor for pretest counseling are completed. Chromosomal microarray is normal, but fragile X southern blot testing shows 250 CGG trinucleotide repeats. Referrals to early intervention and nutrition are made. Parent support resources and education about sleep hygiene are provided. Parents are given training to increase functional communication and use positive behavioral reinforcement. The child's foster family is counseled about the upcoming transition from the early-intervention system of care to a preschool model based in the local school district or through county services. Recommendations are made for follow-up and developmental assessment within 6 months. There is an increased risk of epilepsy in fragile X syndrome, so continued surveillance for seizures is important. Coordination with primary care around continued monitoring of neurodevelopmental status is completed after the visit.

Key Clinical Points

- Detailed history, including early development, informs the diagnostic formulation.
- Speech and language development are important markers for future cognitive abilities.
- Identifying and treating sensory deficits (e.g., hearing, visual) early on is important.

- Neurodiagnostic testing is indicated in cases of focal neurological symptoms or signs, behavioral regression, or suspicion of an underlying genetic condition.
- Genetic testing has become the standard of care in intellectual disability and ASD.
- Early developmental problems increase the risk for future academic or behavioral problems.
- A multidisciplinary therapeutic plan should focus on the context and settings of problem behaviors and provide parent training to foster a supportive environment.

Review Questions

1. In an evaluation for shortness of breath, a 33-year-old woman with epilepsy, autism, and mild intellectual developmental disorder is found to have a cystic lung disease. She has multiple hypomelanotic macules on examination. Which of the following neurocutaneous syndromes is most likely to be present?

   A. Neurofibromatosis type 1
   B. Tuberous sclerosis
   C. Sturge-Weber syndrome
   D. Ataxia-telangiectasia
   E. Epidermal nevus syndrome

2. Which of the following syndromes is associated with the highest risk of childhood-onset schizophrenia?

   A. Angelman syndrome
   B. 22q11 deletion syndrome
   C. Fragile X syndrome
   D. Smith-Magenis syndrome
   E. Williams syndrome

3. Which of the following syndromes is most associated with self-injurious behavior?

   A. Down syndrome
   B. Fragile X syndrome
   C. Smith-Magenis syndrome

D. Angelman syndrome
E. Fetal alcohol syndrome

Answers

Question 1: B. Individuals with tuberous sclerosis complex are often, but not invariably, diagnosed in childhood when presenting with cardiac rhabdomyomas, epilepsy, IDD, or ASD. As adults age with this syndrome, they should be monitored for systemic manifestations, including lymphangioleiomyomatosis, which may present with progressive dyspnea.

Question 2: B. 22q11 deletion syndrome, also known as velocardiofacial or DiGeorge syndrome, may account for up to 6% of childhood-onset schizophrenia. Also, people with 22q11 deletion syndrome have a 25%–30% incidence of schizophrenia.

Question 3: C. Smith-Magenis syndrome is strongly associated with self-injurious behavior. People with this syndrome may be moderately to severely intellectually disabled, compulsively pick at their skin and nails, and compulsively insert foreign objects into their bodies. They often have sleep disturbances and may have seizures, neuropathy, anxiety disorders, or ADHD.

References

American Psychiatric Association: Diagnostic and Statistical Manual of Mental Disorders, 5th Edition, Text Revision. Washington, DC, American Psychiatric Association, 2022

Benjamin S, Lauterbach MD: The neurological examination adapted for neuropsychiatry. CNS Spectr 23(3):219–227, 2018 29789033

Bourgeron T: From the genetic architecture to synaptic plasticity in autism spectrum disorder. Nat Rev Neurosci 16(9):551–563, 2015 26289574

Butler MG, Rafi SK, Manzardo AM: High-resolution chromosome ideogram representation of currently recognized genes for autism spectrum disorders. Int J Mol Sci 16(3):6464–6495, 2015 25803107

Daniel SS, Walsh AK, Goldston DB, et al: Suicidality, school dropout, and reading problems among adolescents. J Learn Disabil 39(6):507–514, 2006 17165618

Danielson ML, Bitsko RH, Ghandour RM, et al: Prevalence of parent-reported ADHD diagnosis and associated treatment among U.S. children and adolescents, 2016. J Clin Child Adolesc Psychol 47(2):199–212, 2018 29363986

DuPaul GJ, Gormley MJ, Laracy SD: Comorbidity of LD and ADHD: implications of DSM-5 for assessment and treatment. J Learn Disabil 46(1):43–51, 2013 23144063

Faraone SV, Larsson H: Genetics of attention deficit hyperactivity disorder. Mol Psychiatry 24(4):562–575, 2019 29892054

Fisher PW, Reyes-Portillo JA, Riddle MA, et al: Systematic review: nonverbal learning disability. J Am Acad Child Adolesc Psychiatry 61(2):159–186, 2022 33892110

Fuller-Thomson E, Carroll SZ, Yang W: Suicide attempts among individuals with specific learning disorders: an underrecognized issue. J Learn Disabil 51(3):283–292, 2018 28635417

Hyman SL, Levy SE, Myers SM; et al: Executive summary: identification, evaluation, and management of children with autism spectrum disorder. Pediatrics 145(1):e20193448, 2020 31843858

Kaufman MD, Geyer HL, Milstein MJ: Kaufman's Clinical Neurology for Psychiatrists, 9th Edition. Philadelphia, PA, Elsevier, 2023

Kuo DZ, Houtrow AJ; Council on Children With Disabilities: Recognition and management of medical complexity. Pediatrics 138(6):1, 2016 27940731

Loo SK, Barkley RA: Clinical utility of EEG in attention deficit hyperactivity disorder. Appl Neuropsychol 12(2):64–76, 2005 16083395

Mayes SD, Calhoun SL: Frequency of reading, math, and writing disabilities in children with clinical disorders. Learn Individ Differ 16(2):145–157, 2006

Mugnaini D, Lassi S, La Malfa G, et al: Internalizing correlates of dyslexia. World J Pediatr 5(4):255–264, 2009 19911139

Mullin AP, Gokhale A, Moreno-De-Luca A, et al: Neurodevelopmental disorders: mechanisms and boundary definitions from genomes, interactomes, and proteomes. Translational Psychiatry 3(12):e329, 2013 24301647

National Center for Education Statistics: Students With Disabilities. Condition of Education. U.S. Department of Education, Institute of Education Sciences, 2021. Available at: nces.ed.gov/programs/coe/indicator/cgg. Accessed May 1, 2022.

Ott D, Siddarth P, Gurbani S, et al: Behavioral disorders in pediatric epilepsy: unmet psychiatric need. Epilepsia 44(4):591–597, 2003 12681010

Reid SM, Meehan EM, Arnup SJ, et al: Intellectual disability in cerebral palsy: a population-based retrospective study. Dev Med Child Neurol 60(7):687–694, 2018 29667705

Sellier E, Uldall P, Calado E, et al: Epilepsy and cerebral palsy: characteristics and trends in children born in 1976-1998. Eur J Paediatr Neurol 16(1):48–55, 2012 22079130

Sporn A, Addington A, Reiss AL, et al: 22q11 deletion syndrome in childhood onset schizophrenia: an update. Mol Psychiatry 9(3):225–226, 2004 14699434

Sprich S, Biederman J, Crawford MH, et al: Adoptive and biological families of children and adolescents with ADHD. J Am Acad Child Adolesc Psychiatry 39(11):1432–1437, 2000 11068899

Srivastava S, Love-Nichols JA, Dies KA, et al: Meta-analysis and multidisciplinary consensus statement: exome sequencing is a first-tier clinical diagnostic test for individuals with neurodevelopmental disorders. Genet Med 21(11):2413–2421, 2019 31182824

Williams CA: The behavioral phenotype of the Angelman syndrome. Am J Med Genet C Semin Med Genet 154C(4):432–437, 2010 20981772

Zablotsky B, Black LI, Blumberg SJ: Estimated prevalence of children with diagnosed developmental disabilities in the United States, 2014–2016. NCHS Data Brief (291):1–8, 2017 29235982

8

Epilepsy

Sonali Sharma, M.D.
Andres M. Kanner, M.D.

Case Example

A 37-year-old woman with a history of mild obesity, hypertension, major depressive disorder, and ADHD, inattentive type, presents to the emergency room after having experienced two focal to bilateral tonic-clonic seizures in the last 2 days. As witnessed, she displayed a sudden arrest of speech and became unresponsive, associated with motionless staring, for a period of 30–45 seconds. This was followed by aversive head deviation to the right, after which she had a generalized tonic contraction of all four extremities followed by generalized clonic activity lasting 2 minutes. The patient was unresponsive for 10–15 minutes afterward and remained confused for another 30 minutes. Her home medications include venlafaxine 150 mg/day and methylphenidate 10 mg twice a day.

Epilepsy is one of the most common brain diseases. According to the International League Against Epilepsy (ILAE), an epileptic seizure is a transient occurrence of signs or symptoms resulting from abnormally excessive synchronous neuronal activity in certain circuits of the brain (Fisher et al. 2005). Epilepsy has been defined as "a disorder of the brain characterized by an enduring predisposition to generate epileptic seizures and by the neurobiological, cognitive, psychological, and social consequences of this condition" (Fisher et al. 2005, p. 476). By definition, a provoked seizure is an acute symptomatic seizure in response to a transient insult to the brain (e.g., acute hemorrhage), whereas an unprovoked seizure occurs spontaneously. A reflex seizure is provoked in that it occurs in response to a particular stimulus (e.g., music) but has a tendency to recur. The practical clinical definition of epilepsy includes any of the following (Fisher et al. 2014):

1. At least 2 unprovoked (or reflex) seizures occurring 24 hours apart.
2. One unprovoked (or reflex) seizure in the presence of one of the following variables that increase the risk of further seizures by at least 60%: (i) occurrence during sleep; (ii) epileptiform discharges identified on electroencephalographic (EEG) recordings; (iii) structural pathology in a neuroimaging study; or (iv) prior brain insult.
3. Diagnosis of an epileptic syndrome.

Epidemiology

Epilepsy affects roughly 70 million people worldwide (Ngugi et al. 2010). There were 126,055 epilepsy-related deaths in 2016 globally (2016 GBD Epilepsy Collaborators 2019).

Approach to Patients With Seizures

Obtaining an accurate history from the patient is paramount to the diagnosis. The history should include seizure semiology (objective signs and symptoms) and frequency, longest seizure-free interval, risk factors (e.g., birth history, developmental history, febrile seizures, head trauma, family history of seizures, prior CNS infections), prior antiseizure medications (ASMs) and side effects, and finally, medical, neurological, and psychiatric histories. Results of a complete neurological examination may be normal or reveal focal/lateralizing signs that point to a structural lesion in the brain. Particular attention should be paid to motor function, language, and verbal/nonverbal recall.

The diagnosis of epilepsy is primarily based on clinical data derived from a careful description of the ictal event by patients and witnesses.

Videos recorded with cell phones have become helpful diagnostic aids. The clinician must address the following basic questions:

1. Is this paroxysmal event an epileptic seizure or a non-epileptic event?
2. If it is an epileptic seizure, what seizure type is it? For example, is it a focal or generalized onset seizure?
3. Given the seizure type, what is the type of epilepsy? For example, is it focal, generalized, or combined epilepsy?
4. Can an epileptic syndrome be identified? (Table 8.1)

The clinical data will dictate the type of auxiliary diagnostic studies, which include different types of EEG, structural and functional neuroimaging, neuropsychological and neuropsychiatric evaluations, and when indicated, genetic studies and evaluations for endocrine, autoimmune, and neurodegenerative disorders. Five to ten percent of people in the general population will have a single seizure in their lifetime (Krumholz et al. 2015). Therefore, the clinician must establish whether this seizure was 1) a provoked seizure, 2) the only unprovoked seizure in the patient's lifetime, or 3) the first seizure of an epileptic disorder.

Neurodiagnostic Studies

Electroencephalography

The goal of the EEG is to confirm the diagnostic hypothesis generated by the clinical information. A diagnosis of epilepsy cannot be made based on EEG data alone. The electrical signal recorded by the EEG is generated by local field potentials from ionic currents flowing in the extracellular space, primarily by the pyramidal neurons in the cortical layers. The electrical activity is recorded with scalp or intracranial electrodes, which transmit it to amplifiers in the EEG recording unit. A synchronous activation of at least 6–10 cm^2 of cortex is required to generate an electrical signal that can be recorded with scalp electrodes, whereas intracranial electrodes can detect electrical activity generated within 1.5 mm^2. Typically, a set of 21 scalp electrodes are used and placed according to predetermined positions (International 10–20 system). However, additional electrodes may be required to better identify the electric field of epileptiform activity. These are known as *double-density electrodes,* which are positioned on the scalp according to the

Table 8.1 Common epilepsy syndromes

Syndrome name	Typical age of presentation	Clinical characteristics
Childhood absence epilepsy (CAE)	2–10 years	Brief impairments of consciousness, unresponsiveness, and interruption of activity lasting less than 10 seconds, occurring several times per day; typically resolves after childhood
Juvenile absence epilepsy (JAE)	9–13 years	Absence seizures and generalized tonic-clonic seizures; requires lifelong treatment
Juvenile myoclonic epilepsy (JME)	Adolescence	Myoclonic seizures that involve one or both upper extremities, head, lower extremities, or the entire body; can result in dropping items from hands and occasional falls; typically occurs early in the morning after awakening; absence and generalized tonic-clonic seizures also occur; requires lifelong treatment
Lennox-Gastaut syndrome (LGS)	Early childhood, typically 3–5 years	Cognitive impairment, multiple generalized and focal seizure types: tonic, atonic, myoclonic, focal seizures, generalized-tonic-clonic, atypical absence; status epilepticus occurs in ≥50% of LGS patients

International 10–10 system. The electrical activity is analyzed and visually displayed in different arrangements known as montages. Bipolar montages compare voltage differences between pairs of electrodes in a chain, and referential montages compare each electrode to a common comparator.

The aim of a routine EEG in seizure evaluations is generally to identify interictal epileptiform discharges. Occasionally, routine EEGs can also record actual epileptic seizures. Routine EEGs for epilepsy evaluation generally last 30–60 minutes and ideally include awake and sleep recordings, particularly during N1 and N2 sleep stages (Hermanet al. 2001).

The absence of epileptiform activity on routine EEG does not rule out a diagnosis of epilepsy. The initial EEG recordings of approximately 50% of patients with known epilepsy may not reveal epileptiform activity (Baldin et al. 2014). However, a second 90–180-minute sleep-deprived EEG will show epileptiform activity in 70% of people with epilepsy (PWE). If the second EEG is negative, a 24–48-hour EEG has a 90%–95% probability of capturing interictal epileptiform activity in PWE.

Prolonged EEG monitoring can be done in an ambulatory (at home) or in-hospital laboratory setting. The former typically lasts 12–72 hours and may or may not have concurrent video recording. Inpatient video-EEG monitoring is best to differentiate epileptic from non-epileptic paroxysmal events. The advantages of an outpatient video-EEG include lower cost and the ability to record in the patient's environment. The disadvantages include more artifacts that may make EEG recordings unreadable and that distinguishing epileptic from non-epileptic events is more difficult without a video accompanying the EEG.

The presence of epileptiform discharges on EEG does not establish a diagnosis of epilepsy. Epileptiform activity may be identified in up to 2% of the general population who have never had an epileptic seizure (Sam and So 2001). This may include people with migraines, first-degree relatives of people with idiopathic generalized epilepsy, and people with autism spectrum disorder. Clinical correlation is paramount for the diagnosis of epilepsy, and ASM therapy should not be started solely based on an abnormal EEG.

Neuroimaging

CT with and without contrast may be useful to rule out large structural abnormalities or emergent etiologies, but CT can miss a variety of pathologies in up to 30% of cases (Bronen et al. 1996). High-resolution brain MRI is recommended for all PWE except for those with certain idiopathic generalized epilepsy syndromes such as childhood absence epilepsy or juvenile myoclonic epilepsy. Ideally, a 3T MRI with thin (1-mm) continuous slices through the regions of interest should be considered in patients with treatment-resistant epilepsy.

CT angiography, MR angiography, or arteriography may be required to investigate vascular malformations associated with seizures. Functional MRI to identify eloquent cortex and positron emission tomography (PET) or single-photon emission computed tomography (SPECT) studies to assist in localizing the epileptogenic zone are part of presurgical evaluations for treatment-resistant focal epilepsy.

Neuropsychological/Psychiatric Evaluation

Cognitive and psychiatric comorbidities are common among PWE and often precede or follow the onset of seizures. Neuropsychological testing should be considered in the initial phases of the epilepsy evaluation, particularly in children and adolescents in whom cognitive disorders can negatively impact their academic performance. Neuropsychological testing is typically included as part of the evaluation for epilepsy surgery, both to determine evidence of lateralized cognitive dysfunction and to establish a cognitive baseline. Furthermore, investigation of current or past cognitive comorbidities plays an important role in the selection of ASMs (Scott et al. 2017).

Classification of Seizures and Epilepsy

The ILAE revised its classification of seizure types, epilepsy types, and epilepsy syndromes in 2017 (Fisher et al. 2017). The classification system divides seizures into three types: 1) focal, 2) generalized, and 3) unknown. Focal seizures are classified as 1) focal seizures with awareness, previously referred to as simple partial seizures; 2) focal seizures with impaired awareness, previously referred to as complex partial seizures; and 3) focal to bilateral tonic-clonic seizures, previously referred to as secondarily generalized tonic-clonic seizures (GTCs). Table 8.2

Table 8.2 Major seizure types

Type	Motor	Nonmotor
Generalized onset	Tonic-clonic, clonic, tonic, myoclonic, myoclonic-tonic-clonic, myoclonic-atonic, atonic, epileptic spasms	Absence: typical, atypical, myoclonic, eyelid myoclonia
Focal onset	Automatisms, atonic, clonic, epileptic spasms, hyperkinetic, myoclonic, tonic	Autonomic, behavior arrest, cognitive, emotional, sensory
Unknown onset	Tonic-clonic, epileptic spasms, unclassified seizures	Behavior arrest

delineates major seizure types (Fisher et al. 2017). Finally, the identification of epilepsy syndromes incorporates the seizure types, EEG data, imaging, and genetics.

After classifying the seizures and epilepsy syndrome, seizure etiology is considered, including structural, genetic, infectious, metabolic, autoimmune, or unknown causes. Provoked seizures are triggered by potentially reversible pathologic processes, such as metabolic (e.g., hyponatremia, hypernatremia, hypocalcemia, hypoglycemia, hyperglycemia), medical (e.g., eclampsia), toxic (e.g., medication adverse effect), or substance-related (e.g., alcohol withdrawal, cocaine, phencyclidine) processes (Moosavi and Swisher 2020). Provoked seizures may require short-term or no treatment with ASMs, depending on the severity, duration, and underlying pathologic process. The risk of recurrence in provoked seizures is lower than in a first unprovoked seizure.

Psychiatric Comorbidity

Although seizures are the primary clinical manifestation of epilepsy, comorbid neurologic, psychiatric, and cognitive dysfunctions are relatively common clinical expressions of the disease, and their early identification and treatment are paramount in PWE. The existence of these comorbidities needs to be investigated at the first visit, as they can have a significant impact on the course of the seizure disorder, selection of the ASMs, and response to treatment. In fact, one of every three PWE will experience a comorbid psychiatric disorder during their life (Tellez-Zenteno et al. 2007). Depression, anxiety, and attention-deficit disorders are the most common psychiatric comorbidities, followed by psychotic disorders. For example, in a systematic review and meta-analysis of 10,527 PWE (≥18 years of age), the prevalence of depression was 32%; in a separate meta-analysis of 3,221 PWE (≥16 years of age), the overall pooled prevalence rates of depressive and anxiety disorders were 22.9% and 20.2%, respectively, and those of suicidality were 7%–9% (Lu et al. 2021). ADHD has been reported in 25%–30% of children with epilepsy; the actual prevalence in adults is yet to be established, as it is often unrecognized (Besag et al. 2016). Psychotic disorders have been reported in up to 9% of PWE (Kanner and Rivas-Grajales 2016).

The relation between these psychiatric disorders and epilepsy is bidirectional, as demonstrated in several population-based studies (Hesdorffer et al. 2012). For example, patients with primary mood and anxiety disorders have a 2- to 3-fold increased risk; children with

ADHD, inattentive type, have a 3.5-fold increased risk; and patients with primary psychotic disorders have a 7-fold risk of developing epilepsy (Kanner and Rivas-Grajales 2016).

In PWE, the type of psychiatric symptoms must be interpreted according to their temporal relation to seizure occurrence to help determine if the psychiatric symptoms are an expression of the seizure disorder, iatrogenic effects of seizure treatment, or unrelated. Events that are independent of seizure occurrence are considered *interictal,* and those that are temporally related to seizures are *peri-ictal* events. The peri-ictal period is further subdivided into *pre-ictal* (preceding the seizure by 1–3 days), *ictal* (an expression of the seizure activity), and *postictal* (after the seizure). Postictal events may include confusion, agitation, or psychosis and can occur in the immediate postictal period (lasting minutes to hours); they can also take place several hours to 7 days after a cluster of seizures and can last from several hours to 3 days or longer (Kanner et al. 2004). Iatrogenic psychiatric symptoms can be caused by epilepsy surgery or changes in ASMs (Kanner 2016). Most of the recognized psychiatric disorders are interictal; whereas peri-ictal and postictal episodes are often mistaken for interictal disorders, leading to unnecessary treatments.

Imitators of Epileptic Seizures

Twenty to twenty-five percent of patients referred for diagnosis of treatment-resistant epilepsy do not suffer from epilepsy. Imitators of epileptic seizures can be the expression of various neurologic events (e.g., migraines, transient ischemic attacks, movement disorders), psychiatric symptoms (e.g., psychogenic non-epileptic events, panic attacks), and other medical disorders (e.g., syncope, endocrinopathies) (Xu et al. 2016).

Psychogenic non-epileptic seizures (PNES), or functional neurological disorder (FND) with seizures and/or attacks, is one of the most frequent imitators of epileptic seizures. PNES are episodes that may involve altered subjective consciousness or motor phenomena and over which patients have no conscious control. They are not caused by abnormal synchronized electrical activity of the brain but are the expression of a variety of neuropsychiatric disorders (LaFrance et al. 2013).

The proposed diagnostic levels of certainty for PNES include possible, probable, and clinically established. The gold standard includes documented history, captured event by video-EEG monitoring, and absence of epileptiform activity during the event. PNES can be the expression of mood, anxiety, or personality disorders; history of traumatic experiences and PTSD; family conflict; or accumulated life stress. In up to 20% of patients, however, no psychogenic cause can be identified at the time of the evaluation (Hingray et al. 2018). The treatment must be tailored to the individual's psychiatric and social profile and often requires multidisciplinary interventions by psychiatrists, psychologists, social workers, and neurologists (Reiter et al. 2015). It is essential to present the diagnosis in a very clear manner, ensuring that the patient and family members have understood and accepted it and working closely with the mental health team to ensure prompt treatment of the psychiatric comorbidities. See Chapter 10 ("Functional Neurological Disorder") for a detailed discussion of FND.

Pathogenic Mechanisms of Epilepsy

The pathophysiology of human epilepsy is complex and incompletely understood. Epileptic activity is thought to be the result of an imbalance between synaptic excitatory and inhibitory activity of neurotransmitters such as glutamate and γ-aminobutyric acid (GABA), respectively. However, other neurotransmitters (such as serotonin, norepinephrine, and dopamine), neuronal abnormalities (such as gap junctions, SV2A synaptic protein vesicles, G protein–coupled receptors, and ionotropic glutamate receptors), and neuronal inflammatory and oncological processes play an important role in the pathophysiology of human epilepsy (Engelborghs et al. 2000). Finally, genetic factors are important, particularly in generalized epilepsy and epilepsy syndromes (Sheidley et al. 2022). Whereas generalized epilepsy disorders are more likely caused by a genetic anomaly, focal epilepsy typically occurs due to an acquired lesion such as ischemic or hemorrhagic stroke, neoplasms, arteriovenous malformations, infections, developmental cortical malformations, CNS trauma, and CNS autoimmune disorders. Kindling is an experimental model of focal epilepsy that has been widely investigated, a process by which repeated subthreshold electrical stimulation of specific neuroanatomical structures leads to developing electrographic seizures that evolve into electroclinical seizures that worsen over time.

The existence of common pathogenic mechanisms operating in psychiatric disorders and epilepsy may explain the bidirectional relationship between the conditions. For example, common pathogenic mechanisms in depression and epilepsy include the following (Kanner et al. 2014):

1. Neurotransmitter disturbances including low GABAergic, low serotonergic, and low noradrenergic activity and high glutamatergic neurotransmission in neuronal circuits.
2. Hyperactive hypothalamic-pituitary-adrenal axis resulting in high levels of cortisol, which in turn causes an increase in glutamatergic and a decrease in serotonergic activity, as well as a decrease in glial and neuronal density in frontal and temporal structures.
3. Inflammatory mechanisms resulting in high secretion of cytokines (e.g., interleukin-β).

Identifying psychiatric disorders is crucial because PWE with mood and anxiety disorders have a twofold higher risk of developing treatment-resistant epilepsy and experiencing psychiatric adverse events when exposed to certain ASMs such as barbiturates, levetiracetam, topiramate, zonisamide, perampanel, and vigabatrin. Conversely, discontinuing ASMs with mood-stabilizing properties (e.g., valproic acid, carbamazepine, oxcarbazepine, and lamotrigine), antidepressant properties (e.g., lamotrigine), or anxiolytic properties (e.g., benzodiazepines, valproic acid, gabapentin, and pregabalin) can result in recurrence of mood or anxiety disorders that were successfully treated by these ASMs (Ribot et al. 2017). Furthermore, patients with mood and anxiety disorders are less likely to tolerate ASMs and more likely to complain of a variety of medication-related neurological and medical adverse events (Kanner et al. 2012). Finally, PWE are two- to threefold more likely to die by suicide than the general population, with the risk increasing by 32-fold in the presence of a concurrent mood disorder and by 12-fold in the presence of a concomitant anxiety and psychotic disorder (Christensen et al. 2007).

The bidirectional relationship between psychiatric disorders and epilepsy plays a role in managing the psychiatric comorbidities. There is evidence that patients started on antidepressants versus placebo will have a lower incidence of epileptic seizures, suggesting a protective role of selective serotonin reuptake inhibitors (SSRIs), serotonin-norepinephrine reuptake inhibitors (SNRIs), and tricyclic antidepressants.

Treatment of Epilepsy

Pharmacology

ASMs are commonly grouped into first-, second-, and third-generation medications. A comprehensive treatment plan requires pharmacotherapy that targets not only the seizure type, epilepsy, or epileptic syndrome but also the medical, neurological, cognitive, and psychiatric comorbidities (Table 8.3). Seizure freedom may be expected in 60%–90% of patients with idiopathic generalized epilepsy and 30%–50% of those with focal epilepsy (Semah et al. 1998). Conversely, patients with symptomatic generalized epilepsy, such as Lennox-Gastaut syndrome (LGS), are unlikely to become seizure-free.

A first spontaneous seizure can be the expression of a seizure disorder with a recurrence rate of 36%–51% within 2 years, particularly in the presence of 1) epileptiform activity on EEG; 2) structural lesions on brain MRI or CT; 3) occurrence in sleep; or 4) family history of epilepsy. This risk increases with a remote (≥7 days) symptomatic seizure and two or more seizures (Marson et al. 2005). The American Academy of Neurology (AAN) and the American Epilepsy Society (AES) published guidelines for the treatment of a first unprovoked seizure and recommended starting pharmacotherapy under the conditions listed above. Treatment after the first seizure decreases the recurrence rate by 30%–60%.

Several population-based studies indicate that 60%–70% will achieve seizure remission with ASMs, but this will depend on the type of epilepsy and epilepsy syndrome (Kwan and Brodie 2001). Nearly 50% of patients with newly diagnosed epilepsy will respond to the first ASM, with an additional 10% achieving seizure freedom with two ASMs.

The ILAE, AAN, and AES have published several guidelines on the use of these ASMs. There is a consensus that antiepileptic efficacy is comparable among the appropriate medications for a given type of epilepsy, but that tolerability differs (Glauser et al. 2006). The choice of ASM depends on 1) type of seizure, epilepsy, and epileptic syndrome; 2) pharmacokinetic properties; 3) pharmacodynamic properties; 4) age; 5) sex; 6) reproductive status and family planning (e.g., birth control, teratogenicity, breastfeeding); 7) potential therapeutic or iatrogenic effects of comorbid medical, neurologic, and psychiatric disorders; and 8) cost.

Table 8.3 Characteristics of commonly used antiseizure medications

ASM	Seizure type/indication	Mechanism of action	Positive effects	Negative effects	Teratogenic effects
First-generation antiseizure medications					
Carbamazepine	Focal, tonic-clonic	Sodium channel blockade	Mood stabilizer, neuropathic pain	Hyponatremia; CYP inducer	Intermediate risk: spina bifida
Clonazepam	Focal, tonic-clonic, myoclonic, LGS	Enhanced GABA activity	Anxiolytic	—	Unknown
Ethosuximide	Absence	Decreased (T type) calcium channel activity	—	—	Unknown
Phenobarbital	Focal, tonic-clonic, absence, perhaps LGS	Increases GABA activity	—	Cognition, CYP inducer	High risk: cardiac malformations, cognitive dysfunction
Phenytoin	Focal, tonic-clonic	Sodium channel blockade	—	Cognition, CYP inducer	Intermediate risk: orofacial clefts, cardiac and genitourinary defects
Primidone	Focal, tonic-clonic	Increases GABA activity	—	Cognition, CYP inducer	Unknown

Table 8.3 Characteristics of commonly used antiseizure medications (*continued*)

ASM	Seizure type/ indication	Mechanism of action	Positive effects	Negative effects	Teratogenic effects
Sodium valproate	Focal, tonic-clonic, absence, myoclonic, LGS	Increases GABA activity; sodium channel blockade	Mood stabilizer, anxiolytic, headache	CYP inhibitor; increases level of lamotrigine; liver toxicity, platelet dysfunction, weight gain	Very high risk: major malformations, reduced verbal IQ, autism
Second-generation antiseizure medications					
Felbamate	Focal, tonic-clonic, LGS	NMDA receptor antagonist, sodium channel blockade	—	Depression, CYP inducer	Unknown
Gabapentin	Focal, tonic-clonic	Unknown, likely increases GABA transmission	Anxiolytic, headache, neuropathic pain	Cognition (in older patients)	Low risk
Lamotrigine	Focal, tonic-clonic, absence, myoclonic, LGS	Sodium channel blockade	Mood stabilizer, antidepressant	Levels decrease with oral contraceptives; levels increase with valproic acid	Low risk

Table 8.3 Characteristics of commonly used antiseizure medications (*continued*)

ASM	Seizure type/ indication	Mechanism of action	Positive effects	Negative effects	Teratogenic effects
Levetiracetam	Focal, tonic-clonic, myoclonic, absence, perhaps LGS	Synaptic vesicle protein (SV2A)	—	Depression, irritability, behavioral disturbance	Low risk
Oxcarbazepine	Focal, tonic-clonic	Unknown, presumed blockade of voltage-sensitive sodium channels	Mood stabilizer, neuropathic pain	Hepatic CYP inducer (>900–1,200 mg)	Low risk
Tiagabine	Focal, tonic-clonic, perhaps myoclonic, LGS	Blocks GABA uptake to presynaptic neurons	—	Depression, cognition, risk of absence status	Unknown
Topiramate	Focal, tonic-clonic, myoclonic, LGS	Sodium channel blockade, increased GABA activity, AMPA/glutamate antagonism, carbonic anhydrase inhibitor	Headache pain	Depression, anxiety, cognition, CYP inducer (>200 mg), decreases oral contraceptive levels	Intermediate risk: cleft lip
Zonisamide	Focal, tonic-clonic, perhaps absence/ myoclonic, LGS	Sodium channel blockade, carbonic anhydrase inhibitor	—	Depression, cognition	Low risk

Table 8.3 Characteristics of commonly used antiseizure medications (*continued*)

ASM	Seizure type/ indication	Mechanism of action	Positive effects	Negative effects	Teratogenic effects
Third-generation antiseizure medications					
Brivaracetam	Focal, generalized tonic-clonic	Synaptic vesicle protein SV2A, 20-fold higher affinity than levetiracetam	—	—	Unknown
Cannabidiol	Focal, LGS	Allosteric modulation of $GABA_A$ receptor	—	—	Unknown
Cenobamate	Focal	Unknown, allosteric modulator of $GABA_A$ receptor, inhibits voltage-gated sodium channels	—	—	Unknown
Clobazam	Focal, tonic-clonic, myoclonic, LGS	Enhanced GABA activity	—	—	Unknown
Eslicarbazepine	Focal	Sodium channel blockade	Mood stabilizer	—	Unknown
Lacosamide	Focal	Sodium channel slow inactivation	—	—	Unknown

Table 8.3 Characteristics of commonly used antiseizure medications (*continued*)

ASM	Seizure type/ indication	Mechanism of action	Positive effects	Negative effects	Teratogenic effects
Perampanel	Focal, generalized tonic-clonic, myoclonic	Noncompetitive AMPA glutamate receptor antagonist	—	Aggression, psychosis, depression	Unknown
Pregabalin	Focal, tonic-clonic, perhaps absence, myoclonic, LGS	GABA analog, binds to calcium channel	Anxiolytic, headache, neuropathic pain	—	Unknown
Rufinamide	Focal, tonic-clonic, LGS, perhaps absence and myoclonic	Unknown, may prolong inactive state of sodium channel	—	—	Unknown
Vigabatrin	Infantile spasms	Unknown, thought to irreversibly inhibit GABA transaminase	—	Irritability, depression	Unknown

AMPA = α-amino-3-hydroxy-5-methyl-4-isoxazolepropionic acid; ASM = antiseizure medication; CYP = hepatic cytochrome P450; GABA = γ-aminobutyric acid; LGS = Lennox-Gastaut syndrome; NMDA = *N*-methyl-ᴅ-aspartate.

The following principles should be applied when selecting an ASM:

1. Initiate oral monotherapy with a stepwise titration targeting moderate doses. Faster titration may be required in hospitalized patients who experience seizure clusters or frequent GTCs. Further dose adjustments can be carried out with persistent seizures until seizure freedom is achieved or adverse events develop.
2. An ASM trial is considered a failure if the patient exhibits undesirable side effects or seizures continue at optimal doses. In a case of toxicity, a rechallenge at a lower dose or an ASM with different pharmacodynamic properties should be considered. In a case of treatment inefficacy, however, a medication with a different mechanism of action is indicated.
3. The plasma concentration of a first-generation ASM is helpful in assessing possible causes of failure to achieve seizure freedom, explaining adverse events, monitoring treatment compliance, and adjusting dosage. However, serum concentration should not be the only criterion for adjusting ASM, especially if the patient is seizure free and without adverse events. There is no advantage to obtaining plasma concentrations for second- and third-generation ASMs, except in the case of pregnancy and co-occurring morbidities (e.g., renal and hepatic failure) that would necessitate dose adjustments.
4. Parenteral ASMs should be considered in cases of GTCs lasting >5 minutes or focal unaware seizures lasting >10 minutes, seizures occurring in clusters, and frequent focal unaware seizures or GTCs over the previous 2 weeks.

Information on teratogenic potential is more readily available for first- and second-generation ASMs than for third-generation ASMs. Lamotrigine and levetiracetam are first-line treatments and safest for pregnant PWE. The next safest drugs include oxcarbazepine and zonisamide (Hernández-Díaz et al. 2012; Tomson et al. 2011). Valproic acid has one of the highest risks for major congenital malformations, including CNS, cardiac, urologic, and facial malformations, as well as developmental cognitive deficits, with an increased risk for autism spectrum disorder. Topiramate is associated with an increased risk of cleft lip and palate; phenytoin and phenobarbital are associated with increased cardiac malformations (Harden et al. 2009). Folate supplementation (1–4 mg/day) is recommended for all women with epilepsy during their childbearing years and especially during pregnancy.

Breastfeeding should be encouraged in women with epilepsy. Phenytoin, phenobarbital, carbamazepine, and valproic acid are not secreted in breast milk in clinically significant amounts. Levetiracetam and gabapentin are transported into breast milk but are eliminated by the infant without any clinical impact. Importantly, continuous breastfeeding during the first 6 months is associated with improved outcomes in all developmental domains regardless of maternal ASM regimen (Pennell 2016).

Treatment-Resistant Epilepsy

Treatment-resistant epilepsy is defined as failure to achieve seizure freedom after two trials of the appropriate ASM at optimal doses (in mono- or polytherapy). Seizure freedom is regarded as the absence of seizures for a period of either three times the prior interseizure interval or 1 year, whichever is longer (Kwan et al. 2010). Despite the development of new ASMs, the rate of treatment-resistant epilepsy has not changed: one-third of people have treatment-resistant epilepsy.

Once a patient is determined to have treatment-resistant epilepsy, they should be referred to a comprehensive epilepsy center for further evaluation to determine whether seizure freedom can be achieved with epilepsy surgery. The AAN, AES, and American Association of Neurological Surgeons have developed formal practice guidelines for epilepsy surgery, but less than 1% of patients with treatment-resistant epilepsy are referred to a comprehensive epilepsy center. The patient also may be a candidate for palliative therapy with neuromodulation or a special diet that can significantly decrease seizure frequency and improve quality of life.

Therapy may be either curative in lesional (abnormal MRI) epilepsy or palliative in nonlesional (normal MRI) epilepsy. Among the curative therapies, resection or laser ablation of the abnormal tissue achieves the greatest seizure freedom (Engel et al. 2012; Gross et al. 2018). Palliative therapies include corpus callosotomy, vagus nerve stimulation, responsive neurostimulation (RNS), and deep brain stimulation (Bergey et al. 2015; Ryvlin et al. 2014; Salanova et al. 2015).

Treatment in PWE With Psychiatric Disorders

Impact of Psychotropics on Seizure Threshold

The majority of psychotropic medications do not cause seizures when used at therapeutic doses. The exceptions include clomipramine, bupropion (in its immediate release formulation at doses >300 mg/day), clozapine, olanzapine, and chlorpromazine at doses >1,000 mg/day.

Pharmacokinetic Interaction Between Psychotropics and Antiseizure Medications

Several first-generation ASMs have enzyme-inducing properties (phenytoin, carbamazepine, barbiturates, topiramate at doses >200 mg/day and oxcarbazepine at doses >900–1,200 mg/day) that can increase the metabolism of psychotropic drugs metabolized in the liver by cytochrome P450 (CYP) isoenzymes and metabolic pathways (e.g., hydroxylation, glucuronidation), thus limiting their efficacy. Conversely, several SSRIs (e.g., fluoxetine, fluvoxamine) can inhibit the metabolism of several ASMs, which are metabolized by common CYP isoenzymes, potentially resulting in iatrogenic adverse events. In these cases, the doses of the ASM or psychotropic drug may need to be adjusted.

Pharmacodynamic Interactions Between Psychotropic Drugs and Antiseizure Medications

Psychotropic and antiseizure medication interactions can result in iatrogenic effects when both types of drugs have similar adverse events. For example, SSRIs and some ASMs such as carbamazepine, oxcarbazepine, and eslicarbazepine can cause hyponatremia, which can be precipitated by their concomitant use.

Case Example, Continued

The patient returns to baseline and has a normal neurological exam. An EEG reveals interictal epileptiform activity in the left temporal region, and brain MRI demonstrates a cavernous malformation in the left lateral temporal region. A diagnosis of focal epilepsy of temporal lobe origin secondary to a cavernous malformation is made. The presence of a structural abnormality on the brain MRI and epileptiform activity on the EEG indicates that she has a 60%–80% risk of recurrent seizures. Thus, an ASM is indicated. The selection of the ASM needs to factor in her psychiatric comorbidities as well as the fact that she is a woman of childbearing age. Accordingly, oxcarbazepine is an ideal option, as it is effective for her type of epilepsy, and it may have mood-stabilizing properties. An alternative option could be lamotrigine. Levetiracetam would be less preferred in this patient because it might worsen the patient's psychiatric symptoms. A basic metabolic panel reveals normal sodium, and oxcarbazepine is started. Monitoring of serum sodium concentrations will be necessary, as hyponatremia is a potential adverse event that can be worsened by the presence of venlafaxine. Her methylphenidate and venlafaxine are not discontinued because they do not increase the risk of seizures at therapeutic dosing.

Key Clinical Points

- Epilepsy is one of the most common neurological disorders.
- Clinical data is paramount in the diagnosis of epileptic seizures.
- EEG helps to confirm the diagnosis of epilepsy, but by itself does not establish the diagnosis of epilepsy.
- When establishing a diagnosis of epilepsy, imitators of epileptic seizures need to be excluded.
- The selection of the ASM is based on the type of seizure; the presence of comorbid medical, neurological, and psychiatric disorders; and concomitant medications prescribed for their treatment.
- Psychiatric comorbidities are very frequent in patients with epilepsy and need to be investigated at the time of seizure evaluation and screened at every follow-up visit.

Review Questions

1. Which of the following is *not* helpful for the localization of a seizure focus?

    A. Clinical semiology
    B. Electroencephalogram
    C. Evoked potentials
    D. Brain MRI
    E. Single-photon emission computed tomography

2. Which of the following psychotropic medications is most likely to decrease the seizure threshold?

    A. Fluoxetine
    B. Venlafaxine
    C. Amitriptyline
    D. Risperidone
    E. Clozapine

3. A 13-year-old begins dropping things. His parents notice that he tends to have muscle jerks upon awakening and intermittently in the mornings. After a few months, following a cluster of muscle jerks, he experiences a generalized convulsive seizure. Which of the following syndromes is most likely present?

   A. Childhood absence epilepsy
   B. Juvenile myoclonic epilepsy
   C. Juvenile absence epilepsy
   D. Lennox-Gastaut syndrome
   E. Focal to bilateral seizures

Answers

Question 1: C. Careful history and observation of a seizure may reveal the approximate origin and spread of the seizure. An interictal EEG may locate the suspected area, and the capture of a seizure on EEG helps determine focal onset. Brain MRI may reveal a structural lesion causing seizures. A SPECT scan will show increased blood flow to the area of the brain where the seizure starts. Evoked potentials measure only a specific pathway (e.g., visual pathway in response to a stimulus) so they are generally not used to localize seizures.

Question 2: E. Most psychotropic medications, especially in therapeutic doses, do not decrease the seizure threshold in a clinically significant way. Exceptions may include clomipramine, bupropion, clozapine, olanzapine, and chlorpromazine, especially at higher doses. Clozapine has the strongest effect on seizure threshold.

Question 3: B. Juvenile myoclonic epilepsy presents with myoclonic jerks on awakening from sleep and often generalized convulsions. The other seizure types do occur in childhood but do not have this semiology.

References

Baldin E, Hauser WA, Buchhalter JR, et al: Yield of epileptiform electroencephalogram abnormalities in incident unprovoked seizures: a population-based study. Epilepsia 55(9):1389–1398, 2014 25041095

Bergey GK, Morrell MJ, Mizrahi EM, et al: Long-term treatment with responsive brain stimulation in adults with refractory partial seizures. Neurology 84(8):810–817, 2015 25616485

Besag F, Gobbi G, Caplan R, et al: Psychiatric and behavioural disorders in children with epilepsy: an ILAE Task Force Report, Epilepsy and ADHD. Epileptic Disord 18(Suppl 1):S8–S15, 2016

Bronen RA, Fulbright RK, Spencer DD, et al: Refractory epilepsy: comparison of MR imaging, CT, and histopathologic findings in 117 patients. Radiology 201(1):97–105, 1996 8816528

Christensen J, Vestergaard M, Mortensen PB, et al: Epilepsy and risk of suicide: a population-based case-control study. Lancet Neurol 6(8):693–698, 2007 17611160

Engel J Jr, McDermott MP, Wiebe S, et al: Early surgical therapy for drug-resistant temporal lobe epilepsy: a randomized trial. JAMA 307(9):922–930, 2012 22396514

Engelborghs S, D'Hooge R, De Deyn PP: Pathophysiology of epilepsy. Acta Neurol Belg 100(4):201–213, 2000 11233674

Fisher RS, van Emde Boas W, Blume W, et al: Epileptic seizures and epilepsy: definitions proposed by the International League Against Epilepsy (ILAE) and the International Bureau for Epilepsy (IBE). Epilepsia 46(4):470–472, 2005 15816939

Fisher RS, Acevedo C, Arzimanoglou A, et al: ILAE official report: a practical clinical definition of epilepsy. Epilepsia 55(4):475–482, 2014 24730690

Fisher RS, Cross JH, French JA, et al: Operational classification of seizure types by the International League Against Epilepsy: position paper of the ILAE Commission for Classification and Terminology. Epilepsia 58(4):522–530, 2017 28276060

GBD 2016 Epilepsy Collaborators: Global, regional, and national burden of epilepsy, 1990–2016: a systematic analysis for the Global Burden of Disease Study 2016. Lancet Neurol 18(4):357–375, 2019 30773428

Glauser T, Ben-Menachem E, Bourgeois B, et al: ILAE treatment guidelines: evidence-based analysis of antiepileptic drug efficacy and effectiveness as initial monotherapy for epileptic seizures and syndromes. Epilepsia 47(7):1094–1120, 2006 16886973

Gross RE, Stern MA, Willie JT, et al: Stereotactic laser amygdalohippocampotomy for mesial temporal lobe epilepsy. Ann Neurol 83(3):575–587, 2018 29420840

Harden CL, Hopp J, Ting TY, et al: Practice parameter update: management issues for women with epilepsy—focus on pregnancy (an evidence-based review): obstetrical complications and change in seizure frequency: report of the Quality Standards Subcommittee and Therapeutics and Technology Assessment Subcommittee of the American Academy of Neurology and American Epilepsy Society. Neurology 73(2):126–132, 2009 19398682

Herman ST, Walczak TS, Bazil CW: Distribution of partial seizures during the sleep-wake cycle: differences by seizure onset site. Neurology 56(11):1453–1459, 2001 11402100

Hernández-Díaz S, Smith CR, Shen A, et al: Comparative safety of antiepileptic drugs during pregnancy. Neurology 78(21):1692–1699, 2012 22551726

Hesdorffer DC, Ishihara L, Mynepalli L, et al: Epilepsy, suicidality, and psychiatric disorders: a bidirectional association. Ann Neurol 72(2):184–191, 2012 22887468

Hingray C, El-Hage W, Duncan R, et al: Access to diagnostic and therapeutic facilities for psychogenic nonepileptic seizures: an international survey by the ILAE PNES Task Force. Epilepsia 59(1):203–214, 2018 29152734

Kanner AM: Management of psychiatric and neurological comorbidities in epilepsy. Nat Rev Neurol 12(2):106–116, 2016 26782334

Kanner AM, Rivas-Grajales AM: Psychosis of epilepsy: a multifaceted neuropsychiatric disorder. CNS Spectr 21(3):247–257, 2016 27322691

Kanner AM, Soto A, Gross-Kanner H: Prevalence and clinical characteristics of postictal psychiatric symptoms in partial epilepsy. Neurology 62(5):708–713, 2004 15007118

Kanner AM, Barry JJ, Gilliam F, et al: Depressive and anxiety disorders in epilepsy: do they differ in their potential to worsen common antiepileptic drug-related adverse events? Epilepsia 53(6):1104–1108, 2012 22554067

Kanner AM, Mazarati A, Koepp M: Biomarkers of epileptogenesis: psychiatric comorbidities (?). Neurotherapeutics 11(2):358–372, 2014 24719199

Krumholz A, Wiebe S, Gronseth GS, et al: Evidence-based guideline: management of an unprovoked first seizure in adults: report of the Guideline Development Subcommittee of the American Academy of Neurology and the American Epilepsy Society. Epilepsy Curr 15(3):144–152, 2015 26316856

Kwan P, Arzimanoglou A, Berg AT, et al: Definition of drug resistant epilepsy: consensus proposal by the ad hoc Task Force of the ILAE Commission on Therapeutic Strategies. Epilepsia 51(6):1069–1077, 2010 19889013

Kwan P, Brodie MJ: Effectiveness of first antiepileptic drug. Epilepsia 42(10):1255–1260, 2001 11737159

LaFrance WC Jr, Baker GA, Duncan R, et al: Minimum requirements for the diagnosis of psychogenic nonepileptic seizures: a staged approach: a report from the International League Against Epilepsy Nonepileptic Seizures Task Force. Epilepsia 54(11):2005–2018, 2013 24111933

Lu E, Pyatka N, Burant CJ, et al: Systematic literature review of psychiatric comorbidities in adults with epilepsy. J Clin Neurol 17(2):176–186, 2021 33835737

Marson A, Jacoby A, Johnson A, et al: Immediate versus deferred antiepileptic drug treatment for early epilepsy and single seizures: a randomised controlled trial. Lancet 365(9476):2007–2013, 2005 15950714

Moosavi R, Swisher CB: Acute provoked seizures: work-up and management in adults. Semin Neurol 40(6):595–605, 2020 33155185

Ngugi AK, Bottomley C, Kleinschmidt I, et al: Estimation of the burden of active and life-time epilepsy: a meta-analytic approach. Epilepsia 51(5):883–890, 2010 20067507

Pennell PB: Use of antiepileptic drugs during pregnancy: evolving concepts. Neurotherapeutics 13(4):811–820, 2016 27502786

Reiter J, Reiter J, Andrews D, et al: Taking Control of Your Seizures: Treatments That Work. New York, Oxford University Press, 2015

Ribot R, Ouyang B, Kanner AM: The impact of antidepressants on seizure frequency and depressive and anxiety disorders of patients with epilepsy: is it worth investigating? Epilepsy Behav 70(Pt A):5–9, 2017 28407526

Ryvlin P, Gilliam FG, Nguyen DK, et al: The long-term effect of vagus nerve stimulation on quality of life in patients with pharmacoresistant focal epilepsy: the PuLsE (Open Prospective Randomized Long-term Effectiveness) trial. Epilepsia 55(6):893–900, 2014 24754318

Salanova V, Witt T, Worth R, et al: Long-term efficacy and safety of thalamic stimulation for drug-resistant partial epilepsy. Neurology 84(10):1017–1025, 2015 25663221

Sam MC, So EL: Significance of epileptiform discharges in patients without epilepsy in the community. Epilepsia 42(10):1273–1278, 2001 11737162

Scott AJ, Sharpe L, Hunt C, et al: Anxiety and depressive disorders in people with epilepsy: a meta-analysis. Epilepsia 58(6):973–982, 2017 28470748

Semah F, Picot MC, Adam C, et al: Is the underlying cause of epilepsy a major prognostic factor for recurrence? Neurology 51(5):1256–1262, 1998 9818842

Sheidley BR, Malinowski J, Bergner AL, et al: Genetic testing for the epilepsies: a systematic review. Epilepsia 63(2):375–387, 2022 34893972

Tellez-Zenteno JF, Patten SB, Jetté N, et al: Psychiatric comorbidity in epilepsy: a population-based analysis. Epilepsia 48(12):2336–2344, 2007 17662062

Tomson T, Battino D, Bonizzoni E, et al: Dose-dependent risk of malformations with antiepileptic drugs: an analysis of data from the EURAP epilepsy and pregnancy registry. Lancet Neurol 10(7):609–617, 2011 21652013

Xu Y, Nguyen D, Mohamed A, et al: Frequency of a false positive diagnosis of epilepsy: a systematic review of observational studies. Seizure 41:167–174, 2016 27592470

9

Movement Disorders

Ashley Paul, M.D., M.Ed.
Ankur Butala, M.D.

Case Example

A 63-year-old woman with a history of major depressive disorder and essential tremor presents with worsening hand tremor despite propranolol 80 mg XL daily. Her hand tremor started 15 years ago, progressing gradually from right unilateral to bilateral. The tremor affects her ability to do her job as a chemist, eat with a spoon, write, and apply makeup. She also complains of morning stiffness. Her family history is positive for tremors in her sister, mother, and maternal uncle, with a maternal grandmother having had a "parkinsonian disorder." The patient rarely drinks alcohol now, but it did improve her tremor in the past.

She denies weakness but occasionally trips while stepping onto a curb and has trouble rising from a chair. Her spouse observes restless sleep with early morning yelling or arm flinging as if interacting with someone in her sleep. Her major depression has been in remission for 5 years on venlafaxine XR 225 mg. She has previously tried fluoxetine, sertraline, and buspirone, with a brief course of aripiprazole and lithium.

Disorders of movement may be related to functional or structural pathology in any of the CNS components of the motor system, including upper motor neurons, the basal ganglia, cerebellum, and lower motor neurons. They are among the most common neurological disorders, occurring in approximately 28% of all people ages 50–89 in one study (Wenning et al. 2005). Disorders of movement frequently include cognitive, emotional, or psychiatric comorbidity and occur frequently in the context of psychiatric symptoms or disorders. In this chapter, we review the more common movement disorders, including tremor, Parkinson disease and related disorders, tics, stereotypies, myoclonus, dystonia, ataxia, chorea, paroxysmal movement disorders, restless leg syndrome, and drug- or substance-induced disorders. For a review of functional neurologic disorders, including functional movement disorders, see Chapter 10, "Functional Neurological Disorder."

Approach to Patients With Movement Disorders

The clinical encounter begins with observation even as the patient walks into the clinic room. The patient's posture and movement are noted during the interview, with special attention to fluctuations. Important features in the history include age at onset; progression; associated features such as autonomic insufficiency, gait apraxia, ataxia, or other co-occurring movements; systemic medical conditions; substance use; occupational exposures; and family history. Important features on neurological examination include movement frequency, amplitude, bodily distribution, and any activation of movements. Given the high prevalence of comorbid psychiatric disorders and co-occurring cognitive and emotional symptoms, a thorough mental and cognitive status assessment is included in the evaluation of movement disorders.

While examining the patient, the examiner considers possible etiologies that may include acquired injury (e.g., post-hemorrhagic, hypoxic), structural (e.g., basal ganglia calcinosis), inherited (e.g., Huntington disease, spinocerebellar ataxia), drug- or substance-induced, and sporadic or idiopathic disorders. With successive examinations, the etiology may become clearer. More than one genotype may be associated with a given phenotypic syndrome, and more than one phenotype may be associated with a given disorder. Evaluation of hyperkinetic movement disorders typically includes assessment for polycythemia, abnormal red blood cell morphology, hyperthyroidism, iron deficiency, abnormal renal or liver functions, abnormal glucose metabolism, and, if clinically indicated, autoimmune and paraneoplastic disorders or specific genetic syndromes.

Tremor

Tremor is an involuntary, rhythmic, oscillatory movement of a body part. In practice, identification of tremor can be difficult because other phenomenologies such as dystonia and myoclonus have features reminiscent of tremors. Comprehensive descriptions and differentiation of tremor subtypes have been published (Bhatia et al. 2018; McAuley and Rothwell 2004; van de Wardt et al. 2020). A practical summary of tremor classification by primary characteristics and possible etiologies is provided in Table 9.1.

Essential Tremor

Essential tremor is the leading cause of tremors, characterized by bilateral upper limb postural and kinetic tremors typically 6–12 Hz. Essential tremor is a chronic condition (more than 3 years) without significant involvement of other body parts. People with essential tremor typically have a family history of the disorder, but its intensity and age of onset may vary. The classification of essential tremor as a benign entity has been questioned, and a new classification, *essential tremor-plus* (ET-plus), has been introduced. ET-plus overlaps with dystonic and cerebellar disorders, leading to hearing loss, ataxia, cognitive impairment, and gait and postural instability (Espay et al. 2017; Louis et al. 2020). Essential tremor occurs during actions or sustained postures and may be suppressed by alcohol. People with essential tremor may also have an increased risk of substance use disorders (Deik et al. 2012). Essential tremor increases the risk of developing Parkinson disease fourfold, making it challenging to differentiate between the two. The DaTscan can distinguish between essential tremor and Parkinson disease by identifying diminished presynaptic dopamine transporters in the striatum in Parkinson disease. Management of essential tremor includes beta-blockers, antiseizure medications, weighted items, tremor-canceling devices, botulinum toxin, deep brain stimulation, and ablative surgeries.

Intention Tremor

An *intention tremor* is a specific feature of an action tremor wherein the tremor worsens on approach to a target, suggesting dysfunction within the Guillain-Mollaret triangle (red nucleus, inferior olivary nucleus, dentate nucleus, and other deep cerebellar nuclei). These nuclei give rise to the cerebellar outflow tract.

Table 9.1 Tremor characteristics and associated etiologies

Moment of occurrence	Primary features	Possible etiologies
At rest	Body part fully supported against gravity	PD, akathisia, RLS
With Parkinsonism	Rest tremor with classic PD features	PD, DIP, atypical PD, VascP, SCA, WD
Without Parkinsonism	Rest tremor without classic PD features	ET (pseudoresting), DysTr, HT, FMD
With action		Ataxia, action myoclonus
Postural	Body part postured against gravity	PhysT, E-PhysT, ET, DysTr, FMD, NT, PD
Kinetic		Drug-induced
• Simple	During entire movement trajectory	ET, FMD
• Intention	Progressively increases toward target	HT, COT, FMD
• Task-specific	Occurs only during specific actions	DysTr
Isometric	Voluntary muscle contraction against stationary resistance	PhysT and above
Combination	Several features above	ET, atypical PD, DysTr, HT

COT = cerebellar outflow tremor; DIP = drug-induced parkinsonism; DysTr = dystonic tremor; E-PhysT = enhanced physiological tremor; ET = essential tremor; FMD = functional movement disorder; HT = Holmes tremor; NT = neuropathic tremor; PD = Parkinson disease; PhysT = physiological tremor; RLS = restless leg syndrome; SCA = spinocerebellar ataxia; VascP = vascular parkinsonism; WD = Wilson disease.

Rubral Tremor

Rubral tremor, also known as *cerebellar outflow tract tremor* or *Holmes tremor* (Holmes 1939), may develop from acquired, sporadic, or hereditary damage. It may be present at rest and while in motion, usually affecting proximal limbs with a lower (2–5 Hz) frequency. Rubral tremors may be particularly difficult to treat and are severely disabling. As the complex neurocircuitry underpinning tremors, dystonia, and ataxias is further studied, it has become harder to distinguish between these phenomena, with some forms of essential tremor being proposed as classes of rubral tremor.

Enhanced Physiologic Tremor

Enhanced physiologic tremor is a very common low-amplitude, high-frequency (8–12 Hz) rhythmic tremor. A normal person may notice this benign tremor when maintaining outstretched hands for a few minutes after a cup of coffee. Fatigue, anxiety, caffeine, stimulants, or sympathomimetic medication may exacerbate the underlying physiological tremor. Occasionally, carrying a heavy object may cause the amplitude to increase and the frequency to decrease, a helpful distinguishing characteristic.

Parkinson Disease and Related Disorders

Idiopathic Parkinson Disease

Idiopathic Parkinson disease (iPD) is the most common reason for referral to a movement disorders neurologist, with increasing prevalence in people older than 45. The global disease burden is projected to reach 17 million individuals by 2040 (Marras et al. 2018). iPD is caused by pathological misfolding and aggregation of the α-synuclein protein, and, at present, the diagnosis may be confirmed only via autopsy—revisions to the criteria for clinical diagnosis are under debate and forthcoming. Clinical manifestations of iPD are shown in Table 9.2. The cardinal symptoms of iPD are bradykinesia in combination with resting tremor or rigidity. The combination of tremor and rigidity produces cogwheel rigidity. Non-motor symptoms may precede motor symptoms by more than 10 years. Supportive findings include beneficial response to dopa-

Table 9.2 Clinical manifestations of idiopathic Parkinson disease (iPD)

Cardinal features for clinically established iPD	Supportive features	
	Motor features	**Non-motor features**
Bradykinesia plus resting tremor and/or rigidity	Postural instability, beneficial response to dopaminergic therapy, development of motor fluctuations, development of levodopa-induced dyskinesias in moderate to advanced stages, dystonia, micrographia, hypophonia, hypomimia	**Cognitive:** word-finding difficulties (early stages), followed by executive dysfunction, and possible dementia (moderate to advanced stages) **Psychiatric:** mood disturbances (depression, anxiety, apathy), psychosis/hallucinations (advanced stages and in association with Parkinson disease dementia) **Autonomic:** orthostatic hypotension, urinary incontinence, sexual dysfunction, constipation **Olfactory:** hyposmia, anosmia **Sleep disorders:** REM sleep behavior disorder, restless leg syndrome, periodic limb movement of sleep, insomnia

minergic therapy, motor fluctuations, dyskinesia, resting tremor, olfactory loss, or cardiac sympathetic denervation (Postuma et al. 2015).

Atypical Parkinsonism

Differentiating mild iPD from mimicking conditions such as dystonia and essential tremor can be challenging, and determining whether iPD will evolve into an atypical parkinsonian disorder remains difficult even after diagnosis. The atypical parkinsonian or "Parkinson plus" disorders include *dementia with Lewy bodies* (DLB), *multiple system atrophy* (MSA), *corticobasal syndrome* (CBS), and *progressive supranuclear palsy* (PSP).

Misfolded α-synuclein aggregates are found in iPD, DLB, and MSA. Tau and TDP-43 disorders have a more complex phenotype and include CBS, PSP, motor neuron disease, primary progressive aphasia, and frontotemporal dementia. Hyposmia and REM sleep behavior disorder (RBD) can develop years before motor onset in synucleinopathies. RBD involves failure to develop normal REM sleep atonia, resulting in dream enactment. Taken together with a decline in motor function, these features can indicate iPD, DLB, or MSA. Distinguishing these entities can be challenging and requires multiple observations over time.

Diagnostic criteria for DLB are reviewed in Chapter 4, "Dementia." Spontaneous fluctuations in cognition, attention, and arousal may result in daytime drowsiness or lethargy. Complex visual hallucinations are prevalent in more than 80% of patients, and a careful history may reveal subtle passage hallucinations or the feeling of a fleeting phantom presence. The onset of cognitive changes usually occurs within 1 year of motor symptom onset. Only one motor feature (resting tremor, rigidity, or bradykinesia) is required. RBD is another core feature found in DLB patients. DLB and Parkinson disease/dementia are considered to be on a clinical spectrum with iPD (McKeith et al. 2017).

MSA is a progressive condition that presents in adults 30 or older with signs of parkinsonism or cerebellar syndrome and dysautonomia, as well as two supportive motor or nonmotor features. Dysautonomia includes unexplained urinary urge incontinence, unexplained voiding difficulty with postvoid residual ≥100 mL, or neurogenic orthostatic hypotension (≥20/10 mmHg drop in blood pressure within 3 minutes). Stridor is a poor prognostic sign and suggests advanced disease. Polysomnography can help detect central sleep apnea, and laryngoscopy can rule out obstruction. Treatment includes continuous positive airway pressure (CPAP) and tracheostomy for severe or persistent stridor (Wenning et al. 2022).

For DLB and MSA, treatment consists of supportive therapies (there are no specific disease-modifying treatments for atypical parkinsonism). Levodopa is often offered, but the response is limited. In patients with severe dysautonomia with neurogenic orthostatic hypotension or severe hallucinations, caution should be used when initiating levodopa because there is a risk of worsening symptoms with little motor benefit. The mainstay of treatment involves physical, speech, and occupational therapies. Swallowing function should be closely monitored to reduce the risk of aspiration pneumonia or other respiratory complications. Conversations with patients often focus on goals of care and how to maintain quality of life.

CBS is a neurodegenerative disorder caused by the accumulation of misfolded tau aggregates in the brain, which can be secondary to multiple types of tau pathology. When symptoms are attributed to hyperphosphorylated tau in specified areas, the diagnosis is corticobasal degeneration. Probable CBS is diagnosed when there is an asymmetric presentation of two or more features, such as limb rigidity or akinesia, limb dystonia, or limb myoclonus, along with two of the following: orobuccal or limb apraxia, cortical sensory deficit, or alien limb phenomenon (Jabbari et al. 2020).

PSP and iPD both include core bradykinesia and rigidity, but tremors are less frequent in PSP. PSP differs from iPD in its early development of postural instability, vertical gaze restriction, and eventual subcortical dementia. PSP has several established and investigational subsyndromes that can affect its evolution and longevity, including PSP–parkinsonism, PSP–pure akinesia with gait freezing, and PSP–corticobasal syndrome (Höglinger et al. 2017; Jabbari et al. 2020).

PSP and CBS are progressive disorders with no known disease-modifying therapies. The prognosis varies, but symptoms can lead to loss of ambulation, anarthria, and choking. Primary causes of mortality include aspiration pneumonia, hip fractures, and neurogenic respiratory failure. Management is symptomatic and palliative, focusing on exercise and rehabilitation. Levodopa may result in some improvement in bradykinesia and rigidity, but effectiveness decreases over time. High-dose coenzyme Q10 has been shown to modestly improve gait and energy. Botulinum toxin can treat eyelid opening dyspraxia, blepharospasm, and dystonia. Multidisciplinary treatment is essential for improving quality of life and palliation.

Vascular Parkinsonism

Vascular parkinsonism may resemble iPD but with primarily lower-extremity symptoms and spasticity instead of cogwheel rigidity. Tremor is rare. Diagnosis requires convergence of clinical features and imaging findings of cerebrovascular disease. DaTscans are negative in most cases.

Tics

Tics, affecting 4%–10% of children, are sudden, recurrent movements or vocalizations. Tics may be voluntary or involuntary, preceded by urges, temporarily suppressed, and influenced by emotional states. Simple motor tics involve random, purposeless movements isolated to one muscle group, and simple vocal tics include altered breathing, sniffing, or other nonlanguage sounds. For most children, isolated simple tics may self-resolve within 12 months (i.e., transient tic disorder). Complex motor tics entail coordinated patterns involving multiple muscle groups. Complex vocal tics involve blurting out words or phrases.

Tourette disorder,[1] which is more common in boys, develops around school entry; diagnosis requires multiple motor and vocal tics before age 18, persisting over a year. It often co-occurs with obsessive-compulsive behaviors and ADHD. Habit-reversal therapy or comprehensive behavioral intervention for tics improves voluntary control when tics affect daily life. Approximately 50% of children with Tourette disorder will outgrow motor and vocal tics. For the rest, motor symptoms often decrease, although other features may persist.

Pharmacological interventions can be used when tics interfere with quality of life. Clonidine or guanfacine may be tried, followed by topiramate, clonazepam, or baclofen before dopamine blockers. Atypical antipsychotics with fewer metabolic side effects are preferred. Vesicular monoamine transporter 2 (VMAT-2) inhibitors have been increasingly used, although randomized controlled trial evidence is more muted. Deep brain stimulation may be tried in refractory cases (Roessner et al. 2022).

---

[1] Tourette disorder was named for Georges Gilles de la Tourette. His correct surname is *Gilles de la Tourette.*

Stereotypies

Stereotypies are purposeless, repetitive movements, postures, gestures, or utterances seen in a number of neuropsychiatric, developmental, or neurodegenerative disorders. These behaviors most commonly occur in autism spectrum disorder or severe intellectual disability but may also be seen secondary to autoimmune or viral encephalitis, stroke, substance use disorders, and other psychiatric conditions (Shukla and Pandey 2020). Stereotypies are thought to be related to dysfunction of the neural networks responsible for inhibition.

Treatment may be attempted if the stereotypies interfere with function. A multidisciplinary approach is helpful. Several treatments, including response interruption and redirection, have been studied that could potentially reduce motor and vocal stereotypic behaviors (Ryan et al. 2022). Increasing one's daily activities may also serve to reduce stereotypies.

Myoclonus

Myoclonus refers to irregular, arrhythmic, and jerky hyperkinetic movements that can affect any part of the body, including the head, neck, limbs, and torso. Myoclonus can occur in a multitude of settings, and the potential causes of myoclonus are extensive. One of the most common causes of myoclonus is polypharmacy or toxicity from the use of medications, including lithium, antipsychotics, antibiotics, narcotics, and certain antiarrhythmic agents (e.g., amiodarone). Other common causes of myoclonus include electrolyte disturbances, renal failure or hepatic disease, and exposure to toxins. Acute-onset myoclonus can occur when starting a new medication or in the setting of anoxic brain injury after cardiac arrest, which is referred to as Lance-Adams syndrome. If the presentation is subacute, consider infectious, inflammatory, autoimmune, or paraneoplastic etiologies. Myoclonus can also occur in the context of genetic disorders, epilepsy, and other movement disorders, such as corticobasal syndrome; consider these etiologies if the presentation is chronic and progressive. Treatment involves addressing the underlying cause, such as discontinuing offending medications or correcting electrolyte abnormalities. Pharmacological treatments may include the use of antiepileptic medications and benzodiazepines. Depending on the severity of myoclonus, treatment may involve multiple medications, limited by the potential side effects of polypharmacy (Caviness 2019).

Dystonia

Dystonia is twisting or posturing of the body resulting from sustained or intermittent contractions of groups of muscles. This may involve specific or isolated bodily regions (e.g., focal dystonia, such as cervical or focal hand dystonia) or multiple bodily regions (generalized or segmental dystonia). It may develop by itself (i.e., isolated) or as part of a larger constellation of symptoms due to an underlying genetic or neurodegenerative disorder (i.e., combined) (Albanese et al. 2013).

Cervical Dystonia

Cervical dystonia is the most common form of dystonia. Cervical dystonia is an adult-onset, focal, isolated, and sporadic dystonia characterized by abnormal neck posturing such as torticollis, neck tremor, and neck pain. The cause is generally unknown, but some patients have a family history (*THAP1*, formerly *DYT6*) or prior neuroleptic exposure (tardive dystonia) or are developing a forme fruste of a neurodegenerative disorder (e.g., iPD). Cervical dystonia features dysfunction of a central head-neck neural integrator. This hypothesized system summates inputs from the frontoparietal cortex, basal ganglia, brainstem, cerebellum, and cervical muscle spindles. The impaired sensorimotor reintegration results in abnormal posturing and a disturbed "resting state" of the body part. In addition, an irregular, jerky dystonic tremor may result when the body part deviates from a *null point* (a position where the tremor stops). Many dystonias also have a *sensory trick*, which is a tactile maneuver (e.g., touching the face in a particular area) that transiently improves dystonic symptoms.

Dystonic Tremor

Like essential tremor, *dystonic tremor* may be distinguished by its variable frequency, amplitude, and directionality. Anticholinergics, such as trihexyphenidyl, may be used to treat isolated dystonia. Benzodiazepines or skeletal muscle relaxants may be titrated as limited by sedation. The mainstay of therapy is botulinum toxin, which is supported by robust safety and efficacy literature for almost all forms of dystonia.

Ataxia

The word *ataxia* comes from the Greek meaning "without order." Ataxia refers to the inability to coordinate voluntary muscle movements unrelated to muscle weakness and is often used to describe gait disorders (Brusse et al. 2007).

Acquired Ataxias

Acquired ataxias may result from various conditions, including peripheral neuropathy, trauma, hemorrhage, ischemia, paraneoplastic syndrome, and infectious, metabolic, toxic, or nutritional causes. For example, thiamine deficiency, typically seen in chronic alcohol abuse or nutritional impoverishment, may cause ataxia.

Primary or Genetic Ataxias

Relatively common genetic etiologies of ataxia include Friedreich ataxia and the spinocerebellar ataxias (SCAs). *Friedreich ataxia* is an autosomal recessive disease that can include ataxia, neuropathy, dysarthria, dysphagia, vision and hearing loss, scoliosis, and cardiomyopathy that begins in young adulthood to early middle age.

Less common causes include ataxia telangiectasia, episodic ataxia, dentatorubral pallidoluysian atrophy (DRPLA), the cerebellar ataxia with neuropathy and vestibular areflexia syndrome (CANVAS) that presents in middle age, and several others. *Ataxia telangiectasia* is a childhood-onset, autosomal-recessive, neurocutaneous syndrome that includes severe ataxia, telangiectasias, dysarthria, dysphagia, and immunocompromise. *Episodic ataxia* presents in the teenage years with spells of ataxia, dysarthria, nystagmus, vertigo, and headache but is asymptomatic between episodes. *DRPLA* is of special interest as an autosomal-dominant ataxia that can present in childhood or young adulthood with ataxia, myoclonus, seizures, choreoathetosis, and psychotic symptoms and can lead to dementia.

SCAs are a heterogeneous collection of genetic ataxias. They are often autosomal dominant and result from repeat expansions, although they may also have autosomal-recessive, X-linked, and mitochondrial inheritance. Cerebellar features include gait and limb ataxia, dysarthria, dysphagia, and abnormal eye movements (hypermetric saccades and nystagmus). Age at onset, rate of progression, and the presence of additional neurological features vary depending on the specific type of SCA. Some SCAs may be exclusively cerebellar (e.g., SCA6/episodic ataxia type 2) or have pyramidal or neuropathic features (e.g., SCA1 or 2, respectively), extrapyramidal manifestations mimicking parkinsonism (e.g., SCA3), or chorea (e.g., SCA17). Genetic testing should be obtained when an SCA is suspected. Codominant drivers of poor quality of life include major depression, dysexecutive symptoms, and impaired reality testing (Klockgether et al. 2019).

The Cerebellum and Cognition

Cerebellar cognitive affective syndrome (CCAS), also known as Schmahmann syndrome, is a constellation of symptoms, presumed to result from cerebellar pathology, resulting in dysmodulation of various connected cortical areas. Deficits include personality changes, along with impairment of executive functions, spatial cognition, language, and mood. CCAS was first observed in pediatric patients with acquired cerebellar injury. *Postoperative pediatric cerebellar mutism syndrome* may be a severe manifestation of CCAS. There is no specific treatment, but occupational, speech/language, cognitive-behavioral, and vocational therapy may improve dysexecutive symptoms, visuospatial function, language, social behavior, and well-being (Argyropoulos et al. 2020).

Choreoathetosis

Dystonia, chorea, and athetosis are all arrhythmic and irregular. Chorea and athetosis, unlike dystonia, are nonstereotyped movements without sustained postures. Chorea and athetosis are both continual, flowing movements, but chorea tends to be of higher frequency; athetosis is of lower frequency and tends to occur more at rest. The distinction between chorea and athetosis is not significant, and they are often referred to as *choreoathetosis.* Chorea can range from subtle movements (raising an eyebrow) to large-amplitude ballistic movements and involves random movements of various body parts. Diagnosing hyperkinetic adult-onset choreoathetoid disorders is challenging. Genetic causes are numerous, but among the most common are Huntington disease and Wilson disease. Huntington phenocopy disorders, chorea gravidarum, and drug-induced choreoathetosis should also be considered in the differential diagnosis of choreoathetosis.

Huntington Disease

Huntington disease is an autosomal-dominant neurodegenerative condition caused by trinucleotide (CAG) expansion beyond 40 repeats in the *HTT* gene on chromosome 4. Huntington disease is the most common cause of adult-onset chorea. Those with 36–39 CAG repeats may be at risk for mild cognitive impairment without obvious motor symptoms. The age of onset is typically in the 40s but ranges from 20 to 60, with some cases beginning before and after that range. Genetic anticipation can lead to earlier and more severe symptoms across generations. Symptoms vary greatly. The family history should include screening for neuropsychiatric, cognitive, substance use, and legal issues. Presymptomatic testing requires informed consent, and counseling from a certified genetic counselor is strongly recommended.

Chorea is the primary motor feature, but cognitive and neuropsychiatric symptoms can be more disabling and appear earlier. Standardized questionnaires can assess motor, psychiatric, and cognitive domains, and treatment should prioritize the most affected domain. Psychiatric symptoms vary widely and can include paranoia, delusions, hallucinations, substance use disorders, mood lability, impulse control disorders, major depression, and OCD. Motor complications include dystonia, parkinsonism, and frequent falls. VMAT-2 inhibitors are first-line treatment. More potent dopamine antagonists may be needed for dual treatment of motor and psychiatric symptoms. Multidisciplinary care and advanced care planning are important. No curative therapies currently exist, but various trials attempt to mitigate neurodegeneration.

Phenocopy disorders resembling Huntington disease include Huntington disease–like disorders, and genetic testing for *C9orf72* and *TBP* (formerly *SCA17*) should be considered. Additional diagnostic clues may include peripheral smear for neuroacanthocytosis, iron-sensitive MRI sequences for neurodegeneration with brain iron accumulation, ataxia for SCA1–3 or Friedreich ataxia, myoclonus or dementia for prion disease or mitochondrial disorders, African ancestry for Huntington disease–like 2 (HDL2), and seizures for DRPLA.

Neurodegeneration With Brain Iron Accumulation

Neurodegeneration with brain iron accumulation is a heterogeneous group of autosomal recessive disorders unified by a signal loss in iron-sensitive or susceptibility-weighted imaging, especially involving deep gray matter regions: globus pallidus, substantia nigra, putamen, thalamus, and red nucleus. Childhood onset is far more common than adult onset, with symptoms including dystonia, chorea, parkinsonism, spasticity, retinopathy, and cognitive decline. Treatment is mainly supportive and includes botulinum toxin injections for dystonia, monitoring for retinopathy, and multidisciplinary care with physical therapy, occupational therapy, and speech therapy (Hogarth 2015).

Neuroacanthocytosis

Neuroacanthocytosis refers to a group of disorders that include basal ganglia degeneration and abnormal red cells (acanthocytes) in the peripheral smear. Included are chorea-acanthocytosis, McLeod syndrome, HDL2, pantothenate kinase–associated neurodegeneration, and abetalipoproteinemia. *Chorea-acanthocytosis* is an autosomal-recessive disorder with psychiatric symptoms and a characteristic presentation of orolingual self-mutilation, seizures, hyporeflexia, and hepatomegaly. *McLeod syndrome* is an X-linked disorder with cognitive decline, myopathy, peripheral neuropathy, neuropsychiatric features, and the risk of sudden death related to cardiomyopathy. Liver dysfunction and hepatomegaly are common.

When considering the cause of chorea, several factors can help refine the differential diagnosis, including the speed and time course of symptom onset, body distribution, and history of drug exposure. Drug-induced chorea can occur with levodopa, dopamine agonists, anticholinergics, antiseizure medications, oral contraceptives, stimulants, and neuroleptics. Treatment may involve termination of the offending agent and the use of VMAT-2 inhibitors.

Wilson Disease

Wilson disease is an autosomal-recessive disorder caused by a mutation in the *ATP7B* gene, resulting in impaired secretion of copper into bile and accumulation of copper in the liver, brain, heart, eyes, and other organs. The resulting copper overload can cause toxicity from oxidative stress, leading to neurological, psychiatric, and hepatic symptoms. Wilson disease can result in cirrhosis, cardiomyopathy, renal failure, and pancreatitis. The movement disorders seen in Wilson disease include parkinsonism, dystonia, dysarthria, gait disturbance, tremor, cerebellar ataxia, myoclonus, and choreoathetosis, with risus sardonicus and proximal wing-beating tremor as distinctive features. Psychiatric symptoms can also occur, including depression, impulsivity, and psychosis. Kayser-Fleischer rings (golden, brown, or green rims around the iris) are present in most patients with neurological symptoms and are best seen by slit lamp examination. Wilson disease is typically considered in the differential diagnosis of adolescent-onset cognitive decline or tardive dyskinesia.

Diagnostic evaluation includes checking for hepatosplenomegaly, jaundice, elevated hepatic enzymes, elevated 24-hour urine copper, and decreased serum ceruloplasmin. Ceruloplasmin is an acute-phase reactant; thus, illness can affect diagnostic accuracy. Pregnancy and estrogen supplementation can increase ceruloplasmin levels and confound the diagnostic workup. Total serum copper is decreased in proportion to ceruloplasmin. In contrast, serum free copper is increased. Genetic testing or liver biopsy may be needed for diagnosis, especially in the setting of normal serum ceruloplasmin. Treatment involves a low-copper diet, zinc salts, low-dose chelation therapy for asymptomatic patients, and full-dose chelation therapy for symptomatic patients. Fulminant hepatic failure may require a liver transplant. Prompt treatment is crucial, as untreated Wilson disease can lead to continued deterioration and death, whereas early diagnosis and treatment can lead to a normal lifespan (Członkowska et al. 2018).

Chorea Gravidarum

Chorea gravidarum is an uncommon movement disorder that occurs during pregnancy. Women with a history of Sydenham's chorea (rheumatic fever–induced basal ganglia dysfunction), antiphospholipid antibody syndrome, or systemic lupus erythematosus or a family history of chorea are at increased risk.

Paroxysmal Movement Disorders

Paroxysmal movement disorders are characterized by episodic involuntary movements that can be isolated or part of a larger condition. These disorders are believed to be caused by neuronal hyperexcitability due to channelopathies and can be primary (genetic) or secondary. Dystonia or chorea secondary to identifiable triggers is the most common presentation of genetic paroxysmal movement disorders. Triggers can include movement (paroxysmal kinesigenic dyskinesia), caffeine, alcohol, or stress. There is no alteration of consciousness, and dyskinesia is not a manifestation of a seizure, despite a robust response to antiseizure medications such as carbamazepine or oxcarbazepine.

Restless Legs Syndrome

Restless legs syndrome (RLS) is a condition that causes discomfort and a strong urge to move the legs, especially at night. The discomfort causes significant sleep disturbance and can be described as numbness, tingling, cramping, or a creepy-crawling sensation, which can be mistaken for muscle cramps or neuropathy. RLS is thought to be related to dopamine dysfunction, as well as iron deficiency. Iron repletion is the first-line treatment for those with ferritin levels <100 μg/L. As ferritin is an acute-phase reactant, levels may be unreliable; therefore, iron saturation <35% is an alternative threshold (Allen et al. 2018). If iron deficiency is excluded, then the first-line pharmaceutical agents are α2δ ligands such as gabapentin or pregabalin. Dopamine agonists were traditionally used as treatment, but they eventually cause patients to experience increased severity of symptoms (augmentation), earlier onset of symptoms, and spread to upper extremities. Patients who have been on dopamine agonists for more than 2 years are at high risk of developing augmentation and having difficulty discontinuing these agents. Refractory RLS can be cautiously treated with opioids (Manconi et al. 2021).

Drug-Induced Movement Disorders

Drug-induced movement disorders may be acute or late occurring (tardive). Acute disorders include tremor, dystonia, akathisia, and parkinsonism. Although dopaminergic blocking agents account for the majority of the drug-induced movement disorders described here, there are other agents in each category that may cause the particular movement disorder. An exception is tremor, which occurs more frequently with lithium and antidepressant agents than with dopamine-blocking agents. Many drug-induced syndromes may persist beyond the discontinuation of the offending agent, especially parkinsonism; in this case, an unmasking of latent iPD must be considered. Tardive disorders include choreoathetoid movements but may also include prominent dystonia or akathisia. Management of any drug-induced movement disorder should include consideration of lowering or discontinuing the offending agent and finding an alternative medication if needed.

Tremor

Psychotropic agents can cause tremors; up to 20% of people taking selective serotonin reuptake inhibitors (SSRIs) and serotonin-norepinephrine reuptake inhibitors (SNRIs) develop them. Antidepressant-provoked tremors often resemble essential tremor or enhanced physiologic tremor and may improve when the medication is stopped. However, tremor may be a feature of 15% of cases of acute withdrawal of SNRI or SSRI medications. Lithium can cause tremors in up to 60% of patients. Tremors from lithium mainly resemble enhanced physiologic tremor, but cerebellar toxicity and associated ataxia have been reported, even at therapeutic doses. If drug-induced tremors are suspected, the first step is to stop the offending medication; if this is not possible, the tremor is managed symptomatically (Hauser et al. 2022).

Acute Dystonic Reaction

Acute dystonic reaction encompasses several types of dystonia that occur with abrupt onset. Examples include oculogyric crisis (fixed upward or lateral gaze), oromandibular dystonia, acute dystonic laryngospasm, blepharospasm, opisthotonos, and truncal or limb dystonia. Dystonic reactions tend to occur within a few days of initiating antidopaminergic therapy or increasing the dosage of the offending agent. Risk factors for acute dystonic reactions include male sex, younger age, use of higher-potency dopamine blockers, history of dystonic reaction, family history of dystonia, and recent use of psychostimulants such as cocaine. Treatment involves cessation or dosage reduction of the offending agent and treatment with intravenous or intramuscular anticholinergics or antihistamines (Rajan et al. 2019).

Akathisia

Akathisia is characterized by an intense urge to move and inner restlessness, resulting in fidgeting and an inability to sit still. It is most frequently caused by antipsychotics but may also occur with antidepressant treatment and occasionally with calcium channel blockers or anesthetics. RLS may co-occur with akathisia. Treatment with beta blockers or benzodiazepines is helpful. If akathisia is persistent, changing antipsychotic medications can also be entertained.

Parkinsonism

Drug-induced parkinsonism was first described in the 1950s, and its incidence has been declining since the 1970s owing to changes in prescribing practices. It is most commonly caused by typical or atypical neuroleptics but can also be caused by gastrointestinal prokinetic agents, antidepressants, calcium channel blockers, antiarrhythmics, and others. The symptoms of drug-induced parkinsonism typically include symmetrical rest tremor, but it can also present with akinetic rigidity or an asymmetric onset. Risk factors include female sex, older age, and neuroleptic potency. A family history of parkinsonism and mood disorders may contribute to risk. Most people with drug-induced parkinsonism develop symptoms within 3 months of exposure to the offending agent, but symptoms can persist for more than 2 years, even with cessation of the medication in question.

Clinicians may find it challenging to differentiate drug-induced parkinsonism from other neurodegenerative disorders. A DaTscan may be considered if symptoms persist 12 months after discontinuing the offending medication, but the limited sensitivity of DaTscans necessitates continued follow-up.

Sudden and severe onset of parkinsonism is a movement disorder emergency with a broad differential diagnosis. Causes to consider include exposure to dopamine receptor blocking agents, structural brain lesions, exposure to toxins, paraneoplastic or autoimmune disorders, and viral encephalitides. Treatment involves treating the underlying cause, but levodopa can be used for symptomatic management (Hauser et al. 2022).

Tardive Dyskinesia

Prolonged exposure to dopamine-blocking agents, such as antipsychotics and antiemetics, can lead to *tardive dyskinesia*. Classic tardive dyskinesia is choreoathetoid, with buccolingual chorea being the most common manifestation. Tardive dyskinesia can refer to any delayed abnormal involuntary movement resulting from dopamine receptor blockade and can be named according to the most prominent symptom, including tardive akathisia, dystonia, parkinsonism, tic, or myoclonus. Tardive dystonia is a common form and is characterized by twisting and posturing of the neck, trunk, or limbs. Symptoms may persist even after the cessation of the offending drug (Hauser et al. 2022). The Abnormal Involuntary Movement Scale is used to screen patients on neuroleptics for tardive movement disorders or to document their progress (Munetz and Benjamin 1988).

Other Movement Disorder Emergencies

Parkinsonism Hyperpyrexia Syndrome

Parkinsonism hyperpyrexia syndrome is a rare condition that can occur when antiparkinsonian, muscle relaxant, or antidystonia medications are suddenly stopped or reduced. It may also develop when deep brain stimulation is deactivated. Symptoms include fever, rigidity, delirium, dysautonomia, and elevated creatine kinase levels, which can resemble neuroleptic malignant syndrome. If left untreated, the syndrome can progress and become fatal. Patients require close observation and admission to critical care units. Treatment involves resuming necessary therapy, such as levodopa (by nasogastric tube if necessary), and providing supportive care (Rajan et al. 2019).

Neuroleptic Malignant Syndrome

Neuroleptic malignant syndrome is a serious complication of treatment with dopamine blockers. It presents similarly to parkinsonism-hyperpyrexia but with additional symptoms such as catatonia (see Chapter 3, "Neurological Approach to Psychiatric Presentations"), mutism, and metabolic derangements including transaminitis, highly elevated creatine kinase, hypocalcemia, hypomagnesemia, and elevated acute-phase reactants. The offending agent should be discontinued promptly and symptomatic treatment provided. Supportive treatment includes cooling measures and intravenous fluids; therapeutic options include benzodiazepines, dantrolene (for hyperthermia and rhabdomyolysis from rigidity), bromocriptine, or amantadine (Rajan et al. 2019).

Serotonin Syndrome

Serotonin syndrome, which can be fatal if not promptly treated, results from excessive serotonin transmission, often due to drug–drug interactions or polypharmacy. It presents with symptoms such as fever, confusion, agitation, shivering, tremor, and diarrhea. Distinguishing features include myoclonus and hyperreflexia. Diagnosis can be aided by the Hunter Serotonin Toxicity Criteria (Dunkley et al. 2003). Treatment involves discontinuing the offending agent and providing supportive care. Cyproheptadine, a serotonin antagonist, may also be considered as a treatment option.

A Word of Caution in the Diagnosis of Functional Movement Disorders

Patients with functional movement disorders experience involuntary movements with characteristics like distractibility and entrainment. It is a clinical diagnosis based on positive signs, not exclusion, with biomarkers supporting but not necessary for diagnosis. Interrater reliability for functional movement disorder diagnosis is more than 90%. Sometimes, however, functional movement disorders are later found to have a neurogenic etiology. For example, individuals with genetic mutations causing paroxysmal movement disorders were often told that their symptoms were functional before the syndrome was identified and the gene isolated. See Chapter 10, "Functional Neurological Disorder."

Case Example, Continued

The patient has a prominent postural tremor and left-greater-than-right action tremor during finger-to-nose testing. The fourth and fifth digits of her right hand tend to splay out. There may be a rest tremor in the right hand. The tone is slightly increased in her right arm greater than the left arm. She has a slightly stooped posture and reduced arm swing with the right arm, and she has trouble taking a sip of water without using both hands. Her tremor is present with action, impedes skilled movements, and responds to alcohol and propranolol, supporting a diagnosis of essential tremor. However, people with essential tremor have an increased risk of developing Parkinson disease. The presence of dream enactment, asymmetric bradykinesia, and rigidity are consistent with parkinsonism, and there are no red flag symptoms for atypical parkinsonism. The preceding 15 years of tremor are inconsistent with pure iPD, so she likely has a concurrent diagnosis of essential tremor.

A levodopa challenge yields improvements in bradykinesia and rigidity, but not the tremor. A DaTScan confirms iPD. Treatment options are directed for both essential tremor and iPD and include propranolol, primidone, amantadine, or deep brain stimulation. The patient is connected to multidisciplinary care and counseled on the importance of aerobic exercise to slow disease progression and maintain quality of life.

Key Clinical Points

- Essential tremor is the most common cause of postural and action tremors but needs to be distinguished from cerebellar outflow, enhanced physiologic, drug-induced, and parkinsonian tremors. It can sometimes evolve into idiopathic Parkinson disease (iPD).
- Non-motor symptoms of iPD can be as debilitating as motor symptoms and can often precede motor symptoms by 10 years.
- iPD, dementia with Lewy bodies, and multiple system atrophy are synucleinopathies. Progressive supranuclear palsy, corticobasal syndrome, motor neuron disease, primary progressive aphasia, and frontotemporal dementia are tauopathies.
- Myoclonus occurs in several neurologic conditions but often reflects medication toxicity.
- The differential diagnosis of choreiform movements includes genetic causes, the most common of which are Huntington disease and Wilson disease; drug-induced dyskinesias; chorea gravidarum; and other less common conditions.
- Always determine whether iron repletion is needed when treating restless leg syndrome (RLS). The $\alpha 2\delta$ ligands, gabapentin and pregabalin, are first-line treatments for RLS. Dopamine agonists will eventually result in symptom augmentation.
- Acute drug-induced movement disorders include acute dystonic reaction, tremor, parkinsonism, neuroleptic malignant, and serotonin syndrome. The latter two can be life-threatening.
- Tardive dyskinesia can manifest as choreoathetosis (most common), akathisia, dystonia, parkinsonism, tics, or myoclonus.

Review Questions

1. A 38-year-old patient whose uncle had dementia and a movement disorder presents with choreiform movements, hepatomegaly, seizures, and depression that have gradually increased over 10 years. On examination, the patient has glossal and perioral scarring and diminished deep tendon reflexes. The complete blood count revealed abnormal-appearing red blood cells. Which of the following diagnoses is most likely?

   A. Huntington disease
   B. Juvenile Parkinson disease

C. Neurodegeneration with brain iron accumulation
D. Neuroacanthocytosis
E. Wilson disease

2. A 21-year-old man being treated with high-dose olanzapine for schizophrenia suddenly develops upward eye movements and retrocollis associated with ocular discomfort. On request, he can bring his eyes down for a few seconds, but they quickly return to the upward position. Which of the following tests should be done before initiating treatment?

   A. Brain MRI
   B. EEG
   C. Lumbar puncture
   D. Genetic testing
   E. None of the above

3. An adolescent patient with schizophrenia who has required high-dose neuroleptic treatment for at least 5 years is being evaluated for choreoathetoid movements that have gradually increased in the past year. The patient has clearly declined from a higher level of function but has also been continuously psychotic. Which of the following disorders is most important to rule out before making the diagnosis of tardive dyskinesia?

   A. X-linked adrenoleukodystrophy
   B. Wilson disease
   C. 22q11 deletion syndrome
   D. Drug-induced parkinsonism
   E. Functional movement disorder

Answers

Question 1: D. Neuroacanthocytosis encompasses a group of conditions that differ from Huntington disease in that some of the red blood cells become acanthocytes (cells with spike-like projections). The syndrome in this vignette appears to represent chorea-acanthocytosis. Unlike Huntington disease, which is caused by a single genetic mutation, a number of different mutations have been associated with neuroacanthocytosis.

Question 2: E. The vignette clearly describes oculogyric crisis, an acute dystonic reaction to neuroleptic medications that is more common in young males. Treatment with intramuscular benztropine or diphenhydramine will resolve the symptoms and should not be delayed while additional tests are ordered.

Question 3: B. Wilson disease can present with psychosis, cognitive decline, and choreoathetoid movement disorder in adolescence. Examination may show hepatomegaly or jaundice. Hepatic enzymes may be elevated, 24-hour urine copper is increased, and serum ceruloplasmin is decreased.

References

Albanese A, Bhatia K, Bressman SB, et al: Phenomenology and classification of dystonia: a consensus update. Mov Disord 28(7):863–873, 2013 23649720

Allen RP, Picchietti DL, Auerbach M, et al: Evidence-based and consensus clinical practice guidelines for the iron treatment of restless legs syndrome/Willis-Ekbom disease in adults and children: an IRLSSG task force report. Sleep Med 41:27–44, 2018 29425576

Argyropoulos GPD, van Dun K, Adamaszek M, et al: The cerebellar cognitive affective/Schmahmann syndrome: a task force paper. Cerebellum 19(1):102–125, 2020 31522332

Bhatia KP, Bain P, Bajaj N, et al: Consensus Statement on the classification of tremors from the Task Force on Tremor of the International Parkinson and Movement Disorder Society. Mov Disord 33(1):75–87, 2018 29193359

Brusse E, Maat-Kievit JA, van Swieten JC: Diagnosis and management of early- and late-onset cerebellar ataxia. Clin Genet 71(1):12–24, 2007 17204042

Caviness JN: Myoclonus. Continuum (Minneap Minn) 25(4):1055–1080, 2019 31356293

Członkowska A, Litwin T, Dusek P, et al: Wilson disease. Nat Rev Dis Primers 4(1):21, 2018 30190489

Deik A, Saunders-Pullman R, Luciano MS: Substance of abuse and movement disorders: complex interactions and comorbidities. Curr Drug Abuse Rev 5(3):243–253, 2012 23030352

Dunkley EJ, Isbister GK, Sibbritt D, et al: The Hunter Serotonin Toxicity Criteria: simple and accurate diagnostic decision rules for serotonin toxicity. QJM 96(9):635–642, 2003 12925718

Espay AJ, Lang AE, Erro R, et al: Essential pitfalls in "essential" tremor. Mov Disord 32(3):325–331, 2017 28116753

Hauser RA, Meyer JM, Factor SA, et al: Differentiating tardive dyskinesia: a video-based review of antipsychotic-induced movement disorders in clinical practice. CNS Spectr 27(2):208–217, 2022 33213556

Hogarth P: Neurodegeneration with brain iron accumulation: diagnosis and management. J Mov Disord 8(1):1–13, 2015 25614780

Höglinger GU, Respondek G, Stamelou M, et al: Clinical diagnosis of progressive supranuclear palsy: The movement disorder society criteria. Mov Disord 32(6):853–864, 2017 28467028

Holmes G: The cerebellum of man. Brain 62(1):1–30, 1939

Jabbari E, Holland N, Chelban V, et al: Diagnosis across the spectrum of progressive supranuclear palsy and corticobasal syndrome. JAMA Neurol 77(3):377–387, 2020 31860007

Klockgether T, Mariotti C, Paulson HL: Spinocerebellar ataxia. Nat Rev Dis Primers 5(1):24, 2019 30975995

Louis ED, Bares M, Benito-Leon J, et al: Essential tremor-plus: a controversial new concept. Lancet Neurol 19(3):266–270, 2020 31767343

Manconi M, Garcia-Borreguero D, Schormair B, et al: Restless legs syndrome. Nat Rev Dis Primers 7(1):80, 2021 34732752

Marras C, Beck JC, Bower JH, et al: Prevalence of Parkinson's disease across North America. NPJ Parkinsons Dis 4(1):21, 2018 30003140

McAuley J, Rothwell J: Identification of psychogenic, dystonic, and other organic tremors by a coherence entrainment test. Mov Disord 19(3):253–267, 2004 15022179

McKeith IG, Boeve BF, Dickson DW, et al: Diagnosis and management of dementia with Lewy bodies: Fourth Consensus Report of the DLB Consortium. Neurology 89(1):88–100, 2017 28592453

Munetz MR, Benjamin S: How to examine patients using the Abnormal Involuntary Movement Scale. Hosp Community Psychiatry 39(11):1172–1177, 1988 2906320

Postuma RB, Berg D, Stern M, et al: MDS clinical diagnostic criteria for Parkinson's disease. Mov Disord 30(12):1591–1601, 2015 26474316

Rajan S, Kaas B, Moukheiber E: Movement disorders emergencies. Semin Neurol 39(1):125–136, 2019 30743298

Roessner V, Eichele H, Stern JS, et al: European clinical guidelines for Tourette syndrome and other tic disorders-version 2.0. Part III: pharmacological treatment. Eur Child Adolesc Psychiatry 31(3):425–441, 2022 34757514

Ryan J, Rosales R, Rowe E: A review of response interruption and redirection: 2007–2021. Behav Interv 37(4):1206–1236, 2022

Shukla T, Pandey S: Stereotypies in adults: a systematic review. Neurol Neurochir Pol 54(4):294–304, 2020 32706097

van de Wardt J, van der Stouwe AMM, Dirkx M, et al: Systematic clinical approach for diagnosing upper limb tremor. J Neurol Neurosurg Psychiatry 91(8):822–830, 2020 32457087

Wenning GK, Kiechl S, Seppi K, et al: Prevalence of movement disorders in men and women aged 50-89 years (Bruneck Study cohort): a population-based study. Lancet Neurol 4(12):815–820, 2005 16297839

Wenning GK, Stankovic I, Vignatelli L, et al: The Movement Disorder Society criteria for the diagnosis of multiple system atrophy. Mov Disord 37(6):1131–1148, 2022 35445419

10

Functional Neurological Disorder

Kevin Kyle, M.B.B.Ch.
David L. Perez, M.D., M.M.Sc.

Case Example

A 39-year-old woman with a history of anxiety, PTSD, and fibromyalgia is referred for assessment of intermittent tremor in the arms, abnormal gait, and numbness. Symptom onset was acute, 1 day after receiving the flu vaccine. She had previously been treated with anxiolytic medication that was discontinued years ago. She had seen a psychologist many years prior. She reports suffering from long-standing anxiety, including panic attacks, although these symptoms have been less active recently. She alludes to childhood maltreatment and more recent stressors at work related to workload and several difficult workplace interactions. On review of systems, she endorses persistent fatigue, diffuse pain, and constipation.

Functional neurological disorder (FND) is a prevalent and disabling biopsychosocially informed condition at the intersection of neurology and psychiatry, with a vast array of presentations. The overarching disorder that we now denote as FND has been known by many different names and iterations. After being of great interest to early clinical leaders in neurology and psychiatry such as Charcot, Freud, Briquet, and Babinski, the disorder was relatively neglected for most of the twentieth century. In recent years, there has been renewed interest in part because of progress in clinical education, the establishment of a dedicated professional society, and advances in the understanding of FND pathophysiology (Aybek and Perez 2022; Stone et al. 2010, 2011). In 2013, DSM-5 (American Psychiatric Association 2013) reframed the diagnosis of FND based on positive "rule-in" clinical signs (DSM-IV [American Psychiatric Association 1994] framed FND as a diagnosis of exclusion). FND is common, at times disabling, and costly in terms of health care utilization (Stephen et al. 2021).

This chapter focuses on four subtypes of FND: functional movement disorder (including functional weakness); functional (psychogenic non-epileptic/dissociative) seizures; functional cognitive disorder; and persistent postural perceptual dizziness (PPPD).

FND Mechanisms

Risk Factors: The Biopsychosocial Model

Risk factors for the development of FND are considered using a biopsychosocial model (Finkelstein et al. 2022; Saxena et al. 2022). An array of predisposing, precipitating, and perpetuating factors within this model have been identified for FND, although these factors can vary substantially from patient to patient. The summary that follows is not exhaustive but does highlight important factors to consider (McKee et al. 2018; Saxena et al. 2020).

Biological predisposing factors include female sex, comorbid neurological disorders (e.g., migraine headaches, mild traumatic brain injury), intellectual disability, and comorbid functional somatic disorders (e.g., fibromyalgia, irritable bowel syndrome). Precipitating biological factors can include essentially any abnormal physiological event, including pain, injury, or surgery. Perpetuating biological factors include increased physiological arousal, chronic pain, fatigue, abnormal motor habits, and deconditioning, in addition to superimposed medical/neurological comorbidities.

Predisposing psychological factors include mood and anxiety disorders, PTSD, dissociation, and maladaptive personality traits. Psychiatric disorders are often biological in nature but in this context are considered a psychological factor. Precipitating psychological factors include emotional responses to injury, acute dissociation, and panic attacks. Perpetuating psychological factors include negative expectation and attentional bias, in addition to the influences of illness beliefs, perception of symptom irreversibility, or attribution to another cause.

Psychosocial predisposition includes chronic illness in the family, abnormal family dynamics, major adverse life experiences (including childhood maltreatment), and poor social support (Ludwig et al. 2018). Precipitating factors can include bereavement, relational stress, divorce, and occupational difficulties, for example (Morsy et al. 2022). Perpetuating psychosocial factors include provider diagnostic uncertainty, limited patient/family/caregiver diagnostic buy-in, social benefits of illness, ongoing litigation, disability claims, and personal or employer urgency to return to work.

Pathophysiology

The understanding of FND pathophysiology has been enhanced in recent years with the use of functional brain imaging: positron emission tomography (PET), functional magnetic resonance imaging (fMRI), and electrophysiologic studies (Baizabal-Carvallo et al. 2019). Key concepts implicated in the neurobiology of FND are disturbances in self-agency, attention, prediction, and threat processing. Myriad anatomical foci and neural circuits have been implicated to date; thus, FND is now portrayed as a multinetwork disorder.

In functional imaging studies, the overriding patterns that have been identified include alterations in brain areas/networks implicated in motor planning, feed-forward monitoring, self-awareness, and interoception, along with patterns of aberrant motor (salience/limbic network and right temporoparietal junction) and sensorimotor network connectivity (Janzen et al. 2012; Perez et al. 2021b).

Identification of abnormal cerebral activation in foci implicated in motor preparation and suppression of planning have included the supplementary motor area (SMA) and the pre-SMA. Variation in left SMA activity has been observed in patients with functional movement disorders by PET. fMRI studies have demonstrated decreased activity of the right temporoparietal junction in patients with functional movement disorders. This brain area detects mismatches between the expected sensory consequences of behavior and actual outcomes, thereby playing a role in self-agency (action-authorship perceptions). The cingulate gyrus, another multimodal integration area implicated in emotion processing and motor inhibition, has been demonstrated to have increased activity. Abnormal patterns of amygdala activation and increased functional connectivity between the amygdala and SMA, as well as the amygdala and periaqueductal gray, have also been reported.

The influence of genetic/epigenetic and structural variation continues to be investigated, including potential roles in predisposing to the development of FND. Other broad concepts implicated include a state of hyperarousal, both physiologically and psychologically, as well as the possibility of alterations in the acquisition, refinement, and use of emotion concepts (Jungilligens et al. 2022). There is evidence of abnormal somatosensory processing in electrophysiological studies showing decreased sensory attention. This may compromise agency since internally generated stimuli can potentially be interpreted as externally generated. More research is needed to comprehensively detail the roles of genetics, epigenetics, and structural neuroanatomy in FND pathophysiology.

Approach to Patients With Functional Neurological Disorder

As with all initial consultations, the interview starts by openly inquiring about the patient's main concerns. A diagnostically open-minded approach is pivotal. If a patient has specifically been referred for an opinion in an FND clinic, framing the consultation at the outset can be helpful. The reason for the referral should be established, followed by gauging patient expectations and goals. The role of the provider can be outlined: help confirm the diagnosis, guide any further investigations if relevant, and ultimately suggest appropriate therapeutic approaches.

Epidemiology

Demographic information can aid in the diagnostic formulation of FND. FND is more common in females but is certainly well recognized in men as well. The incidence rate of functional movement disorders is estimated at 4–5/100,000 per year, and that of functional seizures at 1.5–4.9/100,000 per year (Aybek and Perez 2022). FND usually begins in late teens through middle age, with the most common age distribution from the 20s through the 40s, though it can present in any age group (Lidstone et al. 2022; Perez et al. 2021a). The age at onset of specific symptoms can provide pertinent information for diagnostic formulation; for instance, taking note of atypical late onset of tics or early-onset parkinsonism.

Clinical History

The chronological patient narrative forms the basis of the history of the presenting complaint. Inquiring about the tempo of symptoms is important; FND symptoms often present suddenly, with maximal severity in a narrow time frame. In terms of symptom duration, FND can be endorsed as rather long-lasting, although at times with periods of spontaneous remission.

The phenomenology of both functional movement disorder and functional seizures may fluctuate, evolve, and spread to different body parts. Comorbid neurological disorders, pain, fatigue, sleep, or cognitive symptoms may be endorsed, as well as functional somatic syndromes (e.g., fibromyalgia, irritable bowel syndrome). As stated previously, there may be a coexistent structural neurological disorder (e.g., a subset of patients with Parkinson disease will have a functional movement disorder; 1 in 5 patients with functional seizures also has epileptic seizures) (Kutlubaev et al. 2018; Wissel et al. 2018). As with the review of systems, a history of a multitude of allergies, while nonspecific, is prevalent in FND (Saxena et al. 2020).

There may be a family history of neurological disorder. Furthermore, although it is infrequently identified, there may even be a family history of FND, particularly a functional movement disorder (Stamelou et al. 2013). Family history may also be pertinent regarding certain movement disorders such as tics, whereas a family history of tics may be notably absent in functional tics. Functional tic–like behaviors have been increasingly characterized over the last several years (Martino et al. 2023).

Precipitating events often occur in the categories of biological and psychosocial. Precipitating events are present in many but not all cases (described in as many as 80% of functional movement disorder cases). Emotional and physical triggers can also coexist. Potential triggers may be contemporaneous to FND, occurring within minutes or days, or may be weeks or even months before FND onset. Physical triggers include but are not limited to physical injury, infection, perceived medication reaction, and surgery. In functional dystonia, preceding limb injury or surgery are common. Emotional triggers vary broadly, including major life events, bereavement, and difficult interpersonal interactions.

Psychiatric and Psychosocial History

The clinical interview for a suspected case of FND benefits from a dedicated psychiatric and psychosocial screen. If there is an established history of diagnosed psychiatric conditions, one should outline the duration and course of these symptoms, prior hospitalizations, and significant treatment modalities. One should also clarify whether the patient has a current psychiatrist and psychotherapist.

The most common coexistent psychiatric disorders include mood, anxiety, PTSD, and dissociative disorders. Additionally, there may be a history of suicidal ideation or attempts. Underlying personality disorders may include, but are not limited to, obsessive-compulsive, borderline, and dependent.

In reviewing the psychosocial history, it can be helpful to transparently point out to the patient that such a transition is being made. Consider asking about developmental history, education, work, and relationship histories, and inquire about litigation, disability status, legal concerns, hobbies, driving status, and adverse life experiences.

In terms of psychosocial factors, childhood maltreatment is common, including sexual, physical, and emotional abuse. Other relevant factors can include neglect or parental divorce, among many other major life events. Note that adverse life experiences are not universally present; if inquiring about the possibility of such experiences, it is important to do so sensitively.

Clinical Features

The examination begins before the patient enters the office, with general observation of movements and gait from the waiting room to the office. General signs of FND include suggestibility, variability, and distractibility (Aybek and Perez 2022; Perez et al. 2021a; Stone et al. 2011). Table 10.1 reviews the clinical signs of FND. Suggestibility refers to the onset or worsening of signs when they are being discussed or on approaching the affected area during the clinical exam. Variability refers to changes in the amplitude, velocity, phenomenology, or strength of a movement or change in sensory distribution. Distractibility refers to the tendency for movements to be diminished or abated by cognitive or motor distraction techniques.

Table 10.1 Clinical signs and symptoms of functional neurological disorder

Signs and symptoms	Description
General	
Distractibility	Symptoms can be diminished by motor or cognitive distraction (see Video 10.2)
Variability	Prominent feature fluctuation (see Video 10.2)
Suggestibility	Signs can be precipitated by suggestion, during discussion or examination
Convergence spasm	Transient convergence with miosis followed by dysconjugate gaze pattern that mimics abducens palsy, observed on asking patient to follow finger into midline
Motor	
Give-way weakness	Non-pain-limited weakness, initially fully strong and then rapidly gives out
Arm drift	Downward drift without pronation (see Video 10.1)
Motor inconsistency	A muscle group is weak when tested directly, but voluntary action is strong when tested indirectly via involuntary action
Hoover sign	Weakness of hip extension is overcome by simultaneously testing contralateral hip flexion
Hip abductor sign	Hip abductor weakness is overcome by bilateral simultaneous hip abductor testing
Co-contraction sign	No movement is seen in muscle being tested owing to co-contraction of agonist and antagonist muscles
Movements	
Tremor entrainment	Tremor changes to match the rhythm of finger tapping by the examiner (see Video 10.3)
Weight loading	Amplitude of movement increases when weight is added
Whack-a-mole sign	Tremor spreads to another area of body when tremulous limb is restrained

Table 10.1 Clinical signs and symptoms of functional neurological disorder (*continued*)

Signs and symptoms	Description
Jerks	Axial, distractible, variable
Dystonia	Fixed posture, lack of *geste antagoniste*
Tic	Lack of typical premonition, lack of relief from performing tic, not stereotyped
Gait	
Noneconomic	Demonstrable gait dysfunction that requires intact coordination
Dragging monoplegic	Dragging a leg in a fixed position, like a plank of wood
Knee buckling	Sudden knee give-way without falling
Chair sign	Patient is able to powerfully propel forward while in a chair despite apparent major gait dysfunction
Functional Romberg	Oscillation with Romberg sign is abated with cognitive distraction such as figuring out what number is being drawn on their back
Seizure	
Long duration	Over 2 minutes
Retained awareness	Postictal recall of ictal events; ictal eye contact and response to stimuli
Specific ictal activities	Forced eye closure, pelvic thrusting, asynchronous limb movements, ictal crying
Rapid recovery	Absence of postictal confusion

Functional Movement Disorder

Functional Weakness

The peripheral motor examination can begin with checking for upper-extremity downward drift, typically without pronation (Video 10.1). (To access all videos mentioned in this book, go to https://www.appi.

org/Benjamin.) Functional weakness can have iterations of give-way/collapsing weakness; this entails initially intact strength against resistance for a moment, which then suddenly gives out or decrements. Caution should be taken, however, to screen for pain-limited weakness, which can give rise to a similar pattern.

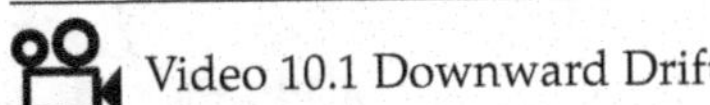

Motor inconsistency is a specific sign of functional limb weakness. This refers to demonstrable variability in motor strength on observation and on performing different examination techniques. The Hoover sign, illustrated in Figure 10.1, is one such technique. It is elicited by first demonstrating apparent hip extensor weakness on isolated limb examination. However, when simultaneously testing hip flexion in the contralateral, strong leg, full strength is now demonstrated in the previously weak limb's hip extension. The hip abductor sign entails apparent weakness of hip abduction when tested unilaterally; however, with bilateral, simultaneous testing, full strength is demonstrated. Motor inconsistency can also be demonstrated on observation, wherein confrontation testing yields weakness or lack of movement, despite voluntary movement of the same limb or muscle group being observed during other actions, such as standing, ambulating, or putting on clothing or shoes. Co-contraction may also be seen in functional limb weakness, wherein no significant gross movement is exhibited in the muscle group being tested due to simultaneous contraction of agonist and antagonist muscles.

Functional Gait

At its core, functional gait (sometimes referred to as "astasia abasia") consists of a non-economical gait pattern. Although objectively abnormal in terms of the apparent degree of deviation or appearance of nearly falling, this gait actually requires intact strength and coordination to achieve. Knee-buckling consists of sudden give-way weakness at the knees without falling. Dragging monoplegic gait may also be observed wherein the weak limb is dragged along the ground rather than circumducted. In the chair sign, there is marked gait dysfunction on ambulating independently; however, the patient is able to propel a chair with wheels better than would be expected, to an extent that is inconsistent with the initial gait exam.

Hoover sign in supine position

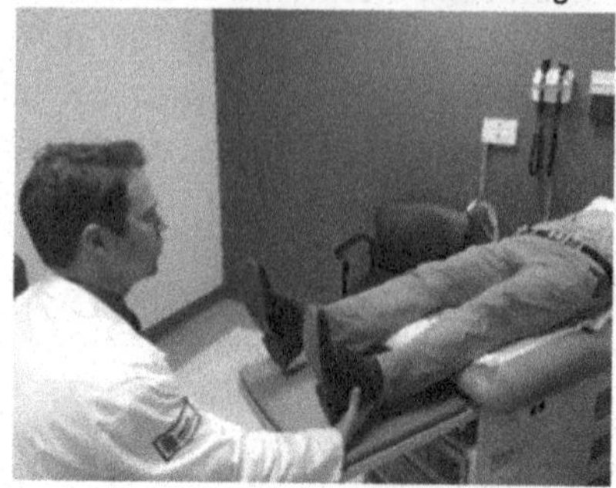

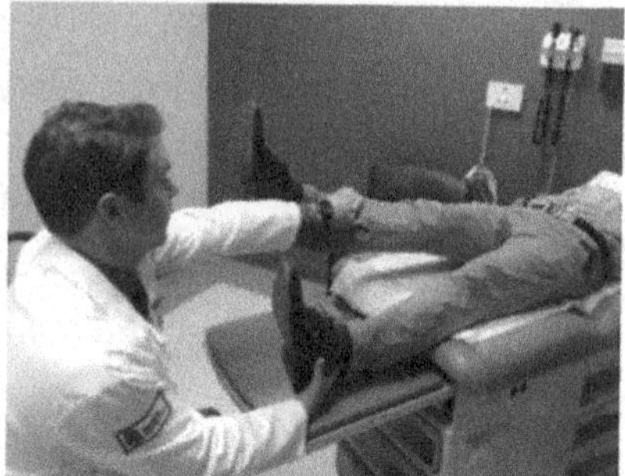

Hoover sign in seated position

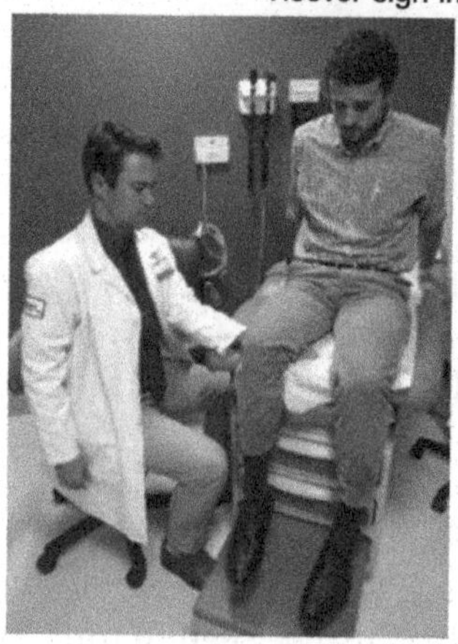

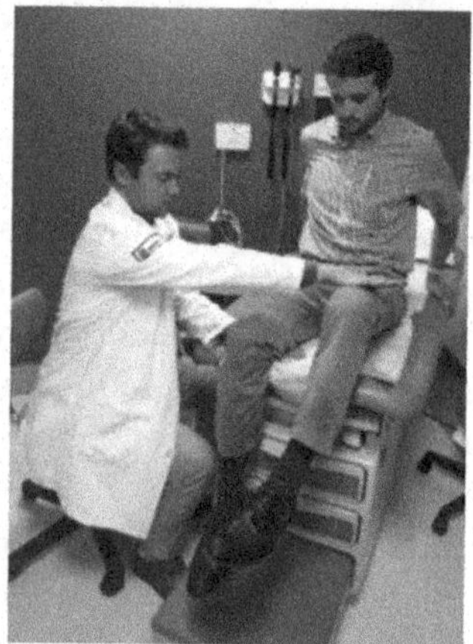

Figure 10.1 Hoover sign.

Source. Anderson JR, Nakhate V, Stephen CD, et al: Functional (Psychogenic) Neurological Disorders: Assessment and Acute Management in the Emergency Department. Semin Neurol 39(1):102–114, 2019. Copyright © 2019. Used with permission.

The functional Romberg sign consists of oscillation while standing with eyes closed, although often without falling. Upon performing this with cognitive distraction of figure or number drawing on the back, the truncal oscillation diminishes or abates. A video library of functional gaits is available (Nonnekes et al. 2020).

Functional Tremor

Functional tremor has variable phenomenology; velocity, amplitude, and position dependence can fluctuate. Functional tremor can be observed in the limbs or trunk or both and can be unilateral, bilateral, or observed in a generalized fashion. It can be increased in amplitude with weight loading. Tremor distraction can be observed by performing contralateral motor tasks such as asking the patient to tap to the examiner's rhythm or by performing more ballistic movements with the contralateral hand (Video 10.2). Cognitive distraction can include performing serial subtraction or performing the Luria task. Entrainment is the phenomenon of the tremor adopting the velocity/rhythm of the examiner's tapping (Video 10.3). The whack-a-mole sign consists of the dispersion of the tremor to other body sites when the tremulous limb is restrained. In particularly challenging cases, surface electromyography (EMG) or accelerometry data may aid diagnosis by demonstrating objective evidence of distractibility and entrainment (Lidstone and Lang 2020).

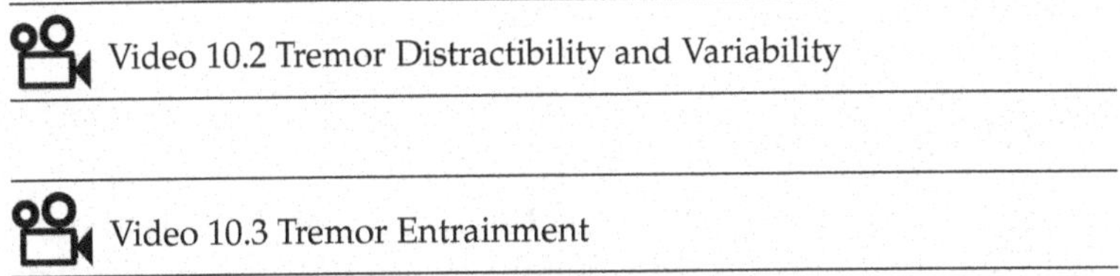

Video 10.2 Tremor Distractibility and Variability

Video 10.3 Tremor Entrainment

Functional Dystonia

Functional dystonia also often presents suddenly with maximal severity, in contrast to neurogenic dystonia (ND) (Frucht et al. 2021). Functional dystonia is frequently associated with preceding limb injury, with considerable overlap with coexistent pain and even complex regional pain syndrome. The dystonia is often fixed, unlike the typically dynamic or task-specific elements of ND. There may be variability in the muscle groups involved between attacks, more so than the stereotyped nature of ND. Rapid spread from focal to multifocal or generalized dystonia can be seen in functional dystonia.

In functional dystonia, there may not be a typical sensory trick, or *geste antagoniste*, that temporarily alleviates the dystonia as in ND. In terms of lower-extremity involvement, foot plantar flexion and inversion does not habituate with walking backward in ND. Specific signs include the "other" Babinski sign (ipsilateral eyebrow raise with eye closure) in neurogenic hemifacial spasm (HFS), which is absent in functional HFS. The striatal toe sign is the dorsiflexion of the great toe classically due to damage to the caudate or putamen. In functional dystonia, passive extension of digits 2 through 5 can give rise to great toe plantar flexion.

Functional Myoclonus

Functional jerks or myoclonus also demonstrate features of variability in velocity, amplitude, and phenomenology that are not typically seen in other forms of myoclonus (Perez et al. 2021a). Functional jerks are more commonly axial. As with other functional movement disorder phenotypes, functional jerks are distractible. Surface EMG can aid the diagnosis of functional myoclonus by demonstrating variability in distal latencies and in muscle recruitment and habituation with repetition. Furthermore, EEG may demonstrate the presence of the *Bereitschaftspotential*, or motor planning potential, objectively exhibiting engagement of voluntary motor pathways in functional jerks.

Functional Tics

The clinical phenomenology of functional tics can be revealing; as opposed to neurogenic tics, functional tics are not usually preceded by a premonitory urge. Furthermore, there is an absence of the typical sense of relief after performing the functional tic (Perez et al. 2021a). Functional tics can vary, lacking the typically stereotyped nature of neurogenic tics. Additionally, functional tics cannot usually be momentarily suppressed in contrast to neurogenic tics.

Functional Seizures

Certain semiological features of functional seizures can be specific and indicative of the diagnosis (Baslet et al. 2021). For example, functional seizures do not tend to occur during physiological sleep. Recall of events or items during the seizure, wherein there was apparent impaired awareness or amnesia, is reported in functional seizures. Functional seizures also tend to be relatively long in duration, without a commensurate postictal period, in contrast to prolonged epileptic seizures or status epilepticus. During the event, specific features of functional seizures include eye closure (including forced closure against resistance), asynchronous limb movements (also seen in supplementary motor seizures), and side-to-side movements (Muthusamy et al. 2022). Pelvic thrusting is more commonly exhibited in functional seizures, but caution should be taken with this sign to not miss a case of frontal lobe epilepsy. Anxiety, PTSD, substance abuse, and personality disorders are more prevalent in functional seizures than in epilepsy.

The aforementioned semiological features can be specific, but sensitivity is variable. Diagnosis can be facilitated by the gold standard method of video EEG (vEEG) capturing one or more events (LaFrance et al. 2013). A brief routine EEG lasting 20–40 minutes may not be sufficient to capture an event; however, sensitivity is greater with a continuous vEEG over 24–72 hours. Induction techniques such as hyperventilation and photic stimulation may be useful and less ethically dubious than placebo injection.

Other FND Phenotypes

Persistent Postural Perceptual Dizziness

PPPD, or functional dizziness, is a phenomenon that has been described relatively recently (Hallett et al. 2022; Staab 2020). It entails a symptom constellation of non-vertiginous, non-syncopal dizziness or disequilibrium. It can be preceded by index dizziness syndromes of vestibular migraine, head injury, or benign positional vertigo. Clinical criteria have been outlined to guide diagnosis. It is described as a non-spinning dizziness or unsteadiness, present on most days for about 3 months, waxing and waning throughout the day, and lasting hours at a time. Symptoms can persist without provocation but are exacerbated by upright posture, active or passive motion, and moving or complex visual stimuli. Dizziness may be triggered by other events that cause dizziness or unsteadiness, including vestibular syndromes, neurological diagnoses, and psychological distress. Symptoms can cause emotional distress and are not better explained by other diseases.

Functional Cognitive Disorder

Functional cognitive disorder (FCD) is likely to be prevalent, though it is contended that this aspect of FND has been underrecognized and underresearched (Ball et al. 2020). The hallmark of FCD is internal inconsistency, marked by the ability to perform cognitive tasks at one time and an impaired ability to perform the same tasks at another time. So-called internal inconsistency can be supported by the observation of inconsistencies during the clinical interview versus performance on exams; the ability to continue performing at a high level professionally or academically; greater concern by the individual than a collateral historian; and evident inconsistencies on formal neuropsychological exams. The diagnostic criteria consist of one or more symptoms of impaired cognitive function, clinical evidence of internal inconsistency, symptoms not being better explained by another medical or psychiatric disorder, and symptoms causing significant distress or impairment.

Management

The initial step in the management of FND is communication of the diagnosis. It is advisable to explain the diagnosis at the outset of patient counseling, once the provider has completed a comprehensive assessment and is confident of the diagnosis (Stone et al. 2016). The current consensus is to lead by discussing why FND is ruled in on the basis of positive signs, symptoms, and supportive data, rather than listing FND as a diagnostic suspicion after reviewing the excluded differential diagnoses (Carson et al. 2016). Framing FND as a diagnosis of inclusion can help increase the patient's diagnostic confidence.

The management of FND should be individualized using a patient-centered, biopsychosocial-informed approach to clinical care. The timing of referral to multidisciplinary team services is highly pertinent and is generally executed when there is a degree of insight or understanding of the FND diagnosis. If the patient agrees with the referral to each team member, they are more likely to engage in the relevant therapy process.

Psychotherapy Approaches

Cognitive-behavioral therapy (CBT) has the most evidence as a psychotherapeutic approach for FND, although there is a smaller body of evidence for psychodynamic therapy and a range of other psychotherapy interventions (Gutkin et al. 2020). In terms of CBT for functional seizures, evidence comes from a multicenter randomized controlled trial that revealed improvement in the longest period of seizure freedom at 12 months, psychosocial functioning, self- and clinician-rated global change, and treatment satisfaction, although no statistically significant improvement in monthly seizure frequency was seen (Goldstein et al. 2020). Certain characteristics, such as a greater burden of psychiatric comorbidities, may predict increased responsiveness to CBT.

In certain circumstances, the choice of psychotherapy may also be tailored to individual patient needs. For instance, there may be a role for prolonged exposure therapy as a specific type of skills-based psychotherapy for patients with functional seizures and PTSD (Myers et al. 2017). In those with functional seizures and co-existing borderline personality disorder, dialectical behavioral therapy may be an appropriate choice (Bullock et al. 2015).

Although CBT has the most evidence at this stage, access to care remains a major issue, secondary to considerable need paired with resource limitations. Self-guided CBT may be an option for some patients (Sharpe et al. 2011). Several psychotherapy manuals are currently available for FND and functional seizures specifically (LaFrance Jr. and Wincze 2015; Reiter et al. 2015; Williams et al. 2017).

Rehabilitation

Neurologic physical therapy is indicated for functional movement disorder. Expert consensus recommendations outline physical therapy for functional motor symptoms, and evidence from randomized controlled trials shows the efficacy of physical therapy in this population (Nielsen et al. 2015; Jordbru et al. 2014).

Important aspects of the physical therapy approaches in treatment include providing patient education and improving understanding of FND. Affirming and demonstrating the patient's positive FND signs as an introduction illustrates the potential for improvement. The principle of retraining normal movement through diverted attention or distraction works most powerfully with a series of task-oriented exercises.

Occupational therapy can be useful for functional motor and sensory symptoms (Nicholson et al. 2020). Patients should understand and agree with the diagnosis and should have identifiable rehabilitation goals. Occupational therapy approaches can broadly include rehabilitation goal setting, FND education, and vocational rehabilitation. The primary focus of occupational therapy is to restore function through rehabilitation. For patients who continue to experience disability despite initial efforts to restore normal movement and motor function, however, time-limited assistance devices may be considered with ongoing monitoring. Aids and other adaptations are generally avoided to mitigate the potential for interrupting normal automatic movement patterns or encouraging maladaptive patterns. Occupational therapy interventions may also have roles for other aspects of FND, such as the assessment and management of sensory processing difficulties (MacLean et al. 2022).

Expert consensus recommendations also exist for speech and language therapy for functional communication, swallowing, and other related upper-airway disorders (Baker et al. 2021). Patient understanding and insight regarding FND is pivotal. In addition to published consensus recommendations for the use of physical therapy, occupational therapy, and speech and language therapy in FND, more clinical research is needed to further refine the rehabilitative therapeutic toolkit for this population. Several published comprehensive reviews discuss treatment interventions in FND (Finkelstein et al. 2022; Hallett et al. 2022; Lafaver et al. 2021).

Case Example, Continued

The patient's clinical examination is significant for right arm posturing and an action tremor present intermittently and becoming more prominent during movement examination. The tremor is variable in amplitude and velocity. When the right hand is restrained, a low-amplitude tremor begins in the left arm. The tremor entrains to the rhythm of the examiner's finger taps. The tremor momentarily ceases while the patient performs contralateral finger taps, contralateral ballistic movements, and serial 7 subtractions. The tremor also increases in amplitude while she holds objects in her right hand. She exhibits left-sided facial and hemibody sensory decrement to pinprick that splits the midline. She stands unassisted and exhibits frequent oscillation with casual and tandem gait, deviating toward the examiner and the wall without falling. She can walk backward more consistently. On Romberg testing, the patient deviates significantly without falling. On repeat Romberg testing while performing graphesthesia testing on the patient's back, the truncal deviation fully abates.

This patient is exhibiting functional tremor and gait disturbance. She has positive signs of suggestibility, marked by tremor on approaching the movement portion of the examination. The tremor is variable in phenomenology, entrainable, and distractible. The tremor also increases in amplitude with weight loading and exhibits a positive whack-a-mole sign. She exhibits a non-economical gait, wherein prominent deviations are seen, without falling, to the extent that coordination must be intact. She exhibits a functional Romberg sign.

The sudden symptom onset is consistent with FND. Predisposing psychosocial factors include anxiety, PTSD, fibromyalgia, and remote history of abuse. Precipitating factors include contemporaneous workplace stress and the temporal proximity to the vaccine, suggesting the potential influence of a nocebo effect.

She was educated about the diagnosis of FND and was shown the positive examination findings. She initially expressed concern and doubt about the diagnosis but was provided with educational resources from www.neurosymptoms.org and offered close follow-up. On follow-up, she reported an improved understanding of FND and wished to commence treatment. Given her symptom complex, she was referred for physical therapy and CBT. She pursued these therapies; on follow-up, she had some initial improvement in tremor and gait.

Key Clinical Points

- Functional neurological disorder (FND) is a common and potentially disabling condition at the intersection of neurology and psychiatry.
- There has been a transition toward diagnostic affirmation using "rule-in" signs.
- Diagnostic formulation should include a neuropsychiatric interview and formulation using the biopsychosocial model.
- A vast array of different presentations of FND include movement, seizure, sensory, speech/voice, dizziness, and cognitive symptoms.
- Education is the first step in treatment.
- Several skills-based psychotherapy manuals have been published for use in FND.
- Rehabilitation is generally recommended for functional motor symptoms, and multidisciplinary care should be implemented whenever possible.

Review Questions

1. A patient presents with weakness of the left arm and leg. Which of the following examination findings is *least* consistent with a functional neurological disorder?

   A. With eyes closed, the left arm pronates and drifts downward.
   B. Left hip abduction is weak when tested in isolation but strong when simultaneously abducting the right hip.
   C. Left hip extension is weak when tested in isolation but strong when simultaneously flexing the right hip.

D. The strength of the left arm is initially strong but then suddenly drops off during testing.
E. When the patient walks, the left foot and leg drag behind them.

2. A patient is diagnosed with psychogenic non-epileptic seizures. Which of the following is a mainstay of treatment?

   A. SSRI
   B. Physical therapy
   C. Occupational therapy
   D. Speech language therapy
   E. Psychotherapy

3. Which of the following factors has been shown to increase the risk for FND?

   A. Male sex
   B. Febrile illness
   C. Currently in puberty
   D. Migraine
   E. Intense anger

Answers

Question 1: A. Pronator drift is a sign of neurogenic weakness. If the left arm did not pronate but only drifted down, this could be consistent with FND. The other choices are exam findings that may be found in FND: b) hip abductor sign, c) Hoover sign, d) give-way weakness, and e) dragging monoplegic sign. In neurogenic weakness, the left leg would circumduct rather than drag behind.

Question 2: E. Psychotherapy including cognitive-behavioral therapy (CBT) is the first line for management. Specialized workbooks have been developed for CBT treatment of non-epileptic seizures. In psychogenic non-epileptic seizures, patients often return to baseline between events, so there may be no deficits to target with physical, occupational, or speech therapy. SSRIs may be used for comorbid depression/anxiety but are not indicated for FND alone.

Question 3: D. Migraine has been shown to increase the risk of FND and to occur as a comorbid symptom in FND. FND is more common in females than males. None of the other answer choices have been shown to increase the risk of FND.

References

American Psychiatric Association: Diagnostic and Statistical Manual of Mental Disorders, 4th Edition. Washington, DC, American Psychiatric Association, 1994

American Psychiatric Association: Diagnostic and Statistical Manual of Mental Disorders, 5th Edition. Arlington, VA, American Psychiatric Association, 2013

Anderson JR, Nakhate V, Stephen CD, et al: Functional (psychogenic) neurological disorders: assessment and acute management in the emergency department. Semin Neurol 39(1):102–114, 2019

Aybek S, Perez DL: Diagnosis and management of functional neurological disorder. BMJ 376:o64, 2022 35074803

Baizabal-Carvallo JF, Hallett M, Jankovic J: Pathogenesis and pathophysiology of functional (psychogenic) movement disorders. Neurobiol Dis 127:32–44, 2019 30798005

Baker J, Barnett C, Cavalli L, et al: Management of functional communication, swallowing, cough and related disorders: consensus recommendations for speech and language therapy. J Neurol Neurosurg Psychiatry 92(10):1112–1125, 2021 34210802

Ball HA, McWhirter L, Ballard C, et al: Functional cognitive disorder: dementia's blind spot. Brain 143(10):2895–2903, 2020 32791521

Baslet G, Bajestan SN, Aybek S, et al: Evidence-based practice for the clinical assessment of psychogenic nonepileptic seizures: a report from the American Neuropsychiatric Association Committee on Research. J Neuropsychiatry Clin Neurosci 33(1):27–42, 2021 32778006

Bullock KD, Mirza N, Forte C, et al: Group dialectical-behavior therapy skills training for conversion disorder with seizures. J Neuropsychiatry Clin Neurosci 27(3):240–243, 2015 25959039

Carson A, Lehn A, Ludwig L, et al: Explaining functional disorders in the neurology clinic: a photo story. Pract Neurol 16(1):56–61, 2016 26769761

Finkelstein SA, Adams C, Tuttle M, et al: Neuropsychiatric treatment approaches for functional neurological disorder: a how to guide. Semin Neurol 42(2):204–224, 2022 35189644

Frucht L, Perez DL, Callahan J, et al: Functional dystonia: differentiation from primary dystonia and multidisciplinary treatments. Front Neurol 11:605262, 2021 33613415

Goldstein LH, Robinson EJ, Mellers JDC, et al: Cognitive behavioural therapy for adults with dissociative seizures (CODES): a pragmatic, multicentre, randomised controlled trial. Lancet Psychiatry 7(6):491–505, 2020 32445688

Gutkin M, McLean L, Brown R, et al: Systematic review of psychotherapy for adults with functional neurological disorder. J Neurol Neurosurg Psychiatry jnnp-2019-321926, 2020 33154184

Hallett M, Aybek S, Dworetzky BA, et al: Functional neurological disorder: new subtypes and shared mechanisms. Lancet Neurol 21(6):537–550, 2022 35430029

Janzen J, van 't Ent D, Lemstra AW, et al: The pedunculopontine nucleus is related to visual hallucinations in Parkinson's disease: preliminary results of a voxel-based morphometry study. J Neurol 259(1):147–154, 2012 21717194

Jordbru AA, Smedstad LM, Klungsøyr O, et al: Psychogenic gait disorder: a randomized controlled trial of physical rehabilitation with one-year follow-up. J Rehabil Med 46(2):181–187, 2014 24248149

Jungilligens J, Paredes-Echeverri S, Popkirov S, et al: A new science of emotion: implications for functional neurological disorder. Brain 145(8):2648–2663, 2022 35653495

Kutlubaev MA, Xu Y, Hackett ML, et al: Dual diagnosis of epilepsy and psychogenic nonepileptic seizures: systematic review and meta-analysis of frequency, correlates, and outcomes. Epilepsy Behav 89:70–78, 2018 30384103

Lafaver K, Lafrance WC, Price ME, et al: Treatment of functional neurological disorder: current state, future directions, and a research agenda. CNS Spectr December 7, 2021 33280634 Epub ahead of print

LaFrance WC Jr, Wincze JP: Treating Nonepileptic Seizures. New York, Oxford University Press, 2015

LaFrance WC Jr, Baker GA, Duncan R, et al: Minimum requirements for the diagnosis of psychogenic nonepileptic seizures: a staged approach: a report from the International League Against Epilepsy Nonepileptic Seizures Task Force. Epilepsia 54(11):2005–2018, 2013 24111933

Lidstone SC, Lang AE: How do I examine patients with functional tremor? Mov Disord Clin Pract 7(5):587, 2020 32626816

Lidstone SC, Costa-Parke M, Robinson EJ, et al: Functional movement disorder gender, age and phenotype study: a systematic review and individual patient meta-analysis of 4905 cases. J Neurol Neurosurg Psychiatry 93(6):609–616, 2022 35217516

Ludwig L, Pasman JA, Nicholson T, et al: Stressful life events and maltreatment in conversion (functional neurological) disorder: systematic review and meta-analysis of case-control studies. Lancet Psychiatry 5(4):307–320, 2018 29526521

MacLean J, Finkelstein SA, Paredes-Echeverri S, et al: Sensory processing difficulties in patients with functional neurological disorder: occupational therapy management strategies and two cases. Semin Pediatr Neurol 41(April):100951, 2022 35450672

Martino D, Hedderly T, Murphy T, et al: The spectrum of functional tic-like behaviours: data from an international registry. Eur J Neurol 30(2):334–343, 2023 36282623

McKee K, Glass S, Adams C, et al: The inpatient assessment and management of motor functional neurological disorders: an interdisciplinary perspective. Psychosomatics 59(4):358–368, 2018 29628294

Morsy SK, Aybek S, Carson A, et al: The relationship between types of life events and the onset of functional neurological (conversion) disorder in adults: a systematic review and meta-analysis. Psychol Med 52(3):401–418, 2022 34819179

Muthusamy S, Seneviratne U, Ding C, et al: Using semiology to classify epileptic seizures vs psychogenic nonepileptic seizures: a meta-analysis. Neurol Clin Pract 12(3):234–247, 2022 35747545

Myers L, Vaidya-Mathur U, Lancman M: Prolonged exposure therapy for the treatment of patients diagnosed with psychogenic non-epileptic seizures (PNES) and post-traumatic stress disorder (PTSD). Epilepsy Behav 66:86–92, 2017 28038392

Nicholson C, Edwards MJ, Carson AJ, et al: Occupational therapy consensus recommendations for functional neurological disorder. J Neurol Neurosurg Psychiatry 91(10):1037–1045, 2020 32732388

Nielsen G, Stone J, Matthews A, et al: Physiotherapy for functional motor disorders: a consensus recommendation. J Neurol Neurosurg Psychiatry 86(10):1113–1119, 2015 25433033

Nonnekes J, Ruzicka E, Serranová T, et al: Functional gait disorders: a sign-based approach. Neurology 94(24):1093–1099, 2020 32482839

Perez DL, Aybek S, Popkirov S, et al: A review and expert opinion on the neuropsychiatric assessment of motor functional neurological disorders. J Neuropsychiatry Clin Neurosci 33(1):14–26, 2021a 32778007

Perez DL, Nicholson TR, Asadi-Pooya AA, et al: Neuroimaging in functional neurological disorder: state of the field and research agenda. Neuroimage Clin 30:102623, 2021b 34215138

Reiter JM, Andrews D, Reiter C, et al: Taking Control of Your Seizures. New York, Oxford University Press, 2015

Saxena A, Godena E, Maggio J, et al: Towards an outpatient model of care for motor functional neurological disorders: a neuropsychiatric perspective. Neuropsychiatr Dis Treat 16:2119–2134, 2020 32982250

Saxena A, Paredes-Echeverri S, Michaelis R, et al: Using the biopsychosocial model to guide patient-centered neurological treatments. Semin Neurol 42(2):80–87, 2022 35114695

Sharpe M, Walker J, Williams C, et al: Guided self-help for functional (psychogenic) symptoms: a randomized controlled efficacy trial. Neurology 77(6):564–572, 2011 21795652

Staab JP: Persistent postural-perceptual dizziness. Semin Neurol 40(1):130–137, 2020 31935771

Stamelou M, Cossu G, Edwards MJ, et al: Familial psychogenic movement disorders. Mov Disord 28(9):1295–1298, 2013 23568243

Stephen CD, Fung V, Lungu CI, et al: Assessment of emergency department and inpatient use and costs in adult and pediatric functional neurological disorders. JAMA Neurol 78(1):88–101, 2021 33104173

Stone J, LaFrance WC Jr, Levenson JL, et al: Issues for DSM-5: conversion disorder. Am J Psychiatry 167(6):626–627, 2010 20516161

Stone J, LaFrance WC Jr, Brown R, et al: Conversion disorder: current problems and potential solutions for DSM-5. J Psychosom Res 71(6):369–376, 2011 22118377

Stone J, Carson A, Hallett M: Explanation as treatment for functional neurologic disorders. Handb Clin Neurol 139:543–553, 2016 27719870

Williams C, Carson A, Smith S, et al: Overcoming Functional Neurological Symptoms: A Five Areas Approach. Boca Raton, FL, CRC Press, 2017

Wissel BD, Dwivedi AK, Merola A, et al: Functional neurological disorders in Parkinson disease. J Neurol Neurosurg Psychiatry 89(6):566–571, 2018 29549192

11

Headache[1]

Melinda A. Thiam, M.D.
Huma U. Sheikh, M.D.
X. Michelle Androulakis, M.D., M.S.
Susan Hutchinson, M.D.
Scott W. Powers, Ph.D.
Mia T. Minen, M.D., M.P.H.

Case Example

A 26-year-old Army veteran with a history of "stress headaches" since her time in the service describes throbbing headaches that cause nausea and make her avoid going outdoors. The headaches increase in intensity, frequency, and severity around her period and improve slightly afterward. She had a brief reprieve from the frequency of the headaches during pregnancy, but the headaches returned with increased intensity, severe nausea, and light sensitivity after delivery. She is struggling to keep up with hydration while trying to breastfeed and care for her

[1] Drs. Thiam and Androulakis are employed by the Department of Veterans Affairs. Although this work pertains to their professional job, it was not undertaken as part of duties assigned by a federal agency and was not funded or endorsed by the Department of Veterans Affairs. Any opinions expressed in this chapter are those of the authors alone and not necessarily the opinions of the U.S. government, U.S. Army, Department of Defense, U.S. Navy, or Defense Health Agency.

6-week-old infant. Her primary care doctor is concerned about possible postpartum depression.

The patient presumes these are the same stress headaches that she had in the service, and says that if the headaches just went away, she would no longer feel depressed and anxious.

Headaches are among the most disabling disorders worldwide. Psychiatric comorbidity is common. Like patients with psychiatric disorders, patients with chronic headaches often struggle with stigma and access to care. Migraine and other headache disorders are underdiagnosed and undertreated (Lipton and Bigal 2005). In this chapter, we first address primary headache disorders including migraine, tension-type headache, and trigeminal autonomic cephalalgias. Discussion of secondary headaches, cranial neuralgias, and headaches in special populations follows. The *International Classification of Headache Disorders,* 3rd Edition (ICHD-3) is used for headache diagnostic criteria (International Headache Society 2018).

Approach to Patients With Headaches

Obtaining a detailed headache history, including information in Table 11.1, is key to headache diagnosis. Asking open-ended questions such as "Can you tell me about your headaches?" and letting the patient tell their story, is important in building rapport.

Key parts of the general neurologic exam such as abnormal fundoscopy or presence of focal neurological signs may help identify important secondary causes of headache. In addition to the standard neurological evaluation, a comprehensive headache examination includes assessing for full range of motion of the neck, a positive occipital Tinel's sign (tapping the occiput to see whether it elicits pain or paresthesias radiating to the apex or ear), and tenderness on the scalp or temporomandibular area.

Primary Headache

Primary headaches constitute up to 90% of headache disorders. There are four major categories of primary headache: migraine, tension-type headache (TTH), trigeminal autonomic cephalalgias (TACs), and other

Table 11.1 Items to include in the headache history

Headache characteristics	Frequency, duration (treated vs. untreated), location, quality of pain, severity, pattern of recurrence (time of day, time of month), time to maximum intensity, precipitating factors and triggers, aggravating factors
Associated symptoms	Neurologic, psychiatric, autonomic, gastrointestinal, hyperactivity, hypoactivity, depression, cravings for particular foods, repetitive yawning, fatigue, neck stiffness or pain
Prodrome	Immediately before headache, during headache, after headache (postdrome)
General health	Nutrition, hydration, sleep
Treatment history	Abortive medication trials, results, side effects, reason for stopping, number used per month; preventive medication trials, results, side effects, reason for stopping; nonpharmacologic treatments
Patient's perceptions	Preconception of diagnosis, fears, concerns
Past headache history	Onset; was patient sent home from school with headaches in childhood?; motion sickness or gastrointestinal issues in childhood; changes in headaches over time; impact of headache
Medical history	Traumatic brain injury, cardiovascular disease, sleep disorders, encephalitis and other infectious disorders, autoimmune disorders, cancer
Psychiatric history	Psychiatric diagnoses, psychopharmacologic treatment, psychotherapy, neuromodulation
Psychosocial history	Living situation, occupational stressors, socioeconomic stressors, life events and transition periods, substance use, toxic exposure
Family history	Headaches, psychiatric disorders

primary headaches (International Headache Society 2018). Although tension-type is the most common type of headache disorder, only 16% of patients with tension-type headache will seek care, versus 56% of patients with migraine (Jensen 2018). Patients with migraine, chronic tension-type headache, and cluster headache are at increased risk for comorbid psychiatric disorders. Chronic migraine increases the risk of insomnia, depression, and anxiety (Lipton et al. 2020). Individuals diagnosed with episodic migraine have a 21.5% lifetime prevalence rate of PTSD compared with only 4.5% in those without headache (Peterlin et al. 2011). Individuals with co-occurring PTSD and depression are also more likely to be diagnosed with migraine (Rao et al. 2015). Risk of suicidal ideation and suicide attempts is almost two and a half times higher in those with cluster, chronic tension, and migraine headaches than in healthy control subjects (Giakas et al. 2023).

Migraine

Epidemiology

Migraine is the second most disabling condition worldwide (after stroke) (Steiner et al. 2020) and occurs about three times more frequently in women than in men. Its prevalence increases in adolescence and peaks from ages 25 to 49. Women of childbearing age are therefore at high risk.

Diagnosis

Migraine is diagnosed based on frequency (episodic vs. chronic) as well as presence or absence of aura. Migraine may have five clinical phases—prodrome, aura, headache, postdrome, and interictal—as illustrated in Figure 11.1 (International Headache Society 2018). For example, prodromal yawning can precede the aura or headache, and postdromal fatigue can follow. About 25%–30% of patients with migraine have aura. Some people with migraines can have aura without a headache. The clinical presentation of each migraine can vary within and between individuals; migraine can even be mistaken for sinus symptoms (Dodick 2018).

Migraine with aura is diagnosed when at least two attacks include a reversible aura of visual, sensory, speech or language, motor, brainstem, or retinal symptoms. The auras should include at least three of the following characteristics: gradual spread over ≥5 minutes, appearance of two or more aura symptoms in succession, duration of each aura symptom 5–60 minutes, at least one unilateral aura, at least one aura includes positive symptoms (e.g., paresthesia, scintillations), or headache occurring within 60 minutes. *Migraine without aura* is diagnosed when the patient has had at least five moderate to severe headaches of 4–72 hours' duration accompanied by nausea/vomiting or photophobia/phonophobia. Additionally, the headache pain is associated with at least two

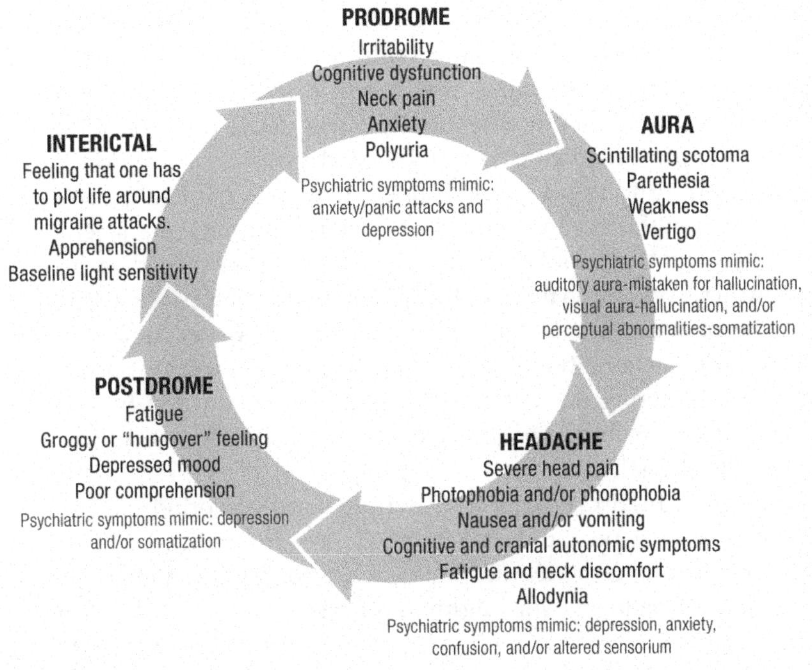

Figure 11.1 Migraine cycle.

of the following four characteristics: unilateral, pulsating, moderate to severe intensity, or aggravated by or causing avoidance of routine physical activity (International Headache Society 2018).

A headache diary can help track attacks and treatment response. This can be done with a paper diary or electronically in a smartphone calendar or app. A diary enables providers to better understand whether a patient has low-frequency episodic migraine (<10 headache days per month), high-frequency episodic migraine (10–14 headache days per month), or chronic migraine, defined as having ≥15 headache days per month for 3 months with at least 8 days per month having migraine features.

Management

The traditional treatment approach has been to target acute therapy in migraine and to begin preventive therapy when patients experience four or more headache days per month. However, the severity of the non-headache symptoms, the length of the migraine symptoms, the comorbid mental health symptoms, and the degree of social-occupational impairment are also critical to consider. Given the high prevalence of co-occurring mental health disorders in patients with migraine, suboptimal migraine management places patients at risk for destabilizing mental health conditions and vice versa. The decreased quality of life and impact of migraine during the interictal period are also important factors to consider for effective migraine management.

Patients who experience more frequent headaches should be offered prophylactic options. Treatment can include pharmacological options and nonpharmacological interventions including neuromodulation devices or behavioral therapies based on Grade A evidence (Silberstein et al. 2012). Studies show that combined medication and behavioral therapy is the treatment of choice in children, adolescents, and adults (Powers et al. 2021)

Given the high prevalence of migraine and comorbid psychiatric disorders, clinicians should be aware of certain medication implications. Some antiseizure medications, such as topiramate and valproate, have Grade A evidence for migraine prevention. Tricyclic antidepressants and the serotonin-norepinephrine reuptake inhibitor (SNRI) venlafaxine have Grade B evidence for prevention. The dosing used for migraine is often lower than for other indications. For example, topiramate may be started at 25 mg with gradual titration to 100 mg twice a day. Amitriptyline may be started at 5–10 mg with slow titration to about 50 mg daily. Selective serotonin reuptake inhibitors (SSRIs) have little evidence for use in migraine but may be used for comorbid psychiatric conditions. SSRIs and SNRIs may be used with a low chance of serotonin syndrome in patients on triptans, as long as they are on a single SSRI or SNRI at standard dose (Orlova et al. 2018).

Antihypertensive medications, including certain beta-blockers, have Grade A evidence for migraine prevention. In addition, angiotensin-converting enzyme inhibitors (ACE-Is) such as lisinopril and angiotensin receptor blockers (ARBs) such as candesartan may be considered for migraine prevention. ACE-Is and ARBs may be good options in patients with psychiatric comorbidities because they are well tolerated, are inexpensive, and do not interact with many other medications.

Other preventive treatments include onabotulinum toxin A for chronic migraine, calcitonin gene-related peptide (CGRP) monoclonal antibodies, and small-molecule receptor antagonists known as Gepants. Gepants may also be used as acute therapy.

Examples of pharmacologic treatments are provided in Table 11.2. Choice of medication often takes into consideration co-occurring dis-

Table 11.2 Pharmacological treatment of migraine

Acute medication treatment	Preventive medication treatment
Over-the-counter: nonsteroidal anti-inflammatory drugs, acetaminophen	**Supplements:** magnesium, riboflavin, feverfew, coenzyme Q10
Dopamine antagonists: prochlorperazine, metoclopramide, promethazine	Tricyclic antidepressants (e.g., amitriptyline)
Triptans: almotriptan, eletriptan, frovatriptan, naratriptan, rizatriptan, sumatriptan, zolmatriptan	Serotonin norepinephrine reuptake inhibitors (e.g., venlafaxine)
Ditan: lasmiditan	Beta-blockers (e.g., propranolol)
Nonselective serotonin-1 agonists: ergotamine, dihydroergotamine	**Other antihypertensive drugs:** candesartan, lisinopril
Other injectables: peripheral nerve blocks, trigger-point injections, sphenopalatine ganglion blocks	**Antiseizure medication:** topiramate, zonisamide, divalproex sodium
Gepants (CGRP receptor antagonists): rimegepant,* ubrogepant	Melatonin
	Memantine
	Onabotulinum toxin A (Botox)
	CGRP antibodies: erenumab, fremanezumab, galcanezumab, eptinezumab

*May also be used as a preventive agent.

orders, side effects, and patient preference. Nonpharmacological treatments can be used for any primary headache and are summarized in Table 11.3. When making treatment recommendations, providers should evaluate the level of evidence, the patient's access to treatment, and the patient's preference. Regarding the advanced therapies, anti-CGRP antibodies have been found to have an antidepressant effect in individuals with co-occurring migraine and depression. Likewise, it has been hypothesized that onabotulinum toxin A injected into corrugator muscles—part of an FDA-approved chronic migraine treatment—may improve depression symptoms.

Tension-Type Headache

TTH is the most prevalent headache disorder, although it may not be as disabling as other headache types (International Headache Society 2018). The average age of onset is 25–30, and the male-to-female ratio is 4:5. Pain may be described as dull, band-like, bilateral, not aggravated

Table 11.3 Nonpharmacological treatment of primary headache

Rest
Hydration
Cognitive-behavioral therapy
Diaphragmatic breathing
Mindfulness, meditation
Guided imagery
Progressive muscle relaxation therapy
Acupuncture
Yoga
Aerobic exercise
Hypnosis
Biofeedback
Neuromodulation
External trigeminal nerve stimulation (E-TNS)
Transcutaneous cervical vagal nerve stimulation (TcVNS)
Single-pulse transcranial magnetic stimulation (STMS)
Remote electrical neuromodulation (REN)
Cranial electrotherapy stimulation (CES)*
Transcranial direct current stimulation (tDCS)*
Transcutaneous auricular vagal nerve stimulation (TaVNS)
Acupressure electrostimulation*
FL-41 tinted eyeglass lenses (blocks certain wavelengths)

*Non-FDA-approved neuromodulatory treatments used in other countries and often with mental health benefit.

by physical activity, and not accompanied by nausea, vomiting, photophobia, or phonophobia. Most often, when a patient with TTH presents to a clinician, it co-occurs with another headache disorder (Jensen 2018).

Trigeminal Autonomic Cephalalgia

TAC refers to a group of four headache disorders characterized by recurrent attacks of unilateral intense pain in the trigeminal distribution, with ipsilateral autonomic symptoms. The latter may include ptosis, miosis, eye redness, lacrimation, periorbital edema, nasal congestion, rhinorrhea, forehead and facial sweating or flushing, and aural fullness (International Headache Society 2018). The headache types are cluster headache, hemicrania continua, paroxysmal hemicrania, and short-lasting unilateral neuralgiform headache attacks (SUNA). SUNA with conjunctival injection/redness and tearing is termed SUNCT (International Headache Society 2018). Although TACs are similar in headache characteristics and associated symptoms, they can be distinguished by headache frequency and duration, as well as associated symptoms.

Epidemiology

Cluster headache accounts for 90% of TACs and 1% of daily headaches, although it occurs in about 1 in 1,000 people age 20–40 (Nahas 2021). Unlike migraine, cluster headache is more prevalent in men. The onset of paroxysmal hemicrania is typically at ages 30–50 and appears more frequently in women (Osman and Bahra 2018). SUNCT and SUNA have a prevalence of 6.6 per 100,000 (Williams and Broadley 2008). Hemicrania continua and paroxysmal hemicrania are even less common, with hemicrania continua being more common in females (Dodick 2001).

Diagnosis

Diagnosis is based on history, including headache characteristics, accompanying symptoms, and duration. Cluster headache can be remembered by the mnemonic SEAR: side-locked unilateral, excruciating pain, agitation, and restlessness (in contrast with migraine). Cluster headache tends to regularly recur with circadian and circannual rhythms, most often in the spring and fall (Nahas 2021).

Paroxysmal hemicrania attacks are similar to cluster headache attacks but are shorter and occur more frequently, sometimes up to 40 times per day. Hemicrania continua is similar, but the pain is continuous and less intense than in cluster headaches. Severity may wax and wane, but the pain never completely resolves. SUNCT and SUNA are characterized by their quick, staccato pattern of sharp stabbing pain lasting a few seconds to 10 minutes. Hundreds of these stabbing sensations may occur each day (Wei and Jensen 2018). SUNCT/SUNA attacks are similar to cranial neuralgia in that they can be provoked by gently touching the skin, chewing, or brushing teeth. The TACs are compared in Table 11.4.

Treatment

The acute treatment of cluster headache includes high-flow oxygen using a non-rebreather mask or subcutaneous sumatriptan. Verapamil and the CGRP inhibitor galcanezumab may be used for cluster headache

Table 11.4 Trigeminal autonomic cephalalgias (all have unilateral autonomic symptoms)

Headache type	Description	Duration and frequency	Treatment
Cluster headache	Excruciating Patient is restless, wants to sit up	15–180 minutes Up to 8/day	Oxygen Triptan
Paroxysmal hemicrania	Excruciating Patient is restless	2–30 minutes >5/day	Indomethacin
Hemicrania continua	Mild/moderate/severe Patient is restless	Continuous ≥3 months	Indomethacin
SUNCT and SUNA	Severe/excruciating Sometimes restless Both conjunctival injection and lacrimation present for SUNCT	1–600 seconds Multiple/hour	Intravenous lidocaine Lamotrigine Oxcarbazepine

SUNA = short-lasting unilateral neuralgiform headache attacks; SUNCT = short-lasting unilateral neuralgiform headache attacks with conjunctival injection and tearing

prevention. Occipital nerve block can also be helpful during an attack and to help shorten a cluster cycle. Noninvasive vagus nerve stimulation (nVNS) can be used alone or combined with the treatment options just described as both acute and preventive therapy for cluster headache.

Hemicrania continua and paroxysmal hemicrania are unique because the response to treatment can help solidify the diagnosis; both headache forms may remit with indomethacin (Burish and Rozen 2019). If this cannot be tolerated, melatonin, verapamil, topiramate, or occipital nerve blocks can be tried (Burish and Rozen 2019). nVNS is recommended for both hemicrania continua and paroxysmal hemicrania.

Secondary Headache

Secondary headaches are a symptom of another primary disorder or medical illness. Changes or variations in previously stable headache patterns can be clues to potential secondary headaches and are important to investigate. A list of causes of secondary headaches is provided in Table 11.5.

Table 11.5 Causes of secondary headache

Posttraumatic headache	Temporomandibular disorder
Ischemic or hemorrhagic stroke	Hypertensive encephalopathy
Giant-cell arteritis	Cervicogenic headache
Chiari malformation	Acute rhinosinusitis
Autoimmune encephalitis	Acute angle glaucoma
Medication overuse	Postvaccination
Alcohol or caffeine withdrawal	Venous sinus thrombosis
Substance-induced	Reversible cerebral vasoconstriction syndrome
Meningitis; viral encephalitis	Subarachnoid hemorrhage
Systemic infection	Pre-eclampsia/eclampsia
COVID-19	Pituitary disease
Sleep apnea	Brain tumor (primary or secondary)

Medication Overuse Headache

A common secondary headache is *medication overuse headache* (MOH). MOH is defined as the overuse of simple analgesics (>15 days per month or >10 days per month for a combination of any triptans, opiates, and analgesics) in parallel with the worsening of a preexisting headache disorder (International Headache Society 2018). Anticipatory anxiety of an impending attack with overuse of acute medications can contribute to MOH. Patients may not be aware that frequent use of an analgesic or triptan can lead to MOH. In particular, overuse of opioid or barbiturate-containing pain medications is associated with an increased likelihood of MOH as well as transformation from episodic migraine to chronic migraine (Schwedt et al. 2018). Effective treatment includes addressing the cause of MOH by tapering the use of acute analgesics while transitioning the patient to a different headache management plan. MOH is one of the reasons that acute medications containing barbiturates are no longer recommended.

Posttraumatic Headache

Posttraumatic headache (PTH) is defined as a headache that develops within 7 days of a traumatic brain injury (TBI) or within 7 days of regaining consciousness after TBI. There are nearly 1.7 million TBIs every year in the United States, and PTH is the most common sequela. PTH semiology can vary; it most often resembles other primary headache disorders such as

TTH or migraine (Kamins and Charles 2018). According to ICHD-3 criteria, "when a *pre-existing* primary headache is made *significantly worse* (usually meaning a twofold or greater increase in frequency and/or severity) in close temporal relation to such a causative disorder, both the primary and the secondary headache diagnoses should be given, provided that there is good evidence that the disorder can cause headache" (International Headache Society 2018). PTH occurring within 3 months of injury is termed acute PTH, and PTH persisting more than 3 months after injury is considered chronic or persistent PTH. Dysautonomia in chronic PTH is often more severe than in primary headache disorders such as migraine (Howard et al. 2018). Few treatments have been studied for acute or chronic PTH. Metoclopramide has been found to be helpful in the emergency department (Friedman et al. 2021); however, there is no FDA-approved therapy for PTH. PTH is often treated based on its headache phenotype but is often refractory to conventional headache treatment.

Red Flag Symptoms

The SNOOP mnemonic (see Table 11.6 for one version) is a way to recall red flag symptoms or warning signs of dangerous secondary headaches (Do et al. 2019). Abnormal neurological examination findings, such as focal deficits, papilledema, confusion, or diplopia, warrant further neuroimaging evaluation. In most cases, a complete neurological examination and brain MRI with or without contrast is indicated. Vessel imaging (cranial magnetic resonance angiography and magnetic resonance venography) and lumbar puncture may also be indicated. If papilledema is suspected or visual defects are described, referral to a neuro-ophthalmologist is recommended.

The sudden onset of a severe headache is termed *thunderclap* and is a neurologic emergency until proven otherwise. If the patient states it is the "worst headache of my life" and is not like their typical headache, emergency evaluation is indicated. The differential diagnosis includes subarachnoid hemorrhage, reversible cerebral vascular syndrome, venous sinus thrombosis, vascular malformation, and hemorrhagic stroke. Workup may include emergency CT, CT angiography, brain MRI, and lumbar puncture.

Table 11.6 Red flags in secondary headaches (SNOOP)

SNOOP mnemonic	Diagnoses to investigate
Systemic signs including fever	Neoplasm, CNS infection, vasculitis
Neurologic deficits or decreased arousal	Stroke, primary neoplasm, brain abscess
Older age (>50)	Giant cell arteritis, glaucoma, cardiac cephalalgia, cerebrovascular disorder, neoplasm
Onset sudden (including "thunderclap" headaches)	Subarachnoid hemorrhage, reversible cerebral vascular syndrome, stroke
Pattern change from previous headache history or progressive	Neoplasm
Postural/positional	Intracranial hypotension or hypertension; cerebrospinal fluid leak; POTS
Pregnancy	Stroke, cerebral sinus thrombosis, post–dural puncture headache, hypertension/preeclampsia, anemia, gestational diabetes, hypothyroidism
Pulsatile tinnitus	Idiopathic intracranial hypertension
Precipitated by valsalva/exertion/sneeze	Posterior fossa pathology such as Chiari malformation, other space-occupying lesion
Papilledema	Neoplasm, intracranial hypertension
Posttraumatic onset	Subdural hematoma, epidural hematoma, other hemorrhage or contusion

CNS = central nervous system; POTS = postural orthostatic tachycardia syndrome.

Headaches With Systemic Symptoms

Headaches accompanied by systemic symptoms such as fever, neck pain or stiffness, nausea, or vomiting should be referred to the emergency department for emergent evaluation to rule out meningitis or subarachnoid hemorrhage. Bacterial meningitis requires antibiotics, and some viral meningitis may require antiviral therapy. Headache is commonly seen in COVID-19 during the prodromal and active stages of the illness. It can persist for months and may be either migraine or TTH. Headache in patients with an underlying condition such as cancer or HIV may indicate metastatic disease or CNS infection. Autoimmune limbic encephalitis can also cause secondary headache.

Giant Cell Arteritis

Onset after the age of 50 is unusual in primary headache disorders and indicates a need for neurologic evaluation. New-onset unilateral temporal headache in the elderly raises concerns for giant cell arteritis. A common laboratory finding is markedly elevated C-reactive protein and erythrocyte sedimentation rate, but definitive diagnosis requires temporal artery biopsy. High-dose steroids are administered as soon as possible to prevent blindness. In most cases, the headache improves within 3 days of high-dose steroid treatment.

Positional Headaches

Headaches described as worse when lying down and better when upright may indicate elevated intracranial pressure due to space-occupying lesions or idiopathic intracranial hypertension (IIH), also known as pseudotumor cerebri. IIH most commonly occurs in women 20–50 years old. Primary symptoms include headache, blurred vision, nausea and/or vomiting, and pulsatile tinnitus. *Pulsatile tinnitus* refers to a rhythmic noise in the ear at the same rate as the heartbeat and represents changes in blood flow in nearby blood vessels. Diagnosis of IIH requires a brain MRI, which may show slit-like ventricles, flattening of the optic globes, empty sella, and narrowing of the transverse sinuses. Additional work-up includes a neuro-ophthalmology referral for evaluation for papilledema, visual field testing, and optical coherence tomography testing. Lumbar puncture, which itself can alleviate the pressure and thus headache, is used to determine whether the opening pressure is abnormally increased.

In contrast, if the headache is described as worse when upright and better when lying down, then a diagnosis of intracranial hypotension should be considered. Low-pressure headaches most commonly occur following lumbar puncture or epidural injection, though they may occur with spontaneous cerebrospinal fluid (CSF) leak. MRI may show pachymeningeal thickening and enhancement, dural venous engorgement, tonsillar herniation, and subdural fluid. Sometimes, more extensive testing with cisternography may be needed to detect slow leaks.

Treatment usually requires a blood patch. In spontaneous CSF leak, an empiric blood patch can be both diagnostic and therapeutic. For refractory cases, a neuroradiologist specialized in CSF leak and fluoroscopic imaging may be consulted.

Secondary Headaches in Pregnancy and Postpartum

New-onset headache, new-onset aura, or worsening of a preexisting headache disorder during pregnancy requires a full evaluation. Risks for secondary headaches vary by timing during pregnancy. There are elevated rates of IIH before 20 weeks' gestation; arterial-venous malformation rupture especially at 15–20 weeks; and pituitary apoplexy, aneurysmal bleeding, reversible cerebral vasoconstriction syndrome, venous thrombosis, pre-eclampsia, eclampsia, and low-pressure headache (e.g., post-epidural headache) in the third trimester or postpartum. Coincident conditions such as symptomatic neoplasm can occur in any trimester (Burch 2019).

Special Populations

Headache in Women

There is a 3:1 ratio of female-to-male prevalence of migraine, and women with migraine are more likely to experience longer headaches with accompanying photophobia, phonophobia, and nausea (Finocchi and Strada 2014). Reproductive hormones can affect the severity of both migraine and mood disorders. A possible explanation for the rate of comorbid depression is a decrease in serotonin uptake and utilization with decreased estrogen levels. Similarly, a drop in estrogen can precipitate or exacerbate migraines (Todd et al. 2018).

The onset of migraine in women commonly occurs around menarche, and migraine frequency can increase just before menstrual periods. *Pure menstrual migraine* refers to migraine occurring exclusively during the premenstrual period, similar to premenstrual dysphoric disorder. In contrast, migraine that occurs throughout the menstrual cycle but is worse immediately before menses is called *menstrual-related migraine,* similar to *premenstrual exacerbation* used to describe mood disorders. Menstrual migraine peaks at approximately 40 years old in women and tends to decline with menopause. Menstrual-related migraines occur in up to 60% of women, although only 7%–35% of women experience pure menstrual migraine (Todd et al. 2018). Women with menstrual migraine participate in fewer social activities and have difficulties performing household chores. About 58% limit family activities, 55% cannot engage in sports, and 45% have work-related disabilities. Menstrual-related migraine is reported to be longer, more painful, and more resistant to treatment than non-menstrual-related migraine (Reddy et al. 2021). Specific treatment strategies include mini-prophylactic medications around menses, and long-term birth control to suppress menstrual cycles.

Pregnancy Planning

Migraine and other primary headache disorders occur in 10%–17% of pregnancies. Studies have shown that one in five women with migraine avoids pregnancy because of concerns that migraine will get worse (Ishii et al. 2020), affect the health of her child, or both (Riggins and Ehrlich 2021). Menstrual migraine is most often migraine without aura and may improve during pregnancy, since estrogen withdrawal can trigger migraine. However, migraine without aura can start during pregnancy, most frequently in the first trimester, in up to 10% of pregnant women (Negro et al. 2017). In comparison, 25% of pregnant women with a history of migraine with aura will continue to have attacks during pregnancy, with hyperemesis, pathological pregnancy course, and increasing frequency and complexity as pregnancy progresses (Burch 2019).

Women with migraine who are pregnant are at increased risk for other medical and neurologic comorbidities. Untreated migraine has consistently been associated with an increased risk of preeclampsia and other hypertensive disorders, low birth weight, preterm birth, and placental abruption. Migraine attacks with associated vomiting can lead to dehydration and electrolyte imbalance, particularly in the setting of poor intake due to pregnancy-associated nausea.

Postpartum Period

The most common cause of postpartum headache is exacerbation of a primary headache disorder, rather than new-onset migraine. Any headache in the postpartum period needs to be evaluated to ensure it is not a secondary headache such as cerebral venous sinus thrombosis. Migraine attacks may occur, typically 2–3 days postpartum, triggered by the precipitous drop in estrogen (Calhoun 2017). Postpartum mood disorders are also common and thought to be due to changes in hormones. Women who breastfeed have a lower recurrence rate of migraine. Although migraine medications can be used under supervision, many women may choose to implement nonpharmacological migraine treatments during pregnancy or breastfeeding (Burch 2019). However, undertreatment of both headache and mental health disorders during the postpartum period can lead to negative consequences for women and mother–child bonding.

Pediatric Headache Disorders

As with many chronic illnesses that can begin in childhood, children with headache disorders are not just "little adults." The focus of diagnosis, management, and care includes the child, family, school, and community. Diagnostic criteria for migraine in children allow for a shorter duration of headache and for symptoms such as avoiding activity to be inferred from observed behavior and caregiver report. Guidelines for the care of youth with migraine have been proposed for both acute and preventive treatment (Oskoui et al. 2019b). Combined cognitive behavioral and pharmacologic therapy is the current recommended approach for migraine prevention (Oskoui et al. 2019a). Despite a high placebo response rate and the need for more pediatric-specific research, youth with headaches generally respond well to therapy and can maintain improvements in headache days and associated disability for several years (Powers et al. 2021). As in adults, headache disorders in youth can be associated with impaired psychological functioning and co-occurring psychiatric conditions. It is important to consider the "whole child" and their lived experiences when developing a comprehensive and interdisciplinary care plan, involving psychiatrists and psychologists as appropriate.

Cranial Neuralgias

Per ICHD-3 criteria, *cranial neuralgias* refer to unilateral or bilateral facial pain associated with dysfunctional nerves. Facial pain is defined as pain in the face, eye, mandible, or oral cavity. Cranial neuralgias are often associated with paroxysmal, lancinating facial pain. The most common is trigeminal neuralgia, but glossopharyngeal and occipital neuralgias are also seen. Cranial neuralgias may also be secondary to medical conditions. Trigeminal neuralgia is very similar to SUNCT/SUNA in that there is unilateral pain lasting from 1 to a few seconds that may repeat for up to 2 minutes at a time. Compared with TACs, however, the autonomic and pain symptoms tend to occur along V2 and V3 distribution (TACs are usually symptomatic in V1) (Nahas 2021). Also, autonomic symptoms can be more prominent in TACs, and trigeminal neuralgia often has trigger zones and a refractory period after attacks.

Case Example, Continued

Especially for the veteran population, it is important to inquire about a history of TBI and PTSD, which the patient denies. A careful evaluation for depression is necessary because of the increased risk of mood disorders in the postpartum period. Although the patient's neurologic examination is normal, the change in headache during the immediate postpartum period is a red flag. Thus, brain MRI and magnetic resonance venography are obtained but do not reveal structural pathology. Headaches "due to stress" are often misdiagnosed as tension headaches, but the severity and presence of light sensitivity and nausea meet criteria for migraine headaches. Sleep hygiene, obviously quite difficult in the postpartum period, is discussed. The importance of hydration is emphasized, and the patient is counseled about the use of medications while breastfeeding. Acute treatment is initiated with acetaminophen and metoclopramide as needed. She is also started on venlafaxine combined with cognitive-behavioral therapy for migraine prevention.

Key Clinical Points

- Headaches frequently co-occur with psychiatric conditions.
- Headache should not be considered "just" a symptom of a psychiatric condition without first conducting a thorough headache history, medical history, and neurologic examination.
- Although tension-type headaches are the most common primary headache type, migraine is the most common headache disorder that will be seen in clinical practice.
- "Red flag" symptoms suggest a secondary headache disorder that requires urgent work-up.
- Headaches and mood may be related during pregnancy and may fluctuate with hormone levels.
- Collaborative care enhances the treatment of both psychiatric and headache diagnoses.

Review Questions

1. Which of the following characteristics is NOT considered a "red flag" in secondary headache?

   A. Fever
   B. Postural component
   C. Unilateral
   D. Maximal pain at onset
   E. Onset at age >50

2. Which of the following medication mechanisms is indicated for both abortive and prophylactic treatment of migraine?

   A. Dopamine antagonism
   B. 5HT-1 agonism
   C. Serotonin norepinephrine reuptake inhibition
   D. CGRP receptor antagonism
   E. Beta blockade

3. A patient with chronic daily headache frequently uses acetaminophen and ibuprofen with only partial relief. By definition, how frequently must the patient use these medications to qualify for the diagnosis of medication overuse headache?

   A. ≥8 days/month
   B. ≥10 days/month
   C. ≥15 days/month
   D. ≥20 days/month
   E. Daily

Answers

Question 1: C. Whereas a strictly unilateral headache might indicate structural pathology, unilateral pain is typical of many primary headache types including migraine, cluster, hemicrania, and SUNCT/SUNA. Fever may be a sign of a systemic issue such as infection. Postural/positional headaches may indicate abnormal intracranial pressure (too high or too low). A headache that is maximal at onset is known as *thunderclap* and can indicate an emergency (e.g., subarachnoid hemorrhage).

A new headache in the elderly is also suspicious for secondary causes, as the risk for giant cell arteritis, strokes, and tumors increases.

Question 2: D. Calcitonin gene-related peptide (CGRP) receptor antagonists (e.g., rimegepant) can be used both as needed for acute treatment and regularly scheduled as a preventive for migraine headaches. Dopamine antagonists (e.g., metoclopramide) are helpful acutely for nausea, and 5HT-1 agonists (e.g., sumatriptan) are a classic first-line abortive medication as well. Serotonin norepinephrine reuptake inhibitors (e.g., venlafaxine) and beta blockers (e.g., propranolol) are used for prophylaxis.

Question 3: C. By definition, the diagnosis of medication overuse headaches due to simple analgesics requires use of the medications for ≥15 days/month. For other analgesics such as triptans, ergots, and opiates, a patient needs to take them only ≥10 days/month to qualify for medication overuse headache.

References

Burch R: Headache in pregnancy and the puerperium. Neurol Clin 37(1):31–51, 2019 30470274

Burish MJ, Rozen TD: Trigeminal autonomic cephalalgias. Neurol Clin 37(4):847–869, 2019 31563236

Calhoun AH: Migraine treatment in pregnancy and lactation. Curr Pain Headache Rep 21(11):46, 2017 28980122

Do TP, Remmers A, Schytz HW, et al: Red and orange flags for secondary headaches in clinical practice: SNNOOP10 list. Neurology 92(3):134–144, 2019 30587518

Dodick D: Hemicrania continua: diagnostic criteria and nosologic status. Cephalalgia 21(9):869–872, 2001 11903278

Dodick DW: A phase-by-phase review of migraine pathophysiology. Headache 58(Suppl 1):4–16, 2018 29697154

Finocchi C, Strada L: Sex-related differences in migraine. Neurol Sci 35(Suppl 1):207–213, 2014 24867868

Friedman BW, Irizarry E, Cain D, et al: Randomized study of metoclopramide plus diphenhydramine for acute posttraumatic headache. Neurology 96(18):e2323–e2331, 2021 33762421

Giakas A, Mangold K, Androulakis A, et al: Risks of suicide in migraine, non-migraine headache, back, and neck pain: a systematic review and meta-analysis. Front Neurol 14:1160204, 2023 37153662

Howard L, Dumkrieger G, Chong CD, et al: Symptoms of autonomic dysfunction among those with persistent posttraumatic headache attributed to mild traumatic brain injury: a comparison to migraine and healthy controls. Headache 58(9):1397–1407, 2018 30156267

International Headache Society: The International Classification of Headache Disorders, 3rd Edition. Cephalalgia 38(1):1–211, 2018 29368949

Ishii R, Schwedt TJ, Kim SK, et al: Effect of migraine on pregnancy planning: insights from the American Registry for Migraine Research. Mayo Clin Proc 95(10):2079–2089, 2020 32948327

Jensen RH: Tension-type headache: the normal and most prevalent headache. Headache 58(2):339–345, 2018 28295304

Kamins J, Charles A: Posttraumatic headache: basic mechanisms and therapeutic targets. Headache 58(6):811–826, 2018 29757458

Lipton RB, Bigal ME: Migraine: epidemiology, impact, and risk factors for progression. Headache 45(Suppl 1):S3–S13, 2005 15833088

Lipton RB, Seng EK, Chu MK, et al: The effect of psychiatric comorbidities on headache-related disability in migraine: results from the Chronic Migraine Epidemiology and Outcomes (CaMEO) study. Headache 60(8):1683–1696, 2020 33448374

Nahas S: Cluster headache and other trigeminal autonomic cephalalgias. Continuum (Minneap Minn) 27(3):633–651, 2021 34048396

Negro A, Delaruelle Z, Ivanova TA, et al: Headache and pregnancy: a systematic review. J Headache Pain 18(1):106, 2017 29052046

Orlova Y, Rizzoli P, Loder E: Association of coprescription of triptan antimigraine drugs and selective serotonin reuptake inhibitor or selective norepinephrine reuptake inhibitor antidepressants with serotonin syndrome. JAMA Neurol 75(5):566–572, 2018 29482205

Oskoui M, Pringsheim T, Billinghurst L, et al: Practice guideline update summary: pharmacologic treatment for pediatric migraine prevention: report of the Guideline Development, Dissemination, and Implementation Subcommittee of the American Academy of Neurology and the American Headache Society. Headache 59(8):1144–1157, 2019a 31529477

Oskoui M, Pringsheim T, Holler-Managan Y, et al: Practice guideline update summary: acute treatment of migraine in children and adolescents: report of the Guideline Development, Dissemination, and Implementation Subcommittee of the American Academy of Neurology and the American Headache Society. Neurology 93(11):487–499, 2019b 31413171

Osman C, Bahra A: Paroxysmal hemicrania. Ann Indian Acad Neurol 21(Suppl 1):S16–S22, 2018 29720814

Peterlin BL, Nijjar SS, Tietjen GE: Post-traumatic stress disorder and migraine: epidemiology, sex differences, and potential mechanisms. Headache 51(6):860–868, 2011 21592096

Powers SW, Coffey CS, Chamberlin LA, et al: Prevalence of headache days and disability 3 years after participation in the childhood and adolescent migraine prevention medication trial. JAMA Netw Open 4(7):e2114712–e2114712, 2021 34251445

Rao AS, Scher AI, Vieira RV, et al: The impact of post-traumatic stress disorder on the burden of migraine: results from the National Comorbidity Survey–Replication. Headache 55(10):1323–1341, 2015 26473981

Reddy N, Desai MN, Schoenbrunner A, et al: The complex relationship between estrogen and migraines: a scoping review. Syst Rev 10(1):72, 2021 33691790

Riggins N, Ehrlich A: The use of behavioral modalities for headache during pregnancy and breastfeeding. Curr Pain Headache Rep 25(10):66, 2021 34668111

Schwedt TJ, Alam A, Reed ML, et al: Factors associated with acute medication overuse in people with migraine: results from the 2017 Migraine in America Symptoms and Treatment (MAST) study. J Headache Pain 19(1):38, 2018 29797100

Silberstein SD, Holland S, Freitag F, et al; Quality Standards Subcommittee of the American Academy of Neurology and the American Headache Society: evidence-based guideline update: pharmacologic treatment for episodic migraine prevention in adults: report of the Quality Standards Subcommittee of the American Academy of Neurology and the American Headache Society. Neurology 78(17):1337–1345, 2012 22529202

Steiner TJ, Stovner LJ, Jensen R, et al: Migraine remains second among the world's causes of disability, and first among young women: findings from GBD2019. J Headache Pain 21(1):137, 2020 33267788

Todd C, Lagman-Bartolome AM, Lay C: Women and migraine: the role of hormones. Curr Neurol Neurosci Rep 18(7):42, 2018 29855724

Wei DY, Jensen RH: Therapeutic approaches for the management of trigeminal autonomic cephalalgias. Neurotherapeutics 15(2):346–360, 2018 29516437

Williams MH, Broadley SA: SUNCT and SUNA: clinical features and medical treatment. J Clin Neurosci 15(5):526–534, 2008 18325769

12

Neuroinfectious Diseases

Lindsey Gurin, M.D.
Deepti Anbarasan, M.D.

Case Example

A 73-year-old woman presents to the emergency department with her wife for evaluation of new-onset mood and behavioral changes. She has no significant medical or psychiatric history and works as a school librarian. Two days ago, she returned home from school in tears, perseverating on "mistakes" she had made while reading *The Velveteen Rabbit*. Since then, she has neither slept nor returned to work and has been at her desk writing continuously. She showers and brushes her teeth multiple times a day, insisting that each time is the first, and this morning she fed their cat six times. During an argument triggered by her wife's attempt to redirect her, she paused mid-sentence, staring vacantly while her wife called her name. On recovering, she accused her wife of being an intruder, then began to cry. The patient does not recall these events and questions her wife's "motives" in having her evaluated.

Neuroinfectious diseases are the clinical syndromes that arise when viruses, bacteria, fungi, or parasites interact with the nervous system. They can appear over any time course, involve any level of the nervous system, and vary in presentation according to the site of infection and the characteristics of both pathogen and host. The protean manifestations of neuroinfectious diseases present substantial challenges for diagnosis and management: diverse pathogens can cause similar clinical syndromes; a given pathogen can produce diverse syndromes under different clinical circumstances; and classic signs of infection may be absent. Patients with neurological infections can deteriorate rapidly. A high index of suspicion, a systematic approach, and a wide clinical lens are crucial to the evaluation of neurological complaints of potential infectious origin so that timely, accurate diagnosis can be accomplished and appropriate treatment pursued (Berkowitz 2021).

Psychiatrists can play a crucial role in this process. Patients with severe mental illness are at increased risk of infections and die from them at disproportionately high rates, even with appropriate treatment (Druss et al. 2018; Ribe et al. 2015). Encephalopathy due to CNS infection can be misattributed to psychiatric illness, especially in patients with preexisting psychiatric diagnoses: in one study, a history of psychotic disorder was a significant risk factor for delayed diagnosis of herpes simplex virus encephalitis (HSVE) (Miller et al. 2021). Familiarity with the risk factors and clinical features of neuroinfectious diseases can thus be critical to optimizing outcomes for patients with these syndromes, with or without co-occurring psychiatric illness.

Whereas the peripheral nervous system (PNS) is relatively accessible to microbes via peripheral nerve endings in body tissues, the CNS is heavily protected by the blood–brain barrier (BBB) and other immune mechanisms. To reach the CNS, microbes pass through breaches in the BBB or hijack physiological processes (e.g., leukocyte migration, retrograde axonal transport from peripheral neurons) to bypass it (Klein and Hunter 2017).

The historical view of the CNS as *immune-privileged,* isolated from normal systemic immune surveillance, is now outdated following the discovery of immune functions served by cerebrospinal fluid (CSF) spaces and a glymphatic system dedicated to the clearance of CNS waste products. Nevertheless, immune surveillance in brain parenchyma is dramatically reduced relative to that in peripheral tissues (Engelhardt et al. 2017). This suppression of CNS immune activity protects neural tissue from the deleterious effects of systemic inflammation, but at a cost: once established, brain-based infections can progress with astonishing speed and may be quite extensive before the systemic immune response is triggered. Neurological injury—which may occur due to the invasion of neural tissue, disruptions to the vasculature, or secretion of neurotoxins—results not only from the pathogen itself but also, frequently, from the inflammation generated to contain it.This complex interplay between protective and pathological immunity dictates the course of CNS infections and forms the basis for their frequent association with autoimmune neurological disorders.

In this chapter, we review the approach to diagnosis and management of suspected neuroinfectious diseases, with emphasis on CNS infections. Persistent infections and postinfectious autoimmune neurological syndromes, both of which frequently manifest with subacute or insidious neurobehavioral changes without overt infectious signs, are also briefly covered.

Approach to Patients With Neuroinfectious Diseases

Key features of the evaluation for neuroinfectious disease include localization; time course; associated non-neurological signs and symptoms; and context, including medical history, travel history, and environmental exposures (Berkowitz 2021).

Localization

Localizing complaints to a specific region of the nervous system confirms the existence of a neurological problem and narrows the differential diagnosis to inform subsequent management. The site of an infection determines its signs and symptoms, although localized syndromes are diagnostically nonspecific, and substantial heterogeneity exists within each one. *Meningitis, encephalitis,* and *myelitis* refer to inflammation of the meninges, brain parenchyma, and spinal cord, respectively. Localization to one or more focal brain regions suggests a bacterial or fungal abscess, a parasitic infection (e.g., neurocysticercosis, toxoplasmosis), or vascular insults caused by infectious vasculitis. PNS infections can involve cranial neuropathies, radiculopathy, peripheral neuropathy, neuromuscular junction disorders, or myopathy.

Timing

Acute onset and rapid progression of neurological dysfunction over hours to days should raise concern for infection, especially bacterial or viral. Infections caused by fungi, spirochetes, mycobacteria, and parasites often have a subacute or chronic presentation, although they can present acutely as well.

Non-neurological Features

Medical review of systems and general physical examination may suggest recent or current infection. Fever is a useful indicator, but it may be absent in very young, very old, or immunocompromised patients. Rashes can indicate specific infections (e.g., bull's-eye rash in Lyme disease, dermatomal vesicular rash in herpes zoster). Otitis and sinusitis can spread locally to produce meningitis or brain abscess. Neurological symptoms appearing soon after a flu-like syndrome suggest either viral meningitis or encephalitis or a postinfectious autoimmune process.

Clinical Context

Historical risk factors include predisposing medical conditions, travel, and environmental exposures. Patients with prior head trauma, recent neurosurgery, or indwelling CNS devices (e.g., CSF shunts) are at particularly elevated risk, and infectious causes must be considered for any new or worsening neurological complaint in these populations. Immunocompromised individuals are at increased risk of infection and may present with deceptively mild or nonspecific symptoms. In patients with HIV, specific $CD4^+$ counts are associated with the risk of opportunistic neurological infections such as cryptococcosis, toxoplasmosis, and progressive multifocal leukoencephalopathy (PML). Congenital heart disease, cardiac valvular disease, and intravenous drug use history confer increased risk of endocarditis and associated complications such as abscess, meningitis, or mycotic aneurysm.

Because some infections are endemic to certain geographic regions, questions about country of origin, place of residence, and travel history can be informative. Exposures to animals, certain foods (e.g. unpasteurized milk, home-canned goods), and outdoor activities (e.g., freshwater swimming) should also be queried.

The clinical assessment provides initial guidance, but definitive diagnosis of infection requires confirmation with microbiological testing. These results are not immediately available, and waiting for them is often infeasible. Neuroimaging can be an essential next step.

Computed Tomography

The most readily available imaging modality is computed tomography (CT), which is typically accessible even in resource-limited settings and takes minutes to complete. Although contrast-enhanced studies are preferred for evaluating infection, noncontrast CT readily identifies acute hemorrhage and can demonstrate focal hypodensities suggestive of edema or leukoencephalopathy. Calcified nodules of neurocysticercosis are also visualized well on unenhanced CT.

Magnetic Resonance Imaging

Brain magnetic resonance imaging (MRI) is more sensitive than CT in diagnosing infections. MRI diffusion-weighted imaging sequences can identify early infectious changes before they appear on T2 or fluid-attenuated inversion recovery (FLAIR) sequences. The use of contrast increases diagnostic sensitivity and specificity. Contrast uptake is not specific to infection, however, and clinical context is needed to distinguish infection from other enhancing lesions.

Cerebrospinal Fluid Analysis

CSF sampling via lumbar puncture (LP) is crucial in the evaluation of suspected neuroinfectious disease and includes cell counts, protein, glucose, and bacterial gram stain/culture. A meningitis/encephalitis polymerase chain reaction (PCR) panel screening for 14 common organisms is now also standard practice, with additional testing added depending on the clinical scenario. Elevations of CSF white blood cells (*pleocytosis*) and protein are nearly universal in neurological infections; the degree of elevation varies by syndrome and pathogen type, and differential cell counts vary by pathogen. Table 12.1 summarizes characteristic CSF findings for selected common syndromes.

Meningitis

Meningitis can be infectious or non-infectious and may have an acute or a chronic presentation. Acute infectious meningitis is usually bacterial or viral, whereas chronic meningitis is more often bacterial or fungal (Aksamit and Berkowitz 2021). Headache and neck pain are core features. Fever, vomiting, and photophobia are also common; seizures,

Table 12.1 Cerebrospinal fluid (CSF) findings by pathogen

CSF Findings	Normal	Bacterial	Viral	Tuberculosis	Fungal
Opening pressure (mm H_2O)	50–200	Elevated	Normal or elevated	Elevated	Normal or elevated
Appearance	Clear	Turbid	Clear	Turbid	Clear
Protein (mg/dL)	15–40	>100	<150	>50	Normal to mildly elevated
Glucose	>40% serum	<40% serum	>40% serum	<40% serum	<40% serum
Gram stain	No microorganisms	Bacteria	No microorganisms	Acid fast bacilli	Negative
White cell count (cells/µL)	0–5	>500	<250	10–1,000	10–50
White blood cell types	Lymphocytes	Neutrophils	Lymphocytes	Lymphocytes	Lymphocytes

cranial neuropathies, and focal neurological deficits can appear late. Symptoms are more severe in bacterial meningitis than in other etiologies. Encephalopathy is not strictly a feature of meningitis but is present in up to 95% of patients; in these cases, the syndrome is technically termed *meningoencephalitis* (Piquet and Lyons 2016). Signs of meningeal irritation (*meningismus*) may be demonstrated via examination maneuvers applying traction to the meninges, eliciting pain or resistance in response. These indications include nuchal rigidity, elicited by passive or active neck flexion; the Kernig sign, elicited by passive knee extension while the hips are flexed; and the Brudzinski sign, in which passive neck flexion elicits reflexive hip flexion. These signs may be absent in older or immunocompromised patients.

Acute Bacterial Meningitis

Incidence rates of bacterial meningitis vary by geographic region and have a strong association with poverty. In high-resource settings, the annual incidence of bacterial meningitis is less than 0.5–1.5 per 100,000 (Wall et al. 2021). The most common cause of acute bacterial meningitis globally is *Streptococcus pneumoniae*, and most community-acquired bacterial meningitis cases are associated with *S. pneumoniae* or *Neisseria meningitidis. Haemophilus influenzae B* remains an important cause of meningitis in countries with limited vaccine programs. *Listeria monocytogenes* is a consideration in infants and individuals who are immunocompromised, pregnant, or older than 50 years. Nosocomial meningitis in the setting of neurosurgery or CSF shunts is associated with a distinct set of pathogens, including the various *Staphylococcus* species found in normal skin flora; *Staphylococcus aureus*; and Gram-negative rods such as *Escherichia coli, Klebsiella* species, and *Pseudomonas aeruginosa*.

Acute bacterial meningitis is a neurological emergency that can result in death if untreated. Early recognition is crucial but can be challenging: only about 41% of patients present with the classic triad of fever, neck stiffness, and a change in mental status (van de Beek et al. 2004). Sensitivity increases when headache is added to the triad, with 95% of patients presenting with at least two of these four cardinal features. Illness onset is typically over 2–3 days, although some cases can emerge over 24 hours.

Once bacterial meningitis is suspected, CSF must be obtained emergently while simultaneously preparing to initiate empiric antimicrobial coverage. Because broad-spectrum antibiotics can rapidly sterilize

CSF, LP should be performed prior to treatment and, in most cases, before neuroimaging; exceptions to this rule are immunocompromised patients and those suspected of having elevated intracranial pressure (ICP). Delays in LP must not delay treatment, however: if LP must be delayed, pretreatment blood cultures should be drawn and antimicrobial therapy started immediately afterward. Delays in antibiotics of even a few hours are associated with worse outcomes in acute bacterial meningitis (van de Beek et al. 2016). CSF findings are reviewed in Table 12.1.

Neuroimaging is not specific for bacterial meningitis. CT may be normal or demonstrate sulcal effacement. MRI may demonstrate T2 hyperintensity and diffusion restriction in the sulci and contrast enhancement of the leptomeninges.

Initial treatment is with multiple antibiotics selected for broad coverage and CSF penetrance. Dexamethasone is initiated with antibiotics; however, the benefits of adjunctive steroids have been demonstrated primarily in streptococcal meningitis, and they are generally discontinued if an alternative etiology is identified (Aksamit and Berkowitz 2021). Standard empiric therapy is summarized in Table 12.2.

Even with treatment, bacterial meningitis is associated with substantial morbidity and mortality: approximately 20%–25% of individuals die, and about half of survivors experience lasting neurological complications such as epilepsy, cognitive impairment, or hearing loss (van de Beek et al. 2016).

Viral Meningitis

Viral meningitis occurs year-round, with peaks in summer and fall. The annual incidence varies by population age and vaccination status but is around 0.26–17 cases per 100,000, with rates highest in young children (McGill et al. 2017). In the United States, viral meningitis cases outnumber cases of all other etiologies of meningitis combined (Rotbart 2000). Enteroviruses, herpes simplex virus 2 (HSV-2), and varicella zoster virus (VZV) are most implicated. Arboviruses, several families of viruses transmitted by arthropod vectors (e.g., mosquitoes, ticks), are a consideration in certain geographic regions: meningitis is the most common neurological presentation of West Nile virus (WNV), tick-borne encephalitis virus, and Toscana virus. Severe acute respiratory syndrome coronavirus 2 (SARS-CoV-2) may also cause meningitis (Berger 2020). Mumps, once the most common cause of viral meningitis, has reemerged as a consideration in the wake of decreased childhood

Table 12.2 Empiric antibiotic treatment for bacterial meningitis

Clinical scenario	Etiologies	Treatment
Adult or child, community acquired	*Streptococcus pneumoniae, Neisseria meningitidis*	Vancomycin + ceftriaxone *or* cefotaxime + dexamethasone
Age >50 years, alcohol use disorder, or immunosuppression	*Streptococcus pneumoniae, Listeria monocytogenes,* Gram-negative rods	Vancomycin + ceftriaxone *or* cefotaxime + ampicillin + dexamethasone
Postneurosurgery, cerebrospinal fluid shunt, or head trauma	*Staphylococcus aureus; S. pneumoniae;* Gram-negative rods	Vancomycin + anti-pseudomonal beta-lactam + dexamethasone

vaccinations. Finally, HIV is an important cause of viral meningitis, most often during the initial seroconversion stage: nearly one-quarter of patients with primary HIV infections present with meningitis, although meningitis can also occur in chronic HIV infection (McGill et al. 2017). In many cases of viral meningitis, no causative pathogen is identified.

Diagnosis

Neuroimaging in viral meningitis is typically normal, although MRI may show leptomeningeal enhancement. CSF abnormalities are less dramatic than those of bacterial meningitis (see Table 12.1). Viral PCR testing is the gold standard for definitive diagnosis except in the case of arboviruses, in which CSF immunoglobulin M (IgM) antibodies are more sensitive than PCR testing (Aksamit and Berkowitz 2021). In HIV meningitis occurring with primary infection, HIV antibodies may not be present yet, and viral load testing is required for diagnosis.

Treatment

Treatment of viral meningitis is primarily supportive except for HSV-2 and VZV meningitis, which are treated with acyclovir. WNV meningitis is sometimes treated with intravenous immunoglobulin; this treatment is based on animal studies and case report data, although no prospective studies support its use.

Parasitic Meningitis

Naegleria fowleri, notoriously nicknamed the "brain-eating amoeba," is a rare but devastating cause of acute meningoencephalitis. *Naegleria*, a free-living amoeba found in warm freshwater that readily infects immunocompetent hosts, enters the nasopharynx during swimming and migrates to the brain via the olfactory nerves. The resulting syndrome of hyperacute purulent meningitis and diffuse hemorrhagic necrosis of brain tissue is nearly always fatal, although rare cases have been treated with combinations of amphotericin B, miconazole, and rifampin (Garcia 2019). Other amoebae capable of causing less severe meningoencephalitis include *Angiostrongylus cantonensis, Balamuthia mandrillaris,* and *Acanthamoeba.* The hallmark of parasitic meningoencephalitis is CSF eosinophilia (Aksamit and Berkowitz 2021).

Chronic Meningitis

Chronic meningitis is inflammation of the meninges persisting for 4 weeks or more (Aksamit 2021). Chronic infectious meningitis is usually bacterial or fungal, with etiologies varying by geographic region. Headache, lethargy, mental status changes, and fever are common, whereas nuchal rigidity occurs less frequently than in acute meningitis. Cognitive changes occur in about 40% of patients and may be the only presenting feature (Aksamit 2021). Evaluation for chronic meningitis is an important element of the diagnostic workup for rapidly progressive dementia, especially in immunocompromised patients. Hydrocephalus and elevated ICP can occur, and seizures or infarcts may result from infectious cerebral vasculitis. The cranial nerves or spinal nerve roots may be affected as they pass through the subarachnoid space, causing cranial neuropathies or radiculopathies.

Tuberculous Meningitis

Tuberculous meningitis (TBM), caused by hematogenous spread of *Mycobacterium tuberculosis* to the meninges, is a common cause of meningitis in lower-income countries. In the United States, TBM occurs primarily in individuals who are immunocompromised, who have been incarcerated, or who have immigrated from regions where tuberculosis is endemic (Aksamit 2021). Headache, stiff neck, and fever are characteristic symptoms, and cranial neuropathies are common. Infarcts or increased ICP may cause focal neurological deficits. TBM can manifest with or without systemic tuberculosis, and skin and serum testing may be negative in isolated CNS disease. Neuroimaging demonstrates hydrocephalus in about half of cases and infarcts related to infectious vasculopathy in about one-quarter; tuberculomas may be visualized along the surface of the brain and spinal cord (Chin 2019). Definitive diagnosis is made in CSF with the PCR-based Xpert MTB/RIF Ultra test, although it has a sensitivity of around 70%, so a negative result does not exclude TBM (Chin 2019). Treatment is with the standard four-medication regimen for medication-sensitive tuberculosis—isoniazid, rifampin, pyrazinamide, and ethambutol—plus adjuvant corticosteroids in the early stage.

Spirochete Meningitis

Neuroborreliosis (Lyme Disease)

Lyme disease is a tick-borne illness caused by any of several species of the spirochete genus *Borrelia*. The majority of the estimated 30,000 cases annually in the United States are caused by *B. burgdorferi* (Ford and Tufts 2021). Lyme involvement of the nervous system—neuroborreliosis—occurs in up to 20% of cases and typically manifests in the early disseminated stage as meningitis associated with cranial neuritis and painful radiculoneuritis. Headache is common; fever and overt meningeal signs are rare; and the facial nerve is the most commonly involved cranial nerve, with bilateral facial nerve palsy occurring in a third of cases (Garcia-Monco and Benach 2019). Serum antibody testing in acute neuroborreliosis is usually positive. CSF demonstrates lymphocytic pleocytosis; approximately 90% of patients have evidence of intrathecal production of antibodies against *B. burgdorferi*. Treatment is with intravenous ceftriaxone, cefotaxime, penicillin G, or oral doxycycline (Lantos et al. 2021).

Neurosyphilis

Treponema pallidum, the spirochete bacterium that causes syphilis, spreads rapidly during the primary (chancre) stage of infection to invade the CNS in at least 30% of infected individuals. The immune system usually clears *T. pallidum* from the CNS before lasting complications emerge, but approximately 0.7% of individuals without HIV and 1.2% of HIV-infected individuals develop neurosyphilis. Among HIV-infected individuals, the risk of neurosyphilis is elevated in those with lower peripheral blood CD4^{+} T cell counts, detectable plasma HIV viral load, or high serum rapid plasma reagin titers, or in those who are not receiving antiretroviral therapy (Gonzalez et al. 2019).

Neurosyphilis syndromes are divided into those occurring early or late in the disease course. Meningitis, the earliest event, occurs in around one-quarter of all syphilis cases (Aksamit 2021). Diagnosis requires serological confirmation of syphilis infection and demonstration of characteristic CSF abnormalities, including lymphocytic pleocytosis, elevated protein, and CSF-Venereal Disease Research Laboratory (CSF-VDRL) test reactivity. Most individuals with early neurosyphilis are asymptomatic (Chow 2021). Early symptomatic syphilis can manifest as syphilitic meningitis, with signs of meningeal irritation or increased ICP, or meningovascular syphilis, which manifests as subacute meningitis complicated by stroke. Late neurosyphilis is discussed later, in the section "Neurological Syndromes Associated With Persistent Infections and Postinfectious Processes."

The prognostic relevance of syphilis-associated CSF abnormalities in asymptomatic individuals is not known. CDC guidelines recommend against routine LP in syphilis-infected patients without neurological symptoms. LP should be considered in HIV-infected patients with high-risk features. Treatment is with penicillin G in combination with probenecid.

Fungal Meningitis

Fungal invasion of the CNS occurs most often in the setting of immunocompromise, although immunocompetent individuals can be affected. Clinical presentation is similar to that of TBM. The most common fungal meningitis is cryptococcosis, caused by *Cryptococcus neoformans* and to a lesser extent by *C. gatti.* Although most patients with cryptococcal meningitis are immunocompromised, up to 20% are immunocompetent (Aksamit and Berkowitz 2021). Fever and meningeal signs are often absent, and patients typically present with symptoms of hydrocephalus. Isolated cognitive impairment can also occur. Neuroimaging demonstrates thick, nodular leptomeningeal enhancement, hydrocephalus, and strokes. Definitive diagnosis requires identification of cryptococcal antigen in CSF. Treatment is with amphotericin B and fluconazole, followed by 1 year of fluconazole maintenance therapy.

Other fungal meningitides are considerations depending on geographic region and immune status. In the southwestern United States, coccidioidomycosis is a common infection that usually causes a benign flu-like syndrome, but patients can present with meningitis. Histoplasmosis and blastomycosis are endemic in the Mississippi and Ohio River valleys, with blastomycosis also found in the Great Lakes region; in both, meningitis is usually accompanied by pulmonary disease. In immunocompromised individuals, *Candida* can invade the CNS in the setting of systemic candidiasis (Aksamit 2021).

Encephalitis

Encephalitis, inflammation of brain parenchyma, may be infectious or autoimmune. The majority of infectious encephalitides are caused by viruses, most commonly herpesviruses, arboviruses, and enteroviruses.

HSV is the leading cause of sporadic encephalitis in the world (Venkatesan 2021). More than 90% of HSV encephalitis is due to HSV-1, a ubiquitous virus that infects sensory neurons and establishes latency in sensory ganglia. During primary or reactivation infection, HSV-1 can reach the brain, where it typically produces mild or no symptoms but can cause devastating acute inflammation in an unfortunate subset of patients (Marcocci et al. 2020). VZV, the second most common cause of sporadic viral encephalitis globally after HSV, similarly can cause encephalitis at the time of primary infection (chicken pox) or during reactivation, where it is often preceded by the painful herpes zoster (shingles) rash. Epstein-Barr virus, cytomegalovirus (CMV), and human herpesvirus 6 (HHV-6) rarely cause encephalitis in immunocompetent adults but can do so in children or immunocompromised patients. CMV is an important cause of encephalitis in patients with AIDS.

Arbovirus transmission rates vary by season and geographic region and are increasingly significant in the context of climate change and global travel. WNV is the most common cause of epidemic viral encephalitis in the United States, whereas Japanese encephalitis virus (JEV) predominates in South and Southeast Asia (Venkatesan 2021).

Enterovirus infections are usually asymptomatic and are rarely associated with neurological complications. However, given their high global prevalence, they are a frequent cause of viral encephalitis. Although most enterovirus encephalitis cases are mild, the EV-71 and EV-D68 strains can cause severe brainstem encephalitis.

Measles virus (MeV) is a rare but potentially devastating cause of acute and chronic encephalitis. Primary measles encephalitis due to neuronal invasion by MeV occurs in about 0.1% of measles infections; 10%–15% of patients die and 25% of survivors have neurological impairments (Fisher et al. 2015). Failure to clear acute MeV infection can result in *subacute sclerosing panencephalitis* (SSPE), a chronic progressive encephalitis discussed later, in the section "Neurological Syndromes Associated With Persistent Infections and Postinfectious Processes." Mumps virus can also cause encephalitis; it is typically mild but rarely can involve the brainstem. Rabies virus, typically transmitted through the bite of an infected animal, causes fulminant encephalitis that is preventable with postexposure prophylaxis but lethal if left untreated. HIV and SARS-CoV-2 can rarely cause acute encephalitis with primary infection (Berger 2020; Eggers et al. 2017).

John Cunningham virus (JCV) is a ubiquitous virus that is asymptomatic in healthy individuals but can reactivate in the setting of impaired T cell–mediated immunity to cause progressive multifocal leukoencephalopathy (PML), a potentially devastating demyelinating disease. Risk factors include immunocompromise due to hematological malignancies; HIV/AIDS; autoimmune disorders; and immunosuppressive or immunomodulatory therapies associated with organ transplants and autoimmune disorders, most notably the multiple sclerosis medication natalizumab (Anand 2021). Reactivated JCV selectively infects and kills brain oligodendrocytes, producing focal demyelinating lesions that spread progressively. Prognosis depends on the underlying condition and is generally best in natalizumab-associated cases, although significant neurological disability is common, and the disease is often fatal. In some individuals, restoration of immune function triggers a damaging inflammatory process within PML lesions known as *immune reconstitution inflammatory syndrome*, which can further compound neurological injury.

Bacteria and parasites infrequently cause encephalitis. Brain inflammation related to bacterial infection is usually a complication of bacterial meningitis. *L. monocytogenes* can cause brainstem encephalitis, more often in immunocompromised individuals.

Clinical Presentation

The clinical manifestations of encephalitis vary according to the focal distribution of brain inflammation. International Encephalitis Consortium consensus criteria for clinical diagnosis of encephalitis require the presence of altered mental status for ≥24 hours plus at least two of the following supportive features: fever within 72 hours of presentation; new-onset seizures or focal neurological deficits; CSF pleocytosis; and neuroimaging or electroencephalography abnormalities consistent with encephalitis (Venkatesan et al. 2013).

Some encephalitides have characteristic clinical syndromes. HSV-1 is the most important infectious consideration in *limbic encephalitis,* features of which may include psychiatric disturbances (psychosis, affective lability, mania/hypomania, aggression); seizures with temporal lobe semiology; and cognitive impairments, especially those involving memory and language. Neurobehavioral alterations typically manifest early and may be the sole presenting feature of HSV-1 encephalitis in immunocompromised individuals (Wiedłocha et al. 2015). HHV-6 can cause limbic encephalitis in hematopoietic stem cell transplant recipients. Arboviruses frequently target the basal ganglia and may manifest with movement disorders (e.g., parkinsonism). Brainstem findings such as cranial nerve palsies, dysarthria, ataxia, and nystagmus occur in *rhombencephalitis* associated with arboviruses, enteroviruses, *L. monocytogenes,* and, rarely, HSV.

Diagnosis

Neuroimaging can suggest specific etiologies based on inflammatory lesion distribution. MRI typically reveals T2/FLAIR hyperintense lesions associated with diffusion restriction and/or contrast enhancement. Abnormalities of the medial temporal lobes or other limbic cortices should prompt consideration of HSV-1. Abnormalities of the basal ganglia and thalamus are most often associated with arboviruses, whereas those of the pons and medulla can be seen with *L. monocytogenes,* arboviruses, neurobrucellosis, and enteroviruses. White matter abnormalities can be caused by microangiopathy, as in VZV encephalitis, or demyelination, as in neuroborreliosis, PML, or CMV encephalitis. Hemorrhage can occur with VZV vasculitis or in the context of acute necrotizing encephalopathy related to some respiratory viruses, including SARS-CoV-2. Historically, hemorrhage was considered a signature feature of HSV-1 encephalitis, but this finding is now less common because of improved early detection and treatment (Venkatesan 2021).

CSF analysis includes gram stain and culture; viral PCR testing; cryptococcal antigen testing; and syphilis testing. Arbovirus IgM testing should be considered on the basis of clinical presentation or geographic region. In the absence of an identified etiology, brain biopsy may be pursued in select patients.

Treatment

Supportive care is the mainstay of treatment for most viral encephalitides, with the exception of HSV-1, which is treated with acyclovir. Because even minor treatment delays are associated with poorer outcomes in HSVE, empiric acyclovir is initiated in all suspected encephalitis cases while CSF HSV-1 PCR results are pending. Adjunctive corticosteroids are used in HSV and other severe infectious encephalitides to reduce brain swelling and mitigate the extent of secondary immune-mediated injury, although data on their benefits are mixed (Gundamraj and Hasbun 2020).

Outcomes

Outcomes in encephalitis vary by causative pathogen, although advancing age and immunosuppression are associated with poorer outcomes. Treatment of HSV-1 encephalitis with acyclovir reduces mortality from 70% to less than 20% (Marcocci et al. 2020). Even with optimal treatment, encephalitis is associated with substantial long-term neurological and psychiatric morbidity. Epilepsy is common, especially after HSV-1 and JEV encephalitis, and persistent movement disorders can follow arbovirus encephalitis (Bohmwald et al. 2021). Many patients experience chronic cognitive impairments. Nearly half of all survivors of HSV-1 encephalitis receive psychiatric diagnoses, including psychosis, emotional dysregulation, and personality disorders (Wiedłocha et al. 2015). Importantly, HSV encephalitis is a robust trigger for antineuronal antibody development: more than a quarter of patients develop postinfectious secondary autoimmune encephalitis despite effective antiviral treatment (Armangue et al. 2018).

Brain Abscess

Brain abscesses arise when bacteria, fungi, or parasites access the brain via contiguous spread (e.g., from sinusitis, otitis), hematogenous spread (e.g., from bacterial endocarditis), or direct inoculation from an external source (e.g., head trauma, neurosurgery). Infection begins as focal encephalitis and develops over weeks into a suppurative lesion surrounded by a fibrotic, vascularized capsule. Brain abscesses in immunocompetent adults are generally bacterial, whereas fungal and parasitic causes predominate in immunocompromised patients (Venkatesan 2021). Aerobic and anaerobic streptococci are most often identified.

Staphylococcus aureus is an important consideration in patients with endocarditis, head trauma, or recent neurosurgery. Immunocompromised patients are vulnerable to abscesses caused by opportunistic fungal species (e.g., *Aspergillus, Candida*) and parasites (e.g., *Toxoplasma gondii*). *M. tuberculosis* typically causes nonsuppurative granulomatous brain lesions (tuberculomas) but can cause abscesses in immunocompromised and, rarely, immunocompetent individuals.

Clinical Presentation

Although edema may surround an abscess, the capsule effectively contains the infection, limiting its impact on surrounding brain tissue and muting the systemic inflammatory response. Fever is absent about half the time; presenting symptoms usually relate to focal mass effect or increased ICP, with seizures in about one-quarter of cases (Venkatesan 2021). Fewer than 25% of patients present with the classic triad of fever, headache, and focal neurological deficits, and symptoms may be present for a week or more before a diagnosis is made. Abrupt worsening of headache, new-onset meningeal signs, or rapid neurological deterioration may signal capsule rupture with infectious invasion of the subarachnoid or intraventricular space. Intraventricular rupture is typically fatal.

Diagnosis

Contrast-enhanced neuroimaging is essential in the diagnosis of brain abscesses. MRI is more sensitive than CT in the early stages. A mature abscess appears as a centrally necrotic lesion, visualized as focal hypodensity on CT or T2/FLAIR hyperintensity and diffusion restriction on MRI, surrounded by a rim of contrast enhancement and variable vasogenic edema. Contiguous spread of cranial infections usually produces solitary abscesses, whereas abscesses due to systemic infections are typically multifocal. Most occur in frontotemporal regions at the gray-white matter junction.

Diagnosis usually requires biopsy. Blood cultures may yield a pathogen in one-quarter of patients (Cantiera et al. 2019). HIV status is important because toxoplasmosis is the most common cause of focal brain lesions in HIV-infected individuals. LP is generally avoided given the risk of herniation with space-occupying lesions.

Treatment

Brain abscesses are treated with a combination of antibiotics and surgical drainage. Most patients require neurosurgical intervention. Needle aspiration is preferred over surgical excision given its lesser association with neurological complications, although excision may be needed in select circumstances such as traumatic abscesses containing foreign material or if clinical deterioration continues despite needle aspiration.

Antibiotics alone may be attempted for abscesses that are small, not yet encapsulated, located in brain regions unfavorable to surgical intervention, or associated with systemic infection, in which case blood cultures may yield a causative organism. Empiric antibiotic regimens are selected on the basis of the presumed infectious source and typically involve a combination of medications that penetrate the BBB and provide broad-spectrum coverage. Standard protocols typically include a third-generation cephalosporin and metronidazole, with vancomycin added if methicillin-resistant *Staphylococcus* coverage is needed. HIV-infected patients should receive empiric treatment for toxoplasmosis. The regimen is narrowed once an organism is identified.

Adjunctive corticosteroids are administered when abscesses are accompanied by significant edema and mass effect, but their use may hamper the immune system's ability to contain the infection by interfering with capsule formation. Corticosteroid treatment of brain abscesses should be time-limited, reserved for patients at risk of brain herniation, and discontinued as soon as clinical improvement occurs.

Outcomes

Mortality from brain abscess is around 10%–20% and is associated with advanced age, medical comorbidities, hematogenous spread of infection, and the number of abscesses (Venkatesan 2021). Epilepsy and chronic focal neurological deficits are common.

Infections of the Spinal Cord and Peripheral Nervous System

A wide range of pathogens can infect the spinal cord and PNS. In the spinal cord, certain microbes preferentially affect the anterior horns (e.g., poliovirus); dorsal columns (e.g., syphilis); or dorsal root ganglia (e.g., herpesviruses). Intramedullary spinal cord abscesses, like brain abscesses, can result from contiguous or hematogenous spread. *Transverse myelitis,* cross-sectional inflammation of a given spinal cord segment, can be caused by infection (e.g., early HIV, Lyme disease, polio). PNS infections can produce cranial neuropathy, radiculopathy, various mono- and polyneuropathies, autonomic neuropathy, motor nerve hyperexcitability, neuromuscular junction dysfunction, and myopathy. The list of organisms capable of infecting the PNS is extensive and is reviewed elsewhere (LoRusso 2021).

Neurological Syndromes Associated With Persistent Infections and Postinfectious Processes

Delayed-onset, chronic, or progressive neurological dysfunction following an initial infection can be caused by low-level persistence of the infection itself or by postinfectious immune dysregulation.

Persistent Infection

The most important pathogen capable of causing chronic neurological dysfunction is HIV, which enters brain parenchyma soon after infection and may replicate there at a low level for years despite antiretroviral therapy (Eggers et al. 2017). Cerebral manifestations of chronic HIV infection include cognitive, behavioral, and motor disturbances collectively referred to as *HIV-associated neurocognitive disorder* (HAND). Insidious onset and slow progression are typical. HAND may respond to antiretroviral therapy.

Lyme disease infrequently causes a chronic encephalomyelitis manifesting months or years after initial infection (Garcia-Monco and Benach 2019). Diagnosis of *late neuroborreliosis* requires demonstration of intrathecal production of anti–*B. burgdorferi* antibodies, and antibiotics can be curative. Late neuroborreliosis, in which there is evidence of active infection, is distinct from *posttreatment Lyme disease syndrome,* which is diagnosed in individuals who previously received antibiotics for symptomatic, laboratory-proven Lyme disease (Roos 2021). Posttreatment Lyme disease can include nonspecific features such as fatigue, chronic pain, sleep disturbances, paresthesias, and cognitive complaints. The syndrome is believed to be related to a dysregulated immune response to the initial infection, and antibiotics are not recommended (Garcia-Monco and Benach 2019).

Late neurosyphilis has two forms: *tabes dorsalis,* caused by infectious demyelination of the posterior columns of the spinal cord; and *general paresis,* a chronic encephalitis that manifests insidiously with cognitive and behavioral changes and can progress to severe dementia. In both forms of tertiary syphilis, the patient may have Argyll Robertson pupils, in which the pupils constrict with accommodation but not in response to light (also referred to as light-near dissociation). Even with treatment with high-dose penicillin G, up to a third of patients may not improve (Chow 2021).

SSPE is a rare, late complication of measles infection believed to be due to incomplete clearance of acute MeV infection. Onset is typically 6–15 years after primary infection. Initial cognitive and behavioral disturbances are followed by progressive neurological deterioration with seizures, movement disorders, and eventually coma. Definitive diagnosis requires demonstration of high MeV antibody titers in CSF. Electroencephalogram (EEG) shows generalized, periodic, high-voltage slow-wave complexes that are bilaterally synchronous and occur every 5–15 seconds. Treatment is supportive. Death occurs within 3 years; the mortality rate is 95% (Diwan et al. 2022).

Postinfectious Autoimmune and Inflammatory Syndromes

A wide range of postinfectious autoimmune neurological syndromes have been described. *Guillain-Barré syndrome,* the most common cause of acute flaccid weakness, is an immune-mediated polyneuropathy that can be triggered by several pathogens, including *Campylobacter jejuni,* influenza, HIV, and SARS-CoV-2 (Blackburn and Wang 2020). Autoimmune encephalitis has been associated with HSV-1, SARS-CoV-2, and WNV, among others. Acute disseminated encephalomyelitis causes multifocal demyelination in the CNS and can follow various infections. Group A streptococcal infections can cause Sydenham's chorea, an autoimmune-mediated hyperkinetic movement disorder.

Many pathogens have been implicated in the development of myalgic encephalomyelitis, also known as chronic fatigue syndrome or postviral fatigue syndrome (Stefano 2021). The association of SARS-CoV-2 infection with chronic symptoms of fatigue, cognitive dysfunction, dysautonomia, and mood disturbances—collectively referred to as *long COVID*—has increased research interest in this area.

Case Example, Continued

The patient reluctantly allows her vital signs to be checked, revealing a temperature of 100.9°F and a heart rate of 124 bpm. She gives the year as 1987, repeatedly asks for the examiner's name, and needs frequent reminders to remain seated. Throughout the examination, she has several brief episodes of speech arrest, repetitive swallowing, and leftward gaze. She cries after each of these events, although she denies awareness of anything amiss.

The patient undergoes head CT, which reveals subtle focal hypodensity in the right anteromedial temporal lobe. She then has a generalized tonic-clonic seizure, prompting the initiation of broad-spectrum antibiotic coverage with intravenous vancomycin, cefepime, and acyclovir. Brain MRI demonstrates gyriform swelling and T2/FLAIR hyperintensity in the right anteromedial temporal lobe (Figure 12.1) with an area of diffusion restriction within the lesion. She undergoes an urgent LP. CSF reveals lymphocyte-predominant pleocytosis with 14 white cells/µL and 3 red cells/µL, mildly elevated protein of 53 mg/dL, normal glucose of 68 mg/dL, and a negative gram stain. Vancomycin and cefepime are stopped; acyclovir is continued. The meningitis-encephalitis PCR panel subsequently is positive for HSV-1, confirming the final diagnosis of HSV encephalitis.

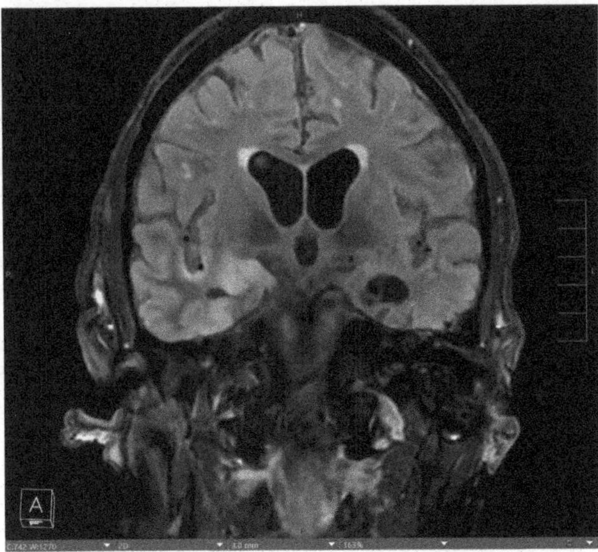

Figure 12.1 Brain MRI of herpes simplex virus type 1 encephalitis.

Key Clinical Points

- Neurological infections can manifest over any time course and involve any level of the neuraxis. They can be caused by viruses, bacteria, fungi, or parasites.
- Although some pathogens cause specific clinical symptoms or have unique radiological correlates, most resulting diseases can manifest with a wide variety of clinical presentations and/or radiological abnormalities.
- A high index of suspicion for infection should be exercised in immunocompromised populations because these patients may present with atypical clinical symptoms and radiological findings because of reduced inflammatory reaction.
- Classic symptoms of acute infectious meningitis include fever, headache, neck stiffness, and altered mental status. If there is high clinical suspicion for meningitis, the patient should be given broad empiric treatment while awaiting results of further testing to narrow antimicrobial coverage.
- Most infectious encephalitides are viral. Treatment is supportive for most viral encephalitides except for HSV, which should be treated expeditiously with acyclovir.
- Most brain abscesses require biopsy for definitive diagnosis and often require combination treatment with both antibiotics and surgical drainage.
- Neurological infections of the peripheral nervous system may lead to infectious myelitis, cranial neuropathies, radiculopathies, peripheral neuropathies, neuromuscular junction disorders, and myopathies.

Review Questions

1. An acutely ill patient in the ICU with fever and nuchal rigidity is found to have abnormalities in the basal ganglia and thalamus on FLAIR MR images. While awaiting the results of CSF analysis, which of the following encephalitides is a likely presumptive diagnosis?

   A. HSV-1.
   B. Neurobrucellosis.
   C. VZV.

D. SARS-CoV-2.
E. Arbovirus.

2. A 23-year-old patient becomes acutely ill with behavior changes that rapidly progresses to seizures, catatonia, and coma. EEG reveals bilaterally synchronous high voltage slow wave complexes occurring at 10-second intervals. Which of the following conditions is likely?

   A. Subacute sclerosing panencephalitis.
   B. General paresis.
   C. Creutzfeldt-Jakob disease.
   D. Arbovirus encephalitis.
   E. HSV-1 encephalitis.

3. A patient with a stiff neck and recent low-grade fever undergoes a diagnostic LP. The CSF findings are opening pressure 110 mm H_2O, clear colorless fluid, protein 35, glucose 80 (serum 105), gram stain negative, 2 WBCs (lymphocytes). Which of the following conditions is most likely?

   A. Normal CSF examination.
   B. Bacterial meningitis.
   C. Viral meningitis.
   D. Tubercular meningitis.
   E. Fungal meningitis.

Answers

Question 1: E. MRI can help in identifying possible etiologies of encephalitis. Arboviruses such as West Nile virus may cause hyperintensities on T2/FLAIR in the thalamus, basal ganglia, and midbrain. Medial temporal abnormalities are seen in HSV-1. Microangiopathic changes can be seen in varicella zoster virus encephalitis, and pontomedullary abnormalities may be seen in neurobrucellosis.

Question 2: A. Subacute sclerosing pan encephalitis (SSPE) is a progressive, usually fatal complication of measles virus occurring 6–15 years following the initial infection. EEG findings combined with the clinical symptoms are usually sufficient for presumptive diagnosis. Like SSPE, Creutzfeldt-Jakob disease is also a rapid dementia that can include myoclonic jerks, but the typical EEG findings are triphasic or biphasic sharp wave complexes occurring every second.

Question 3: A. In bacterial meningitis, the opening pressure might be elevated, the fluid may be turbid, protein may be elevated, and glucose may be decreased, and polymorphonuclear cells may be present in the CSF. With viral meningitis, test results might be normal except for lymphocytes in the CSF. Tubercular meningitis can include CSF lymphocytosis, elevated opening pressure, moderately elevated protein, and acid-fast bacilli on gram stain. The CSF in fungal meningitis may be normal except for elevated WBCs that are lymphocytic.

References

Aksamit AJ: Chronic meningitis. N Engl J Med 385(10):930–936, 2021 34469648

Aksamit AJ Jr, Berkowitz AL: Meningitis. Continuum (Minneap Minn) 27(4):836–854, 2021 34623095

Anand P: Neurologic infections in patients on immunomodulatory and immunosuppressive therapies. Continuum (Minneap Minn) 27(4):1066–1104, 2021 34623105

Armangue T, Spatola M, Vlagea A, et al: Frequency, symptoms, risk factors, and outcomes of autoimmune encephalitis after herpes simplex encephalitis: a prospective observational study and retrospective analysis. Lancet Neurol 17(9):760–772, 2018 30049614

Berger JR: COVID-19 and the nervous system. J Neurovirol 26(2):143–148, 2020 32447630

Berkowitz AL: Approach to neurologic infections. Continuum (Minneap Minn) 27(4):818–835, 2021 34623094

Blackburn KM, Wang C: Post-infectious neurological disorders. Ther Adv Neurol Disord 13:1756286420952901, 2020 32944082

Bohmwald K, Andrade CA, Gálvez NMS, et al: The causes and long-term consequences of viral encephalitis. Front Cell Neurosci 15:755875, 2021 34916908

Cantiera M, Tattevin P, Sonneville R: Brain abscess in immunocompetent adult patients. Rev Neurol (Paris) 175(7-8):469–474, 2019 31447060

Chin JH: Neurotuberculosis: a clinical review. Semin Neurol 39(4):456–461, 2019 31533186

Chow F: Neurosyphilis. Continuum (Minneap Minn) 27(4):1018–1039, 2021 34623102

Diwan MN, Samad S, Mushtaq R, et al: Measles induced encephalitis: recent interventions to overcome the obstacles encountered in the management amidst the COVID-19 pandemic. Diseases 10(4):104, 2022 36412598

Druss BG, Chwastiak L, Kern J, et al: Psychiatry's role in improving the physical health of patients with serious mental illness: a report from the

American Psychiatric Association. Psychiatr Serv 69(3):254–256, 2018 29385957

Eggers C, Arendt G, Hahn K, et al: HIV-1-associated neurocognitive disorder: epidemiology, pathogenesis, diagnosis, and treatment. J Neurol 264(8):1715–1727, 2017 28567537

Engelhardt B, Vajkoczy P, Weller RO: The movers and shapers in immune privilege of the CNS. Nat Immunol 18(2):123–131, 2017 28092374

Fisher DL, Defres S, Solomon T: Measles-induced encephalitis. QJM 108(3):177–182, 2015 24865261

Ford L, Tufts DM: Lyme neuroborreliosis: Mechanisms of B. burgdorferi infection of the nervous system. Brain Sci 11(6):789, 2021 34203671

Garcia HH: Parasitic infections of the nervous system. Continuum (Minneap Minn) 27(4):943–962, 2021 34623099

Garcia HH, Nath A, Del Brutto OH: Parasitic infections of the nervous system. Semin Neurol 39(3):358–368, 2019 31378871

Garcia-Monco JC, Benach JL: Lyme neuroborreliosis: clinical outcomes, controversy, pathogenesis, and polymicrobial infections. Ann Neurol 85(1):21–31, 2019 30536421

Gonzalez H, Koralnik IJ, Marra CM: Neurosyphilis. Semin Neurol 39(4):448–455, 2019 31533185

Gundamraj S, Hasbun R: The use of adjunctive steroids in central nervous infections. Front Cell Infect Microbiol 10:592017, 2020 33330135

Klein RS, Hunter CA: Protective and pathological immunity during central nervous system infections. Immunity 46(6):891–909, 2017 28636958

Lantos PM, Rumbaugh J, Bockenstedt LK, et al: Clinical Practice Guidelines by the Infectious Diseases Society of America, American Academy of Neurology, and American College of Rheumatology: 2020 Guidelines for the Prevention, Diagnosis, and Treatment of Lyme Disease. Neurology 96(6):262–273, 2021 33257476

LoRusso S: Infections of the peripheral nervous system. Continuum (Minneap Minn) 27(4):921–942, 2021 34623098

Marcocci ME, Napoletani G, Protto V, et al: Herpes simplex virus-1 in the brain: the dark side of a sneaky infection. Trends Microbiol 28(10):808–820, 2020 32386801

McGill F, Griffiths MJ, Solomon T: Viral meningitis: current issues in diagnosis and treatment. Curr Opin Infect Dis 30(2):248–256, 2017 28118219

Miller AC, Koeneman SH, Arakkal AT, et al: Incidence, duration, and risk factors associated with missed opportunities to diagnose herpes simplex encephalitis: a population-based longitudinal study. Open Forum Infect Dis 8(9):ofab400, 2021 34514018

Piquet AL, Lyons JL: Infectious meningitis and encephalitis. Semin Neurol 36(4):367–372, 2016 27643906

Ribe AR, Vestergaard M, Katon W, et al: Thirty-day mortality after infection among persons with severe mental illness: a population-based cohort study in Denmark. Am J Psychiatry 172(8):776–783, 2015 25698437

Roos KL: Neurologic complications of Lyme disease. Continuum (Minneap Minn) 27(4):1040–1050, 2021 34623103

Rotbart HA: Viral meningitis. Semin Neurol 20(3):277–292, 2000 11051293

Stefano GB: Historical insight into infections and disorders associated with neurological and psychiatric sequelae similar to long COVID. Med Sci Monit 27:e931447, 2021 33633106

van de Beek D, de Gans J, Spanjaard L, et al: Clinical features and prognostic factors in adults with bacterial meningitis. N Engl J Med 351(18):1849–1859, 2004 15509818

van de Beek D, Brouwer M, Hasbun R, et al: Community-acquired bacterial meningitis. Nat Rev Dis Primers 2:16074, 2016 27808261

Venkatesan A: Encephalitis and brain abscess. Continuum (Minneap Minn) 27(4):855–886, 2021 34623096

Venkatesan A, Tunkel AR, Bloch KC, et al: Case definitions, diagnostic algorithms, and priorities in encephalitis: consensus statement of the International Encephalitis Consortium. Clin Infect Dis 2013;57(8):1114–1128 23861361

Wall EC, Chan JM, Gil E, Heyderman RS: Acute bacterial meningitis. Curr Opin Neurol 34(3):386–395, 2021 33767093

Wiedłocha M, Marcinowicz P, Stanczykiewicz B: Psychiatric aspects of herpes simplex encephalitis, tick-borne encephalitis and herpes zoster encephalitis among immunocompetent patients. Adv Clin Exp Med 24(2):361–371, 2015 25931371

13

Neuro-oncology

Oluwatosin Akintola, M.D.
L. Nicolas Gonzalez Castro, M.D., Ph.D.

Case Example

A 58-year-old right-handed male attorney is brought to an emergency department by a colleague after erratic behavior during court proceedings. Over the past 6 weeks, the patient has been reported to have shown progressive paucity of speech, delay in answering questions, and increased use of inappropriate language. He also has been noted to submit his legal briefs with significant delays and lower quality than usual. In addition, the patient reports significant fatigue, not improved by increased sleep time, as well as lack of interest in his work and other activities. On evaluation 3 weeks prior, the patient was diagnosed with major depressive disorder and started on citalopram.

Neoplastic brain lesions that arise from brain parenchyma or the meninges are classified as primary brain tumors. Secondary brain tumors result from metastasis of cancers originating outside the brain. Both primary and metastatic brain tumors can lead to disruption of brain function, with signs and symptoms that correlate with the anatomical location of the tumor. Disruption of brain function results from direct infiltration and destruction, by mass effect mediated by the tumor, or by peritumoral edema. Metastatic brain tumors are generally malignant, fast-growing tumors within the brain parenchyma. Leptomeningeal metastases result from dissemination of cancer into the arachnoid mater, pia mater, and cerebrospinal fluid (CSF).

Primary brain tumors are further divided into low-grade (slow-growing) and high-grade (fast-growing) tumors. Tumors are graded according to the WHO scale based on cellularity, mitotic counts, presence of brain invasion, and evidence of spontaneous necrosis (Louis et al. 2021). Primary brain tumor subtypes include tumors that arise from glial cells (astrocytomas, oligodendrogliomas, glioblastomas, ependymomas) and tumors that arise from intracranial supportive structures such as the meninges (meningiomas), glands (pituitary adenomas), and lymphatic tissue (CNS lymphomas). The relative incidence of these tumors may be found in Table 13.1. Gliomas, meningiomas, primary CNS lymphomas, and brain metastases are discussed in this chapter.

Cancers may lead to indirect pathologic states in the CNS. Paraneoplastic neurological syndromes may occur when the immune system, activated by the underlying cancer, also attacks parts of the nervous system. Autoimmune effects of cancer on the brain, spinal cord, peripheral nerves, neuromuscular junction, or muscle may cause problems with muscle movement or coordination (e.g., myasthenia gravis); sensory perception (peripheral neuropathy); and memory, orientation, language, and executive skills (autoimmune encephalitis).

It is important to note that nonneoplastic conditions may appear similar to primary brain tumors or secondary brain tumors on cranial imaging. The differential diagnosis of brain masses includes abscesses/ infections, demyelination, subacute infarction, subacute hemorrhage, vascular malformations, and inflammatory disorders such as neurosarcoidosis. Neuropsychiatric paraneoplastic syndromes are discussed later in this chapter and in Chapter 14, “Neuroimmunology.”

Approach to Patients With Brain Tumors

Common Clinical Presentations

Brain tumor patients generally present with subacute symptoms unless they present with a seizure. Most brain tumor patients present with progressive headache and seizures. Headache is usually holocephalic, progressive, and worse in the morning and fails to respond to symp-

Table 13.1 Incidence of brain tumors

CNS tumor type	AAIR per 100,000	Percentage of brain tumors
Primary malignant		
Glioma	—	24.5[a]
Oligodendrogliomas	0.40	1.5[a]
Diffuse astrocytomas	0.88	3.5[a]
Glioblastomas	3.23	14.3[a]
CNS lymphoma	0.4	2[a]
Primary nonmalignant		
Meningioma	9.49	39[a]
Pituitary tumors	4.36	17.1[a]
Secondary		
Brain metastases	24.2	>50[b]

AAIR = average annual age-adjusted incidence rate.
[a]Percentage of primary brain tumors.
[b]Percentage of all brain tumors.
Source. Adapted from Habbous et al. 2020; Ostrom et al. 2021.

tomatic analgesic treatment. Behavioral symptoms develop over weeks and months and are often best described by collateral information, especially if the patient has limited insight into their condition. Other symptoms include decreased level of arousal, abulia, anhedonia, irritability, dysregulation of executive function, memory loss, and language impairments.

Neurologic Examination Considerations

Fundoscopic examination to evaluate for blurring of the optic disk margins—a sign of increased intracranial pressure (ICP)—should be performed in all patients reporting headaches. Focal weakness develops over weeks and months unless experienced transiently after focal motor seizure (postictal paralysis). Weakness can be subtle but is frequently unmasked by evaluating for pronator drift or loss of dexterity (bilateral finger tapping).

Imaging Considerations

After obtaining a careful history and performing a detailed neurologic examination, neuroimaging is the next step to rule out other etiologies and confirm the presence of a brain lesion. MRI ordered with and without gadolinium is the most sensitive imaging study for brain tumors. One should systematically survey soft tissues, bone structures, meninges, and fluid-filled spaces in addition to evaluating the brain parenchyma. Start with T2-weighted sequences, particularly T2-fluid-attenuated inversion recovery (FLAIR), as many lesions are visible only in these sequences and may not enhance after the administration of gadolinium. Then, compare T1 with and without contrast side by side to identify areas of contrast versus areas of intrinsic T1 hyperintensity. Review diffusion-weighted imaging and apparent diffusion coefficient sequences to identify areas of increased cellularity; review gradient recalled echo or susceptibility-weighted images to identify areas of hemorrhage. Note the size, morphology, number, and location (extra- vs. intra-axial; supra- vs. infratentorial) of lesions, as well as the pattern of contrast enhancement, to find clues as to the origin of the tumor (primary vs. metastatic) and its potential clinical behavior (high-grade vs. low-grade).

Gliomas

Epidemiology

Gliomas are the most common malignant primary brain tumors (Ostrom et al. 2021). The most common and aggressive glioma subtype is glioblastoma, WHO grade 4, with a median age at diagnosis of 65. Isocitrate dehydrogenase (IDH) mutant gliomas are diagnosed in younger patients (median age at diagnosis of 35 for diffuse astrocytoma, WHO grade 2–4, and 40 for oligodendroglioma, WHO grade 2–3) and have a better prognosis than glioblastoma (10–15 years vs. 16 months). A few rare genetic syndromes (Li-Fraumeni, Turcot, neurofibromatosis type I) are associated with a greater probability of developing gliomas. The only known environmental risk factor for glioma is prior exposure to ionizing radiation.

Diagnosis

Glioma diagnosis is suspected based on MRI findings and established after review of histological features and molecular alterations via biopsy or tumor resection. Diffuse astrocytic gliomas can be low-grade, slow-growing tumors (grade 2) or higher-grade, fast-growing malignant tumors (grade 3–4). Low-grade gliomas are associated with *IDH* mutations, and *IDH* mutations are often required for a diagnosis of low-grade glioma. Although specific mutations are outside the scope of this chapter, it is important to note that the grading and subtyping of gliomas depends on their genetic profile. Gliomas are often graded based on the genetic signature, regardless of histological appearance (Gritsch et al. 2022; Louis et al. 2021).

Management

All diffusely infiltrating gliomas progress after treatment and are invariably terminal. According to National Comprehensive Cancer Network guidelines, enrollment in a therapeutic clinical trial is the leading recommendation for management. For patients unable to enroll in a clinical trial, the standard of care after maximal safe resection involves radiation and alkylating chemotherapy (temozolomide for high-grade gliomas; temozolomide vs. procarbazine/lomustine/vincristine for low-grade tumors). The use of targeted therapy with IDH inhibitors (e.g., vorasidenib) is also an option for patients with low-grade *IDH*-mutant glioma after resection. An external, alternating electric field device (tumor-treating fields) is also available to be used in combination with chemotherapy for the treatment of glioblastoma. Bevacizumab, an anti-angiogenic monoclonal antibody, is indicated for the management of recurrent glioblastoma.

Neuropsychiatric Complications

Gliomas can often present with behavioral changes, particularly when tumors involve the frontal or temporal lobes or when there is diffuse cerebral infiltration, such as in the gliomatosis cerebri pattern of glioma growth (Rhee and Gonzalez Castro 2022). Patients with temporal lobe gliomas often experience behavioral changes that may be subtle and intermittent, affecting their observation and diagnosis. Involvement of other limbic structures can lead to aggressive and even homicidal behavior. An emblematic case is Charles Whitman (the "Texas Tower Sniper"). He committed multiple homicides, prompting an autopsy upon his demise. He was found to have glioblastoma affecting his left amygdala, a brain structure crucial for aggression and behavioral control (Eagleman 2011).

Depression is more prevalent in patients with glioma than in the general population. Although it is unclear whether this results from tumor involvement, it is important to screen and treat, as it can markedly affect patient survival (Rooney et al. 2011; Shi et al. 2018). Patients presenting with seizures are often managed with levetiracetam. However, this agent should be avoided in patients with a history of mood disorder, as it can cause irritability, worsen depressive symptoms, or even cause psychotic symptoms. Other antiseizure agents with better behavioral symptom profiles (lacosamide) or mood-stabilizing properties (lamotrigine, valproic acid) may be preferred (Gonzalez Castro and Milligan 2020). Dexamethasone, often used to reduce peritumoral edema, may cause steroid-induced mania or psychosis. Hence, dexamethasone should be used at the lowest effective dose and tapered off as soon as clinically possible.

Meningiomas

Epidemiology

Meningiomas are the most commonly diagnosed CNS tumor, comprising 39% of all primary CNS tumors. Most meningiomas are benign, and meningiomas represent more than half (54.5%) of all nonmalignant CNS tumors. The median age of diagnosis in the United States is 66, with a female-to-male ratio of 2.27:1 (Ostrom et al. 2021). Meningiomas are a common feature of neurocutaneous syndromes, specifically neurofibromatosis type 2 (NF2) and schwannomatosis (Asthagiri et al. 2009). Other risk factors for meningiomas include childhood cranial irradiation (one in eight childhood cancer survivors); lifetime exposure to progesterone and estrogen; and high body mass index (BMI) (Kok et al. 2019; Ostrom et al. 2019).

Diagnosis

Most meningiomas are asymptomatic and are first discovered on radiologic imaging (CT or MRI) for other unrelated complaints. MRI is the gold standard modality of radiological diagnosis of meningiomas. Radiological features of meningiomas may include intralesional calcifications, adjacent bony changes including hyperostosis and skull remodeling, CSF cleft (rim between tumor and brain), and the hallmark "dural tail" (tapered thickening of the surrounding dura). Overall, meningiomas have homogeneous enhancement and are well-demarcated tumors. Most patients with meningiomas present with a solitary tumor. Multiple meningiomas may be seen in syndromes such as NF2 or in radiation-induced meningiomas. The majority of meningiomas are WHO grade 1 (75%–80%), approximately 15%–20% are atypical WHO grade 2, and less than 5% are anaplastic WHO grade 3 (Hollec-zek et al. 2019; Ostrom et al. 2020). Alteration of the tumor-suppressor gene *NF2* is the most commonly observed mutation in meningiomas in NF2 syndrome, as well as in approximately 60% of sporadic meningiomas (Brastianos et al. 2013; Zang 2001).

Management

Surgery is the mainstay of treatment for symptomatic meningiomas and those that measure ≥3 cm in diameter. Meningiomas that are incidentally discovered, asymptomatic, and <3 cm may be monitored with annual MRI head surveillance scans. If surgery is required, the extent of resection is predictive of outcomes in patients with meningioma. The Simpson grading system indicates the degree of resection. Gross total resection (Simpson Grades I–III) is associated with a lower risk of recurrence and can be curative for grade 1 meningiomas, with a <10% recurrence rate. About 40%–50% of gross totally resected grade 2 meningiomas and >75% of gross totally resected grade 3 meningiomas eventually recur (Aghi et al. 2009). Adjuvant radiation is the standard of care following resection of grade 3 meningiomas, regardless of extent of resection. For patients with incomplete resection of grade 2 meningiomas, adjuvant radiation improves local control.

Neuropsychiatric Complications

Although most meningiomas are indolent extra-axial tumors, their capacity to exert pressure on neighboring brain structures often leads to neuropsychiatric symptoms. Headaches are often a reflection of elevated ICP due to direct mass effect or blockage of CSF or venous drainage. Anterior skull base tumors represent 9% of meningiomas (Abbassy et al. 2016). Because of the slow-growing nature of these tumors, quite large frontal or bilateral frontal masses may be discovered in patients presenting with depressive episodes, disorganization, abulia, disinhibition, and hyperactivity. The middle cranial fossa is a common location for meningiomas. Meningiomas in this location often manifest with symptoms related to the compression or invasion of the temporal lobes (seizures, auras, memory changes). In regard to treatment effects, cognitive impairment is a recognized adverse effect of cranial irradiation. Elderly patients are particularly vulnerable in the short term. Given the increased chances of prolonged survival in patients with lower-grade meningiomas, cognitive impairment may present as a complication later in life.

Primary CNS Lymphoma

Epidemiology

Primary CNS lymphoma (PCNSL) is a rare form of extranodal non-Hodgkin's lymphoma involving the brain, spine, CSF, or eyes only. The incidence of PCNSL in the United States is 0.4 per 100,000 per year (Ostrom et al. 2020). Primary CNS lymphomas are generally B cell lymphomas, with <5% being T cell–derived lymphomas. PCNSL may present as part of end-stage disease in immunosuppressed patients with AIDS, posttransplant patients, and people with congenital immunodeficiency.

Clinical Presentation

Patients with CNS lymphoma may present with nonspecific behavioral and mental status changes in 40%–50% of cases (Bataille et al. 2000). Cognitive changes in these patients often result from tumor involvement in structures critical for cognition, such as the frontal lobes, corpus callosum, and deep white matter structures. Because the incidence of primary CNS lymphoma is higher in the elderly, disease onset is often mistaken for symptoms of dementia. Focal neurological symptoms such as aphasia, dysarthria, or cranial nerve palsies may occur, depending on the nervous system structures affected by the disease.

Diagnosis

PCNSL often appears as multifocal, homogeneously enhancing lesions within the deep brain structures on MRI. Stereotactic or open brain biopsy for tissue sampling is required for effective diagnosis. As lymphomas may be partially treated with corticosteroids, steroid use should be avoided until a biopsy is completed to limit the risk of diagnostic failure. Exceptions include patients who present with significant edema and mass effect. Complete neuraxis evaluation is required, with MRI scans of the cervical, thoracic, and lumbar spine. Lumbar puncture for CSF testing (including cell count, glucose, and protein levels, cytology, flow cytometry, and immunoglobulin heavy chain gene rearrangement assay) should be obtained. Complete ophthalmologic work-up with slit lamp evaluation is required for assessment of ocular lymphoma. Evaluation of the extent of disease for the presence of systemic lymphoma is required, with whole-body positron emission tomography (PET)-CT scans or CT chest, abdomen, and pelvis scans. Males should have testicular ultrasound. On pathological review, diffuse large B cell lymphoma is the most common type of PCNSL, although rarer types exist (Pina-Oviedo et al. 2020).

Management

The treatment of primary CNS lymphoma involves two phases—induction therapy and consolidation therapy. Antimetabolite chemotherapies such as high-dose methotrexate or high-dose cytarabine form the backbone of the most-used PCNSL induction regimens. These chemotherapies are often combined with additional agents such as temozolomide, rituximab, etoposide, procarbazine, and vincristine. Consolidation therapy is given after the induction phase to help maintain response to the induction treatment. Consolidation strategies include whole-brain radiotherapy (WBRT), nonmyeloablative high-dose chemotherapy, and myeloablative conditioning with autologous stem cell transplantation.

Neuropsychiatric Complications

Methotrexate is associated with acute encephalopathy (confusion, disorientation, hallucinations, and seizures). Symptoms usually occur within hours to a few days after methotrexate administration. Stroke-like episodes of alternating hemiparesis associated with speech arrest have also been reported with methotrexate use. Delayed leukoencephalopathy is a particular concern in patients treated for CNS lymphoma. Symptoms develop over the course of months to years. Patients may report mild to moderate cognitive deficits, personality changes, motor and coordination deficits, and urinary incontinence. Brain MRI findings often reveal subcortical and periventricular confluent T2/FLAIR hyperintensities consistent with delayed leukoencephalopathy. Cerebellar dysfunction has been the most reported side effect (10%–20%) with cytarabine (Herzig et al. 1987). The cerebellar syndrome is characterized by acute to subacute onset of ataxia, tremors, dysmetria, nystagmus, and imbalance. Encephalopathy, somnolence, and nausea may also be part of the clinical presentation. Most patients recover after discontinuation of cytarabine; however, permanent cerebellar dysfunction has been reported in 20%–30% of patients who develop this syndrome (Di Francia et al. 2021). MRI findings are initially unremarkable, but cerebellar atrophy may be detected after several months.

Brain Metastases

Epidemiology

Brain metastases are the most common malignant neoplasms of the CNS. Approximately 20%–40% of patients with cancer will develop CNS metastases in their lifetime (Mehta et al. 2005). The incidence of brain metastases has been increasing over the years owing to advances in cancer care resulting in longer-term cancer survival. Brain metastases are often a sign of late-stage disease. The most common sources of brain metastases include lung (50%–60%), breast (15%–25%), and melanoma (5%–20%) (Taillibert and Le Rhun 2015); these frequencies reflect the prevalence of these common cancers in the general population. Among all solid tumor subtypes, small cell lung cancer and melanoma have the highest propensity to metastasize to the CNS.

Leptomeningeal metastases, a subset of multifocal CNS metastases, are disseminated in the leptomeninges (pia mater, arachnoid) or subarachnoid space, with cancer cells detected in CSF. Lung cancer, breast cancer, and melanoma have the highest prevalence of leptomeningeal metastases. Leptomeningeal metastases can occur with or without brain parenchymal metastases, and the prognosis is very poor (<6 months). Pachymeningeal metastases, also known as dural metastases, are common in advanced breast and hematological cancers. The prognosis of intracranial and spinal dural metastases is also poor.

Clinical Presentation

The clinical presentation of brain metastases is similar to the presentation of any brain tumor. Metastatic brain lesions are often associated with brain compression and mass effect. Headache is a presenting symptom in up to 50% of patients (Christiaans et al. 2002). Headaches are more common in patients with leptomeningeal metastasis, multiple brain metastases, or posterior fossa metastases. Papilledema (optic disc swelling) may present with headaches in 15%–25% of patients. About 40% of patients with brain metastases present with focal neurological deficits, such as focal motor weakness or sensory loss. Focal seizures based on the location of the lesion occur in 15%–20% of patients, and some patients present with progression to secondary generalized seizures. Another 5%–10% of patients have an acute stroke-like presentation due to spontaneous intratumoral hemorrhage (most likely to occur in individuals with melanoma, renal cell carcinoma, thyroid cancer, and choriocarcinoma) (Kondziolka et al. 1987; Schrader et al. 2000).

Diagnosis

As in primary brain tumors, MRI is superior to CT scan in evaluating individuals with brain metastases. MRI can detect a greater number of lesions and better define their characteristics. Many patients with a single lesion visible on cranial CT scan are ultimately found to have multiple metastases on cranial MR imaging. Contrast-enhanced chest and abdomen CT and/or whole-body PET-CT are used to detect the primary tumor outside the CNS. Systemic pan scans are also useful to quantify the extent of disease involvement in the patient. Common radiographic findings of brain metastases on contrast-enhanced MRI include peripheral enhancement with prominent peritumoral edema, gray–white junctional location, spherical well-encapsulated shape, and presence of multiple lesions. However, these findings are not specific to metastases. Systemic primary neoplasms can readily be biopsied or resected to provide a histological diagnosis for the cancer. If there are no systemic tumors identified at presentation, surgical resection or stereotactic biopsy of the brain lesion for diagnostic confirmation may be offered. Often, surgical resection of single or oligometastatic brain lesions is offered for therapeutic and diagnostic purposes despite an identifiable primary systemic tumor. Histopathological characteristics of brain metastases depend on the histological features of the underlying cancer.

Leptomeningeal Disease

The presentation of leptomeningeal metastasis depends on the location of involvement. Leptomeningeal disease often represents widespread CNS dissemination; therefore, clinical presentation may be nonspecific. The index of suspicion must be high, particularly in individuals with high-risk cancers that have tendencies for leptomeningeal involvement such as triple-negative (estrogen, progesterone, HER2 receptor negative) breast cancer, HER2-positive breast cancer, and hematologic malignancies. Complaints of headaches, nausea, and vomiting are often attributable to increased ICP or meningeal irritation. Cranial nerves VI, VII, and VIII are commonly affected, resulting in diplopia, facial weakness, and hearing loss. Spinal leptomeningeal signs include dermatomal sensory loss, radicular pain, bowel and bladder dysfunction, and motor weakness.

MRI of the brain and entire spine is recommended for evaluation of leptomeningeal disease. MRI scans may show leptomeningeal enhancement, which is often irregular and nodular. Hydrocephalus, due to subependymal deposits or arachnoid granulations obstructed by diffuse leptomeningeal carcinomatosis, may also be seen. MRI findings should be interpreted with caution if a lumbar puncture was recently performed, as resulting low intracranial pressure or inflammation may lead to transient enhancement. The sensitivity of gadolinium-enhanced MRI is approximately 70%, with a specificity of 77%–100% (higher for solid tumors than hematologic malignancies). In the presence of typical radiologic signs of leptomeningeal metastases (increased signal in the sulci, cerebellar folia, cauda equina) and high clinical suspicion, an abnormal MRI is sufficient to make the diagnosis. If neuroimaging is negative and clinical suspicion remains high, lumbar puncture is recommended. CSF findings include mild pleocytosis with elevated protein and hypoglycorrhachia. An elevated opening pressure may be seen in 50%–70% of cases depending on the extent of leptomeningeal involvement. To avoid false negatives, a sufficient CSF volume of up to 30 mL should be obtained for cytologic analysis. CSF samples for cytological evaluation must be processed as soon as possible to maintain sample viability. Lumbar puncture should be repeated at least once if the initial sample is negative and leptomeningeal metastasis is suspected. CSF cytology is positive in >90% of patients with suspected leptomeningeal metastasis after three high-volume lumbar punctures, and specificity is >95%. Flow cytometry and additional molecular studies increase sensitivity over cytomorphologic analysis alone.

Management

Corticosteroids such as dexamethasone can greatly improve the symptoms of brain metastases in the short term. Typically, an improvement in neurological symptoms is shown within the first day after the introduction of steroid treatment. In patients without signs of intracranial hypertension, lower doses of dexamethasone have efficacy similar to that of higher doses. The dose of dexamethasone is modulated according to the response to treatment and the patient's condition, and the aim is to identify the lowest effective dose. Prophylactic antiseizure medication does not reduce the onset of seizures, so there is no indication for its use. Antiseizure medication should be started only in patients presenting with seizures.

The treatment of brain metastases typically involves a combination of surgery and adjuvant radiotherapy with or without systemic therapy. In select cases, stand-alone radiotherapy or systemic medical therapies are offered. Systemic medical therapies include chemotherapy, targeted therapy, and immunotherapy. A single brain metastasis is generally treated with radiotherapy after resection. Limited intracranial metastatic disease (one to three brain lesions) may be treated with focal radiation such as stereotactic radiosurgery or fractionated stereotactic radiotherapy. WBRT is the standard treatment for patients with multiple metastatic lesions (Minniti et al. 2021). Local control of brain metastases using radiotherapy is often combined or followed by systemic therapy such as chemotherapy, immunotherapy, or targeted therapy. Targeted therapies include agents that inhibit tumor-driving mutations in cancers (Robert et al. 2015; Thomas et al. 2022).

Immunotherapies have produced clinically significant outcomes in the management of patients with brain metastases. Immunotherapy is now the standard of care for melanomas with CNS involvement, and immunotherapies are often a mainstay of treatment for other cancer types with brain or leptomeningeal metastases (Akintola and Reardon 2021).

Neuropsychiatric Complications

Patients with multiple metastases or large metastasis with cerebral edema may develop intracranial hypertension. This could cause an altered mental state and cognitive slowing. Management of cerebral edema with high-dose steroids may lead to steroid mania with delirium. WBRT for multiple brain metastases is associated with worsening neurocognitive function. Radiation neurotoxicity evolves in a biphasic pattern, with a subacute transient decline peaking at 4 months and a late delayed irreversible impairment of neurocognition several months or years after completion of WBRT. Hippocampal avoidance and administration of memantine are strategies to protect neurocognitive function. Immune checkpoint blockade leads to systemic immune activation and can mediate central neuroinflammation in patients with brain tumors (Akintola and Reardon 2021). Neuroinflammation due to immunotherapies may worsen neurocognitive function despite a good brain metastasis response (McGinnis and Raber 2017; Parsons et al. 2021).

Neuropsychiatric Paraneoplastic Syndromes

In their most general senses, *paraneoplastic syndromes* are autoimmune conditions in which the immune system's response against an antigen expressed by a tumor leads to some form of organ dysfunction. Paraneoplastic antibodies, associated with specific tumors, have been described to affect all levels of the nervous system, from cortical neurons to muscle. A number of antibodies affecting membrane receptors (NMDA, AMA, LGI-1, GABA-B, GABA-A), synaptic proteins (GAD65), and intracellular proteins (ANNA-1, ANNA-2, PCA-1) are known to cause limbic encephalitis, a syndrome characterized by subacute behavioral changes, progressing to memory loss and seizures (often with status epilepticus). Although immunosuppression can also lead to symptomatic improvement, the treatment of neuropsychiatric paraneoplastic syndromes is directed at the underlying tumor, as this is the most effective way to reduce the antigenic burden (Flanagan 2021).

Case Example, Continued

On neurologic examination, the patient is awake but oriented only to self. He answers questions and follows commands with significant delay. Fluency is decreased. Cranial nerve, motor, and sensory exams are without abnormalities. His gait is slow and has decreased stride length. The patient also has a Myerson's sign and bilateral grasp reflex. Together, the clinical symptoms, exam findings, and poor executive function point to compromise of frontal subcortical structures. MRI brain with gadolinium reveals a large bifrontal, cystic, peripherally enhancing mass with increased surrounding T2-FLAIR signal. The lesion is biopsied, and pathology confirms a diagnosis of glioblastoma, WHO grade 4.

After a maximal safe debulking resection, the patient is treated with radiation and temozolomide followed by four cycles of adjuvant temozolomide. During cycle 4, he experiences clinical decline, with worsening headache, fatigue, and decreased level of arousal. Repeat brain MRI demonstrates evidence of radiographic progression. High-dose corticosteroids improve his level of arousal but cause sleep disruption and agitation, necessitating treatment with low-dose quetiapine. Corticosteroids are stopped after a taper, and he is given palliative treatment with bevacizumab, which leads to symptomatic improvement over a period of 6 weeks. The patient was subsequently transitioned to hospice care and died 10 months after his diagnosis.

Key Clinical Points

- The most common brain tumors in adults are brain metastases, which are secondary brain cancers originating from other cancers in the body. The most common adult primary brain tumors are meningiomas, followed by gliomas.
- Common neuropsychiatric complaints in patients with brain tumors include cognitive impairment, personality changes, delirium, psychosis, depression, headaches, and seizures.
- Brain tumors produce symptoms and signs through brain invasion, compression of adjacent structures, cerebral edema, and increased intracranial pressure (ICP). Clinical manifestations of brain tumors are determined by the location of involved brain structures.
- MRI with contrast is the gold standard for evaluation of brain tumors. CT has much lower resolution, but a contrast-enhanced CT can be useful in patients with a contraindication to MRI. A CT of the chest, abdomen, and pelvis is often required for a complete assessment of patients with brain metastases and CNS lymphoma.
- Corticosteroids, particularly dexamethasone, are used to decrease tumor-associated cerebral edema and elevated ICP in patients with significant deficits or impending herniation. Steroid-induced mania is a common adverse effect of corticosteroids.
- Individuals with primary or secondary brain neoplasms may present with neuropsychiatric symptoms as a direct result of tumors or as a resultof the toxicity of cancer treatment.

Review Questions

1. Which of the following management strategies is not a disease-directed therapy in glioma?

   A. Surgical resection
   B. Chemotherapy
   C. Radiation therapy
   D. Alternating electric field device
   E. Steroids

2. Which of the following is the most common type of malignant primary brain tumor?

   A. Glioma
   B. Metastasis
   C. Meningioma
   D. Pituitary tumor
   E. Lymphoma

3. Which of the following is *not* a typical risk factor for developing meningiomas?

   A. Childhood cranial radiation
   B. Lifetime exposure to testosterone
   C. Higher BMI
   D. Neurofibromatosis type 2
   E. Schwannomatosis

Answers

Question 1: E. Although steroids may be used to decrease surrounding edema, especially when imminent herniation is a concern, steroids do not have a cytotoxic effect on glioma cells. All other choices eliminate, reduce, or prevent the growth of the tumor.

Question 2: A. The most common malignant primary brain tumor is glioma, followed by lymphoma. If all primary brain tumors, including nonmalignant ones, are included, meningioma is the most common. The next most common nonmalignant tumor is a pituitary tumor. If all types of brain tumors are included, then secondary brain tumors from metastatic disease are the most common.

Question 3: B. There is some evidence that higher progesterone and estrogen exposure (but not testosterone exposure) is associated with meningiomas, and this may also be related to the link with higher BMI. Childhood radiation exposure is a well-established risk factor for meningiomas as well as other tumor types later in life. Neurofibromatosis type 2 (*NF2*) and related genes that cause bilateral vestibular schwannomas are also associated with the development of meningiomas.

References

Abbassy M, Woodard TD, Sindwani R, et al: An overview of anterior skull base meningiomas and the endoscopic endonasal approach. Otolaryngol Clin North Am 49(1):141–152, 2016 26614834

Aghi MK, Carter BS, Cosgrove GR, et al: Long-term recurrence rates of atypical meningiomas after gross total resection with or without postoperative adjuvant radiation. Neurosurgery 64(1):56–60, discussion 60, 2009 19145156

Akintola OO, Reardon DA: The current landscape of immune checkpoint blockade in glioblastoma. Neurosurg Clin N Am 32(2):235–248, 2021 33781505

Asthagiri AR, Parry DM, Butman JA, et al: Neurofibromatosis type 2. Lancet 373(9679):1974–1986, 2009 19476995

Bataille B, Delwail V, Menet E, et al: Primary intracerebral malignant lymphoma: report of 248 cases. J Neurosurg 92(2):261–266, 2000 10659013

Brastianos PK, Horowitz PM, Santagata S, et al: Genomic sequencing of meningiomas identifies oncogenic SMO and AKT1 mutations. Nat Genet 45(3):285–289, 2013 23334667

Christiaans MH, Kelder JC, Arnoldus EP, et al: Prediction of intracranial metastases in cancer patients with headache. Cancer 94(7):2063–2068, 2002 11932910

Di Francia R, Crisci S, De Monaco A, et al: Response and toxicity to cytarabine therapy in leukemia and lymphoma: from dose puzzle to pharmacogenomic biomarkers. Cancers (Basel) 13(5):966, 2021 33669053

Eagleman D: The brain on trial. The Atlantic, July/August 2011. Available at: www.theatlantic.com/magazine/archive/2011/07/the-brain-on-trial /308520/. Accessed June 1, 2022.

Flanagan EP: Paraneoplastic disorders of the nervous system. J Neurol 268(12):4899–4907, 2021 33904967

Gonzalez Castro LN, Milligan TA: Seizures in patients with cancer. Cancer 126(7):1379–1389, 2020 31967671

Gritsch S, Batchelor TT, Gonzalez Castro LN: Diagnostic, therapeutic, and prognostic implications of the 2021 World Health Organization classification of tumors of the central nervous system. Cancer 128(1):47–58, 2022 34633681

Habbous S, Forster K, Darling G, et al: Incidence and real-world burden of brain metastases from solid tumors and hematologic malignancies in Ontario: a population-based study. Neurooncol Adv 3(1):vdaa178, 2020 33585818

Herzig RH, Hines JD, Herzig GP, et al: Cerebellar toxicity with high-dose cytosine arabinoside. J Clin Oncol 5(6):927–932, 1987 3585447

Holleczek B, Zampella D, Urbschat S, et al: Incidence, mortality and outcome of meningiomas: a population-based study from Germany. Cancer Epidemiol 62:101562, 2019 31325769

Kok JL, Teepen JC, van Leeuwen FE, et al: Risk of benign meningioma after childhood cancer in the DCOG-LATER cohort: contributions of radiation dose, exposed cranial volume, and age. Neuro-oncol 21(3):392–403, 2019 30099534

Kondziolka D, Bernstein M, Resch L, et al: Significance of hemorrhage into brain tumors: clinicopathological study. J Neurosurg 67(6):852–857, 1987 3316531

Louis DN, Perry A, Wesseling P, et al: The 2021 WHO classification of tumors of the central nervous system: a summary. Neuro-oncol 23(8):1231–1251, 2021 34185076

McGinnis GJ, Raber J: CNS side effects of immune checkpoint inhibitors: preclinical models, genetics and multimodality therapy. Immunotherapy 9(11):929–941, 2017 29338610

Mehta MP, Tsao MN, Whelan TJ, et al: The American Society for Therapeutic Radiology and Oncology (ASTRO) evidence-based review of the role of radiosurgery for brain metastases. Int J Radiat Oncol Biol Phys 63(1):37–46, 2005 16111570

Minniti G, Niyazi M, Andratschke N, et al: Current status and recent advances in resection cavity irradiation of brain metastases. Radiat Oncol 16(1):73, 2021 33858474

Ostrom QT, Adel Fahmideh M, Cote DJ, et al: Risk factors for childhood and adult primary brain tumors. Neuro-oncol 21(11):1357–1375, 2019 31301133

Ostrom QT, Patil N, Cioffi G, et al: CBTRUS statistical report: primary brain and other central nervous system tumors diagnosed in the United States in 2013–2017. Neuro-oncol 22(12)(Suppl 2):iv1–iv96, 2020 33123732

Ostrom QT, Cioffi G, Waite K, et al: CBTRUS statistical report: primary brain and other central nervous system tumors diagnosed in the United States in 2014–2018. Neuro-oncol 23(12)(Suppl 2):iii1–iii105, 2021 34608945

Parsons MW, Peters KB, Floyd SR, et al: Preservation of neurocognitive function in the treatment of brain metastases. Neurooncol Adv 3(Suppl 5):v96–v107, 2021 34859237

Pina-Oviedo S, Bellamy WT, Gokden M: Analysis of primary central nervous system large B-cell lymphoma in the era of high-grade B-cell lymphoma: detection of two cases with MYC and BCL6 rearrangements in a cohort of 12 cases. Ann Diagn Pathol 48:151610, 2020 32889391

Rhee JY, Gonzalez Castro LN: Glioblastoma with gliomatosis cerebri growth pattern presenting as rapidly progressive dementia. Neurohospitalist 12(2):395–399, 2022 35419153

Robert C, Karaszewska B, Schachter J, et al: Improved overall survival in melanoma with combined dabrafenib and trametinib. N Engl J Med 372(1):30–39, 2015 25399551

Rooney AG, Carson A, Grant R: Depression in cerebral glioma patients: a systematic review of observational studies. J Natl Cancer Inst 103(1):61–76, 2011 21106962

Schrader B, Barth H, Lang EW, et al: Spontaneous intracranial haematomas caused by neoplasms. Acta Neurochir (Wien) 142(9):979–985, 2000 11086806

Shi C, Lamba N, Zheng LJ, et al: Depression and survival of glioma patients: a systematic review and meta-analysis. Clin Neurol Neurosurg 172:8–19, 2018 29957299

Taillibert S, Le Rhun É: Epidemiology of brain metastases [in French]. Cancer Radiother 19(1):3–9, 2015 25636729

Thomas NJ, Myall NJ, Sun F, et al: Brain metastases in EGFR- and ALK-positive NSCLC: outcomes of central nervous system-penetrant tyrosine kinase inhibitors alone versus in combination with radiation. J Thorac Oncol 17(1):116–129, 2022 34455066

Zang KD: Meningioma: a cytogenetic model of a complex benign human tumor, including data on 394 karyotyped cases. Cytogenet Cell Genet 93(3–4):207–220, 2001 11528114

14

Neuroimmunology

Mattia Wruble Clark, M.D.
Shamik Bhattacharyya, M.D.

Case Example

A 65-year-old man presents to the emergency department with his partner, who describes several weeks of short-term memory loss, irritability, and apathy. The partner also notes occasional, brief synchronous contractions of his left facial and arm muscles. The patient experienced fever and malaise 2 weeks before symptom onset. Examination identifies deficits in attention and working memory but is otherwise nonfocal. Serum studies show mild hyponatremia. Brain MRI is normal. EEG shows nonspecific slowing but no epileptiform activity. He is discharged home. Two weeks later, he returns to the hospital after a generalized tonic-clonic seizure.

Inflammatory diseases of the nervous system frequently cause neuropsychiatric symptoms. The pathophysiology of these symptoms can be direct, from inflammation of the CNS, or indirect, from medication side effects, secondary complications of disease (such as pain), or psychological reactions to chronic illness. Although presentations can overlap, each inflammatory disease has a distinct spectrum of neurological manifestations. In this chapter, we briefly cover the presentations, diagnostic evaluation, management, and prognosis of demyelinating diseases, autoimmune encephalitides, and systemic autoimmune disorders that affect the CNS.

Multiple Sclerosis and Other Demyelinating Disorders of the CNS

Demyelinating disorders describe a spectrum of pathologies characterized by damage to the myelin sheaths that insulate nerve axons, thus interrupting signal transmission along neurons. Although inflammatory injury primarily targets myelin, secondary axonal damage and atrophy can follow.

Multiple sclerosis (MS)—the most common demyelinating disorder of the CNS—is a leading cause of disability in young adults. With growing recognition of the demyelinating spectrum, however, some patients originally misdiagnosed with MS have since been rediagnosed with other demyelinating disorders, such as acute disseminated encephalomyelitis (ADEM), myelin oligodendrocyte glycoprotein-associated disease (MOGAD), and neuromyelitis optica spectrum disorder (NMOSD). Accurate diagnosis is important because treatment and prognosis differ between diseases.

Approach to Patients With Demyelinating Disorders

History and Presentation

Demyelinating disorders should be suspected in patients with classic demyelinating syndromes—such as optic neuropathy or focal supratentorial, brainstem, cerebellar, or myelopathic syndromes—who have supportive diagnostic tests. Syndrome severity, distribution, and frequency vary between disorders. Supratentorial syndromes can be focal (e.g., aphasia and hemianopia), as seen in MS, NMOSD, and MOGAD, or diffuse (e.g., encephalopathy), as seen in ADEM and MOGAD. Brainstem syndromes can involve diplopia, facial droop, trigeminal neuralgia, facial numbness, vertigo, and dysphagia. Patients with cerebellar syndromes may describe incoordination, gait disturbance, dizziness, dysarthria, or oscillopsia and have ataxia, nystagmus, or other eye movement abnormalities on examination. Myelopathic symptoms include weakness, sensory deficits, bladder dysfunction, Lhermitte's sign (electric shock sensation with flexion of the neck), and a band-like sensation around the trunk. Examination may reveal a sensory level, spasticity, and hyperreflexia. Whereas MS is typically associated with partial myelopathy, complete myelopathy should raise suspicion for MOGAD or NMOSD. Optic neuritis causes vision loss or blurring, color desaturation, periorbital or retro-orbital pain, and pain with eye movement. Examination findings include optic disc edema, optic disc pallor, and an afferent pupillary defect. Optic neuritis is usually unilateral, with mild to moderate vision loss in MS. Bilateral or severe vision loss is more suggestive of MOGAD, NMOSD, or other neuroimmunologic conditions.

When a demyelinating syndrome is identified, interviewers should elicit information pertaining to demyelinating disorders and disease mimics. Practitioners should assess for risk factors (e.g., demographic characteristics, tobacco use, obesity, and vitamin D deficiency) and inquire about symptoms that suggest prior demyelinating events. Demyelination typically progresses over hours to days and lasts days to weeks, so hyperacute symptoms and symptoms lasting less than 1 day point to an alternative diagnosis. A history of a different autoimmune disease, malignancy, infection (e.g., HIV), migraines, fibromyalgia, or functional neurologic disorder may raise suspicion for a disease mimic but does not exclude the possibility of co-occurring demyelinating disease.

Diagnostic Testing

When demyelinating disease is suspected, further evaluation with serum testing, cerebrospinal fluid (CSF) analysis, and MRI is needed to confirm the diagnosis and rule out alternative diagnoses. Serum studies typically include complete blood count (CBC), basic metabolic panel (BMP), and inflammatory markers. Thyroid function tests and antinuclear antibody (ANA) tests are also commonly performed. Serum testing for MOGAD-associated anti-MOG-IgG1 antibodies and NMOSD-associated anti-aquaporin-4(AQP4)-IgG antibodies should be conducted in cases concerning MOGAD or NMOSD.

CSF analyses should include cell counts, protein, glucose, gram stain, culture, immunoglobulin G (IgG) index, and kappa free light chain (κFLC) index and/or oligoclonal bands (OCBs) (the latter three require concurrent serum testing). Depending on the clinical setting, opening pressure and additional CSF testing for autoimmune antibodies, malignancy, and infection may be recommended. Of note, CSF anti-MOG-IgG1 and anti-AQP4-IgG tests are not typically recommended (even when NMOSD and/or MOGAD are suspected). CSF analyses often show mild CSF pleocytosis (usually lymphocytic or monocytic), normal glucose, and normal or elevated protein. CSF-specific OCBs and/or κFLC are present in most patients with MS and, although not specific to MS, are less common in other demyelinating processes (Montalban et al. 2025). Unusual CSF findings—including neutrophil predominance, very high white blood cell count, very low glucose, very high protein, or presence of atypical cells—should raise suspicion for an alternative diagnosis (Thompson et al. 2018).

Evaluation also involves brain MRI with gadolinium contrast and, in many cases, additional MRIs of the orbits and cervical or thoracic spine with contrast. Demyelinating lesions are characterized by T2 or T2-fluid-attenuated inversion recovery (FLAIR) hyperintensity, which may be contrast enhancing in the acute phase. Lesion distribution and appearance vary between disorders. In the brain, MS lesions are usually well-demarcated with ovoid, open-ring, or ring-like shapes and typically affect the optic nerve, cortical or juxtacortical regions, periventricular white matter (including the corpus callosum), and infratentorial structures (Thompson et al. 2018). Periventricular elongated lesions called "Dawson fingers" are a classic finding for MS (Figure 14.1). 2024 updates to the MS diagnostic criteria also incorporated MS-specific MRI biomarkers—namely, the central vein sign and paramagnetic rim lesions on specific susceptibility-weighted imaging sequences—as supportive, but not required, for MS diagnosis.

In contrast to MS, ADEM (which can be MOGAD-asociated) is characterized by large, patchy, poorly circumscribed lesions that are often bilateral and involve deep gray matter structures (Pohl et al. 2016). In ADEM and non-ADEM MOGAD, brain lesions are classically "fluffy" and ill-defined; they are sometimes confluent with involvement of both white and gray matter and supra- and infratentorial structures. Brain lesions in NMOSD often involve the area postrema, periependymal white matter, and subcortical structures. Optic nerve abnormalities are best evaluated on dedicated orbital MRIs, which are more likely to show longitudinally extensive or bilateral optic nerve involvement in MOGAD or NMOSD than in MS. On spine MRIs, MS-associated myelitis is short-segmented and may be multifocal, whereas longitudinally extensive transverse myelitis spanning at least three vertebral segments should raise suspicion for MOGAD, NMOSD, infection, malignancy, rheumatologic, or other autoimmune processes (Banwell

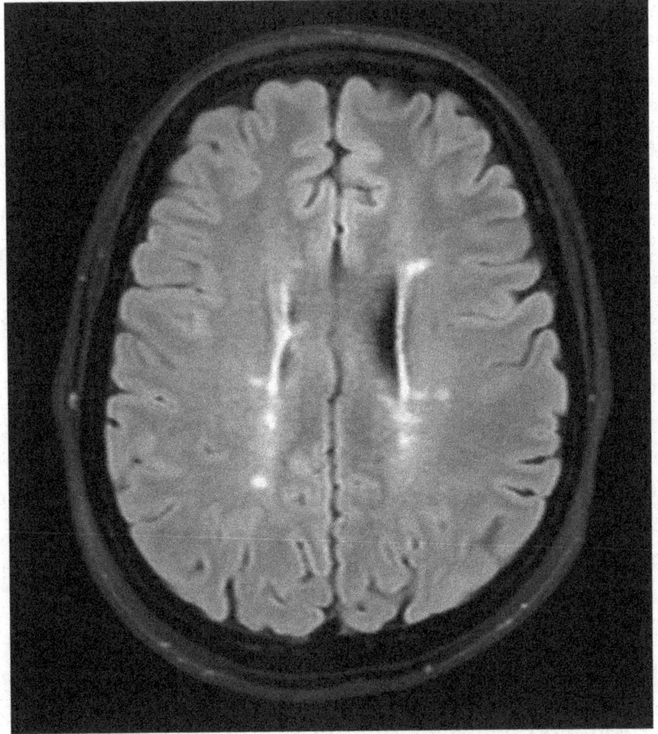

Figure 14.1 Dawson fingers.

T2/FLAIR hyperintensities that are perpendicular to the ventricle are representative of demyelination seen in multiple sclerosis.

et al. 2023). CNS imaging can be normal in early stages of disease. Brain MRI can remain normal in cases of isolated optic neuritis or myelitis. In these cases, repeat imaging, CSF analysis, or evoked potentials can aid in diagnosis.

Management

Treatment often involves a multimodal, interdisciplinary approach to symptom management, acute flares, and long-term disease. High-dose corticosteroids are typically used to treat acute flares in MS, alone or in combination with plasmapheresis in NMOSD, and alone or in combination with plasmapheresis or intravenous immunoglobulin (IVIg) in ADEM and MOGAD. Long-term treatment, when indicated, varies by disease but may involve immunosuppressive agents or serial

IVIg. Disease-modifying therapies (DMTs) decrease rates of relapse and disability in relapsing forms of MS but are generally less effective in progressive forms. DMTs differ by mechanism of action, routes of administration, and side effect profiles. Side effects are typically mild, but severe complications such as malignancy and infection (e.g., progressive multifocal leukoencephalopathy) can occur (Cross and Riley 2022). Corticosteroids and other treatments have well-established psychiatric complications; the relationship between other agents and psychiatric symptoms (e.g., between interferon- and depression) is less well defined. Psychiatric symptoms can be managed by limiting these iatrogenic contributions, adding psychotropic medications, and introducing therapeutic interventions. Other symptoms—such as fatigue, cognitive fog, headaches, trigeminal neuralgia, neuropathic pain, bladder and bowel dysfunction, spasticity, and immobility—may also be managed with a combination of lifestyle intervention, rehabilitation therapies, and medication. When considering psychotropic and other medications, care should be taken to avoid drugs that can worsen other disease symptoms (Murphy et al. 2017).

Multiple Sclerosis

The most common demyelinating disease of the CNS, *multiple sclerosis* classically presents in young adult females with a typical clinical syndrome, such as a focal supratentorial syndrome, focal brainstem syndrome, focal cerebellar syndrome, partial myelopathy, or unilateral optic neuritis (Thompson et al. 2018; Montalban et al. 2025). Realistically, however, MS is a heterogeneous disease that can present with a broad range of symptoms in the young and old. Although its cause remains unknown, genetic and environmental factors have been implicated.

MS subtypes vary by clinical course. *Relapsing remitting multiple sclerosis* (RRMS), the most common initial form of the disease, is marked by discrete clinical attacks with periods of improvement and stability between attacks. RRMS is defined by dissemination in time and space (e.g., evidence of at least two demyelinating events by history and diagnostic testing). Patients who develop a typical syndrome but do not have evidence of dissemination in time or space may instead be diagnosed with clinically isolated syndrome, whereas patients with characteristic imaging findings in the absence of associated signs or symptoms may be diagnosed with radiologically isolated syndrome. In contrast, progressive forms of MS are characterized by slowly deteriorating function independent of disease relapse. Most cases of

RRMS later transition into *secondary progressive MS* (SPMS), defined by an early relapsing-remitting course followed by progressive disease. Unlike SPMS, *primary progressive MS* is marked by progressive disease from the time of disease onset (Thompson et al. 2018).

Most patients with MS experience psychiatric symptoms, which can affect quality of life and functional status. Psychiatric symptoms can occasionally be the presenting sign of MS but typically develop later in the disease course. Unfortunately, rates of anxiety, depression, bipolar disorder, psychosis, and suicide are markedly higher in patients with MS than in the general population. Pseudobulbar affect and substance use disorder can also occur. The pathophysiology of these psychiatric symptoms in MS likely involves a combination of structural brain lesions, medication side effects, and psychosocial factors (Murphy et al. 2017).

Acute Disseminated Encephalomyelitis

ADEM is a heterogeneous autoimmune syndrome characterized by widespread demyelination in the brain and spinal cord; the peripheral nervous system (PNS) can also be affected. ADEM is more common in children than in adults and is among the most common pediatric demyelinating disorders. Although its pathophysiology remains under investigation, ADEM is often preceded by infection and, rarely, by vaccination, suggesting an immunologic response to antigen exposure. There is also a strong association between ADEM and MOGAD, wherein ADEM is the most common presentation of MOGAD in young children (Banwell et al. 2023), but not all patients with ADEM have MOGAD. Diagnosis of pediatric, monophasic ADEM requires encephalopathy characterized by behavioral changes or impaired consciousness (which can range from irritability to coma); an initial clinical event suggestive of a multifocal, demyelinating CNS process; and characteristic brain MRI abnormalities within 3 months of symptom onset. There are no consensus diagnostic criteria for adults; thus, the pediatric criteria are often extrapolated to the adult population. ADEM often begins with a prodrome of fever, fatigue, headache, and nausea. Patients then experience rapidly progressing encephalopathy and neurologic deficits, which reach maximal intensity within days. Associated syndromes can include optic neuritis, language deficits, brainstem syndromes, pyramidal signs (including hemiparesis), ataxia, and seizures. Although ADEM is typically monophasic, polyphasic disease can occur. ADEM once carried a poor prognosis, but outcomes have improved with widespread vaccination, and prognosis today is generally favorable. Yet, one-quarter of patients still require intensive care, and many suffer long-term behavioral and cognitive sequelae, with lower IQ scores and deficits in domains of executive function, attention, and verbal processing (Pohl et al. 2016).

Myelin Oligodendrocyte Glycoprotein-Associated Disease

The first consensus diagnostic criteria for MOGAD were published in 2023. These criteria established MOGAD as a distinct disease associated with anti-MOG-IgG antibodies, which reclassified many patients with anti-MOG-IgG antibodies who were previously diagnosed with seronegative NMOSD or MOG-associated ADEM. According to these criteria, the diagnosis of MOGAD requires at least one core demyelinating event, a clear positive serum MOG-IgG test, and exclusion of alternate diagnoses (including MS). The six core demyelinating events include optic neuritis, myelitis, cerebral syndrome, brainstem or cerebellar syndrome, cerebral cortical encephalitis, and ADEM. A subset of these patients develop FLAIR-hyperintense lesions in anti-MOG-associated encephalitis with seizures ("FLAMES"). Although uncommon, progressive white matter damage in MOGAD can also mimic leukodystrophy. MOGAD can be monophasic or relapsing, but unlike MS is rarely progressive (Banwell et al. 2023).

Neuromyelitis Optica Spectrum Disorder

Originally termed Devic disease, NMOSD was initially thought to be a subtype of MS involving optic neuritis and transverse myelitis. The later discovery of anti-AQP4-IgG in patients with this presentation established NMOSD as a unique disease entity. We now recognize that most patients with NMOSD have anti-AQP4-IgG antibodies and are thus considered seropositive, while a minority are seronegative. The diagnosis of NMOSD requires the presence of one core clinical syndrome (in seropositive patients) or two syndromes (in seronegative patients). The six core syndromes of NMOSD are optic neuritis, myelitis, area postrema syndrome (refractory hiccups, nausea, and/or vomiting), brainstem syndrome, diencephalic syndrome (e.g., narcolepsy or endocrinopathy), and cerebral syndrome. Although attacks can be severe, the disease does not progress between attacks. Preventing disability in NMOSD thus hinges on relapse prevention. As in MS, patients with NMOSD suffer from high rates of depression, suicidality, and cognitive sequelae (Moore et al. 2016). Compared with MS, NMOSD presents slightly later in life and disproportionately affects people of Afro-Caribbean and Asian ancestry (Wingerchuk and Lucchinetti 2022).

Autoimmune Encephalitis

Autoimmune encephalitis describes a spectrum of conditions in which immune-mediated inflammatory injury leads to brain dysfunction. Increasing rates of autoimmune encephalitis diagnosis, along with discovery of new antineural antibodies and associated syndromes, suggest that autoimmune encephalitis may be just as prevalent as infectious encephalitis (Abboud et al. 2021). Patients with autoimmune encephalitis frequently present with neuropsychiatric symptoms that can mimic primary psychiatric disease, often prompting initial evaluation by psychiatrists and other non-neurologists.

Autoimmune encephalitides are named according to their associated antibody or target antigen, which may be located on the neuronal cell surface, in the synapse, or within the neuron cell body. Antibodies against neuronal surface antigens (NSAs) or synaptic antigens can cause receptor internalization (as seen in anti-*N*-methyl-D-aspartate receptor [NMDAR] encephalitis) or ion channel dysfunction (as seen in anti-leucine-rich glioma inactivated protein 1 [LGI1] encephalitis), which may be reversible early in the disease. In contrast, autoantibodies against intracellular antigens might not be directly pathogenic but rather markers of an autoimmune process involving cytotoxic T cell–mediated pathways that cause neuronal injury. These differing mechanisms may explain better outcomes in patients with antibodies against NSAs and synaptic antigens versus patients with antibodies against intracellular antigens (Dalmau and Graus 2018).

Autoimmune encephalitis can be idiopathic or triggered by an immune response to infection (e.g., viral encephalitis), immune-modulating agents (e.g., immune checkpoint inhibitors [ICIs]), or cancer. Autoimmune encephalitis that develops in response to cancer is termed paraneoplastic autoimmune encephalitis (PNAE). In seronegative autoimmune encephalitis, autoantibodies may not be identifiable or have yet to be discovered (Graus et al. 2016). Clinical presentations of autoimmune encephalitis, PNAE, and seronegative autoimmune encephalitis can overlap.

Diagnostic Criteria

Diagnosis of autoimmune encephalitis requires the presence of subacute neuropsychiatric symptoms; new focal neurologic deficits or seizures; associated brain MRI, electroencephalography (EEG), or CSF findings; and exclusion of other etiologies (see Table 14.1) (Graus et al. 2016).

Approach to Patients With Autoimmune Encephalitis

History and Presentation

Although some autoimmune encephalitides are associated with unique clinical presentations, there is clinical heterogeneity both within and across different types (see Table 14.2). Patients with autoimmune encephalitis typically present with subacute neuropsychiatric symptoms that progress rapidly over a 3-month period. More indolent presentations are reassuring against autoimmune encephalitis. Although autoimmune encephalitis occasionally presents with isolated neuropsychiatric symptoms, patients usually have additional signs or symptoms to prompt further evaluation. Red flag signs include a viral-like prodrome, disproportionate cognitive decline, psychiatric symptoms refractory to antipsychotics, adverse responses to antipsychotics (e.g., neuroleptic malignant syndrome), new seizure disorder, seizures refractory to antiseizure medications (ASMs) even in a patient with a known seizure disorder, new or worsening headaches, new autonomic dysfunction, new focal neurologic deficits, decreased level of consciousness, new language or speech disturbance, new movement disorder (e.g., chorea, catatonia), unexplained hyponatremia, the presence of other autoimmune conditions, and current or recent cancer (Pollak et al. 2020).

Autoimmune encephalitis can present with a broad spectrum of clinical syndromes, including limbic and other encephalitides, encephalomyelitis, rapidly progressive cerebellar degeneration, opsoclonus-myoclonus syndrome (OMS), movement disorders, diencephalic syndromes, and autonomic dysfunction (see Table 14.2). Limbic encephalitis is characterized by subacute short-term memory loss, altered mental status, behavioral changes, mood changes, and seizures. Psychiatric symptoms can also include hallucinations, delusions,

Table 14.1 Diagnostic criteria for autoimmune encephalitis and anti-NMDAR encephalitis[a]

Diagnosis	Criteria
Definite autoimmune limbic encephalitis	1. Subacute, rapidly progressive working memory deficits, seizures, or psychiatric symptoms that suggest limbic system involvement 2. Brain MRI with bilateral T2/FLAIR hyperintensities restricted to the medial temporal lobes 3. At least one of the following: • CSF pleocytosis[b] • EEG with slowing or epileptiform activity in the temporal lobes
Possible autoimmune encephalitis	1. Subacute, rapidly progressive working memory deficits, altered mental status, or psychiatric symptoms 2. At least one of the following: • New focal CNS findings • Seizures not explained by a known seizure disorder • CSF pleocytosis • Brain MRI suggestive of encephalitis[c]
Autoantibody-negative, probable autoimmune encephalitis	1. Subacute, rapidly progressive short-term memory loss, altered mental status, or psychiatric symptoms 2. Exclusion of well-defined autoimmune encephalitis syndromes[d] 3. Absence of autoantibodies, with at least two of the following: • Brain MRI suggestive of autoimmune encephalitis[b] • CSF pleocytosis, CSF-unique OCBs, or elevated IgG index • Brain biopsy with inflammatory infiltrates not due to other diagnoses

Table 14.1 Diagnostic criteria for autoimmune encephalitis and anti-NMDAR encephalitis[a] (*continued*)

Diagnosis	Criteria
Definite anti-NMDAR encephalitis	1. Presence of at least one of the six major symptom groups: • Cognitive dysfunction or abnormal behavior • Speech disturbance • Movement disorder, abnormal postures, or dyskinesias • Seizures • Decreased level of consciousness • Central hypoventilation or autonomic dysfunction 2. Anti-NDMAR (GluN1) IgG antibodies
Probable anti-NDMAR encephalitis	1. Rapid onset of at least four of the six major symptom groups (see previous cell) 2. One or more of the following: • Abnormal EEG • CSF pleocytosis or CSF-specific OCBs OR 1. Rapid onset of at least three of the major symptom groups 2. Presence of a systemic teratoma

ADEM = acute disseminated encephalomyelitis; AE = autoimmune encephalitis; CNS = central nervous system; CSF = cerebrospinal fluid; EEG = electroencephalography; FLAIR = fluid-attenuated inversion recovery; IgG = immunoglobulin G; NMDAR = *N*-methyl-D-aspartate receptor; MRI = magnetic resonance imaging; OCBs = oligoclonal bands.

[a]Reasonable exclusion of other causes is required for all diagnoses.

[b]Defined as white blood count >5 cells/mm^3.

[c]T2/FLAIR hyperintensities in unilateral or bilateral temporal lobes or multifocal patterns suggestive of demyelination or inflammation in gray and/or white matter.

[d]Limbic encephalitis, Bickerstaff's brainstem encephalitis, ADEM.

Source. Adapted from Graus F, Titulaer MJ, Balu R, et al: A Clinical Approach to Diagnosis of Autoimmune Encephalitis. Lancet Neurol 15(4):391–404, 2016. Copyright © 2016. Used with permission.

Table 14.2 Autoimmune encephalitis targets, syndromes, paraneoplastic risk, and associated neoplasms

Antigen target (antibody/autoantigen)	Clinical syndromes	Paraneoplastic risk	Associated neoplasms
Intracellular antigen			
Hu (ANNA-1)	EM, LE, SNN/PN, EN, AD	High	SCLC >> NSCLC, neuroendocrine
Ri (ANNA-2)	EM, BE, CD, OMS	High	Breast > SCLC, NSCLC
Ma (PNMA-1) and Ma2 (PNMA-2, Ta)	LE, CD, BE, DS, PN	High	Testicular, NSCLC
Yo (PCA-1)	CD	High	Ovarian, breast
PCA-2 (MAP1B)	CD, OE, EM, PN, AD	High	SCLC, NSCLC, breast
CRMP5, formerly CV2	EM, SSN	High	SCLC, thymoma
SOX-1	LEMS, CD	High	SCLC, NSCLC
KLHL11	BE, CD	High	Testicular
GFAP	ME	Low	Teratoma, adenocarcinoma
ANNA-3	PN, myelopathy, BE, LE	Unknown	Lung
Synaptic intracellular antigens			
Amphiphysin	EM, PN, SPS	High	SCLC, breast

Table 14.2 Autoimmune encephalitis targets, syndromes, paraneoplastic risk, and associated neoplasms (*continued*)

Antigen target (antibody/autoantigen)	Clinical syndromes	Paraneoplastic risk	Associated neoplasms
GAD65	LE, CD, SPS	Low	SCLC, neuroendocrine, thymoma
NSAs and surface antigens			
Tr/DNER	CD	High	Lymphoma
NMDAR	LE, OE, MD, AD	Intermediate	Teratoma
AMPAR	LE	Intermediate	SCLC, thymoma
$GABA_BR$	LE	Intermediate	SCLC
P/Q VGCC	CD, LEMS	Intermediate	SCLC
mGluR5	OE	Intermediate	Hodgkin's lymphoma
Caspr2	LE, Morvan syndrome	Low/intermediate	Malignant thymoma
$GABA_AR$	OE, seizures	Low	Malignant thymoma
LGI1	LE, seizures (e.g., FBDS), hyponatremia, Morvan syndrome	Low	Thymoma, neuroendocrine
DPPX	OE, PERM, CNS hyperexcitability	Low	Hematologic
GlyR	LE, PERM	Low	Thymoma, lymphoma

Table 14.2 Autoimmune encephalitis targets, syndromes, paraneoplastic risk, and associated neoplasms (*continued*)

Antigen target (antibody/autoantigen)	Clinical syndromes	Paraneoplastic risk	Associated neoplasms
mGluR1	CD	Low	Hematologic
Homer-3	CD	Unknown	Uncommon

AD = autonomic dysfunction; AMPAR = α-amino-3-hydroxy-5-methyl-4-isoxazolepropionic acid receptor; ANNA = antineuronal nuclear antibody; BE = bacterial encephalitis; Caspr = contactin-associated protein-like; CD = cerebellar degeneration; CNS = central nervous system; CRMP = collapsin response mediator protein; DNER = δ/notch-like epidermal growth factor-related); DPPX = dipeptidyl-peptidase-like protein; DS = diencephalic syndrome; EM = encephalomyelitis; EN = enteric neuropathy; FBDS = faciobrachial dystonic seizures; GABAR = γ-aminobutyric acid receptor; GAD = glutamic acid decarboxylase; GFAP = glial fibrillary acidic protein; GlyR = glycine receptor; KLHL = Kelch-like protein; LE = limbic encephalitis; LEMS = Lambert-Eaton myasthenic syndrome; LGI = leucine-rich glioma inactivated protein; MAP = microtubule-associated protein; MD = movement disorder; ME = myalgic encephalomyelitis; mGluR = metabotropic glutamate receptor; NMDAR = *N*-methyl-D-aspartate receptor; NSA = neuronal surface antigen; NSCLC = non-small-cell lung cancer; OE = other encephalitis; OMS = opsoclonus-myoclonus syndrome; PCA = Purkinje cell antibody; PERM = progressive encephalomyelitis with rigidity and myoclonus; PN = peripheral neuropathy; PNMA = paraneoplastic Ma antigen family-like; P/Q VGCC = P/Q type voltage-gated calcium channel; SCLC = small cell lung cancer; SNN = sensory neuronopathy; SOX = Sry-like high mobility group box; SPS = stiff person syndrome; SSN = subacute sensory neuropathy.

Source. Adapted from Graus et al. 2021; Lancaster 2015.

paranoia, catatonia, mood changes, and personality changes. Patients with brainstem encephalitis may develop eye movement abnormalities, vertigo, dysarthria, and dysphagia. Encephalomyelitis presents with encephalopathy and myelopathy. Rapidly progressive cerebellar degeneration can lead to disabling gait changes, limb or truncal ataxia, tremor, nystagmus, and dysarthria. OMS involves abnormal movements of the eyes and body and can be accompanied by encephalopathy or cerebellar dysfunction. Movement disorders can range from dyskinesia (e.g., orofacial dyskinesias in anti-NMDAR encephalitis) to dystonia, chorea, parkinsonism, oculogyric crisis, posturing, and catatonia. Diencephalic syndromes include sleep disorders, endocrine dysfunction, hyperthermia, hypersexuality, and hyperphagia. Autonomic dysfunction can cause orthostatic hypotension, cardiac arrhythmias, bowel or bladder dysfunction, hyperhidrosis, and gastrointestinal dysmotility (Graus et al. 2016, 2021).

Providers should assess autoimmune encephalitis risk factors, including exposure to triggers, history of prior CNS infections (including herpes simplex virus [HSV] encephalitis), and a personal or family history of autoimmunity. Paraneoplastic disease should be considered in patients with current or recent cancer, B symptoms (fevers, night sweats, and weight loss), or risk factors (e.g., tobacco use, alcohol use, delayed or abnormal cancer screenings, family history of cancer).

Diagnostic Testing

Diagnosis of autoimmune encephalitis and exclusion of alternative diagnoses involves serum testing, CSF analysis, EEG, brain MRI, and systemic imaging. Autoantibody tests should be performed in the serum and CSF, as some antibodies are found more commonly in one or the other (Graus et al. 2016). To decrease the risk of false-positive and -negative results, practitioners should ensure that comprehensive autoantibody tests are performed (standard panels may not be exhaustive) and use validated tests for IgG autoantibodies (IgA and IgM are of unclear significance). Antibody testing is negative in seronegative autoimmune encephalitis. Results should be interpreted with caution, as autoimmune encephalitis diagnosis also requires the presence of an associated clinical syndrome, and overdiagnosis of autoimmune encephalitis can lead to harm, subjecting patients to invasive testing and immunosuppression (Flanagan et al. 2023).

Serum testing should include basic chemistries to evaluate for hyponatremia, which is associated with several types of autoimmune encephalitis. Additional studies to rule out alternative diagnoses include CBC, BMP, liver function tests, thyroid function tests, ammonia, vitamin B_{12}, folate, copper, syphilis, HIV, ANAs, antiphospholipid antibodies, lupus anticoagulant antibodies, extractable nuclear antigen antibodies panel, anti-thyroid antibodies, and toxicology screens (Abboud et al. 2021). Ceruloplasmin and porphyrin tests may also be considered when psychosis is present.

CSF analyses should include autoimmune encephalitis antibody tests, cell counts, glucose, protein, bacterial culture, OCBs, and IgG index. Lymphocytic pleocytosis and elevated protein are common. When present, an elevated IgG index and CSF-unique OCBs also support the diagnosis. Viral studies (e.g., HSV, human herpesvirus 6 [HHV-6], and varicella zoster virus PCR) are often recommended to exclude alternative diagnoses. Opening pressure, fungal cultures, cytology, flow cytometry, and prion testing may be indicated in select cases (Abboud et al. 2021).

EEG is fairly sensitive, as most patients with autoimmune encephalitis will have nonspecific slowing or epileptiform discharges. However, autoimmune encephalitis–associated seizures can be EEG negative. In some cases, long-term EEG monitoring may be recommended to rule out subclinical seizures.

Brain MRI with contrast often shows T2/FLAIR hyperintensities in affected regions (often the limbic system), with or without enhancement (see Figure 14.2) (Graus et al. 2016). However, brain MRI can be normal, particularly early in the disease course. In these cases, repeat brain MRI and/or brain positron emission tomography (PET) are recommended. Systemic imaging to evaluate for an underlying malignancy—including full-body CT, PET, or MRI; mammogram or breast MRI; and testicular or transvaginal ultrasounds—may also be indicated, particularly when paraneoplastic disease is suspected (Abboud et al. 2021).

Management

When history and evaluation are otherwise suggestive of autoimmune encephalitis, empiric treatment should begin before antibody test results return, as antibody test results can take weeks. Early treatment initiation is associated with better outcomes (Titulaer et al. 2013). First-line treatment in the acute setting involves several days of intravenous methylprednisolone (IVMP) followed by a steroid taper, although IVIg or plasmapheresis may be added in severe or steroid-refractory cases.

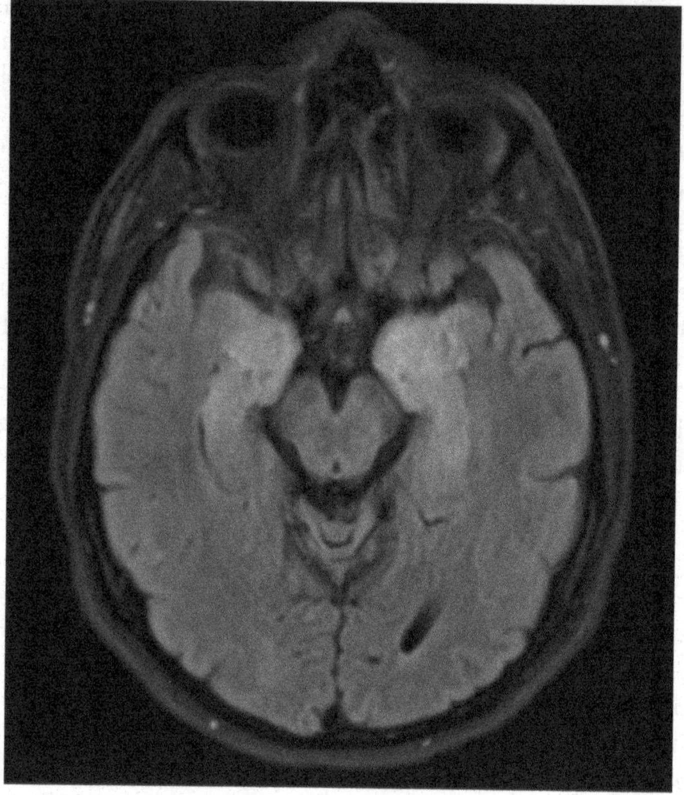

Figure 14.2 MRI of limbic encephalitis

Rituximab is recommended in cases of primary autoimmune encephalitis that require long-term treatment, whereas cyclophosphamide is usually preferred in PNAE (Abboud et al. 2021). Management of PNAE also involves treating the underlying cancer. Autoimmune encephalitis–associated seizures can be difficult to treat and often respond better to immunosuppression than ASMs. Recovered patients may not need lifelong ASMs (de Bruijn et al. 2019).

Anti-NMDAR Encephalitis

Anti-NMDAR encephalitis is among the most common causes of immune-mediated encephalitis, second only to ADEM. Anti-NDMAR encephalitis is most common among young adult women, although men account for a relatively higher proportion of cases in young children and older adults (Titulaer et al. 2013).

Despite its prevalence, anti-NMDAR encephalitis was discovered as recently as 2007, when a case series reported a cohort of women with neuropsychiatric symptoms, altered levels of consciousness, hypoventilation, and ovarian teratomas found to have anti-NMDAR antibodies (Dalmau et al. 2007). We now recognize that neoplasms, most commonly teratomas, are present in nearly 40% of all cases and are even more prevalent in female patients (Titulaer et al. 2013). Some nonparaneoplastic cases appear to be triggered by infection, namely HSV encephalitis (Dalmau and Graus 2018).

Anti-NMDAR encephalitis is mediated by autoantibodies against NMDAR, a synaptic, neuronal cell-surface receptor that binds glutamate. More specifically, antibodies target the extracellular component of the NMDAR's NR1 subunit, which results in NMDAR internalization, lower NMDAR surface density, and glutamate pathway hyperactivity. In this way, the pathophysiology of anti-NMDAR encephalitis may parallel NMDAR hypoactivity in schizophrenia (Dalmau et al. 2011).

History and Presentation

Anti-NMDAR encephalitis often progresses in a stepwise fashion, heralded by a prodromal phase, followed by rapidly progressive neuropsychiatric symptoms, then decreased responsiveness. Prodromal symptoms can include nonspecific malaise, headache, and fever. Neuropsychiatric features typically develop shortly thereafter. Cognitive changes can manifest with amnestic syndromes, speech dysfunction (e.g., pressured speech, echolalia, speech paucity, mutism), or rapidly progressive cognitive impairment. Psychiatric changes can include irritability, psychosis, hallucinations, delusions, mania, paranoia, grandiosity, hyperreligiosity, and catatonia. Although affective psychiatric symptoms predominate, negative symptoms including depression and suicidality are often present (Pollak et al. 2020). Seizures can be focal or generalized, and status epilepticus can occur. The next phase is characterized by decreased levels of responsiveness, which can range from fatigue to coma. During this phase, patients can also develop abnormal movements (classically orofacial dyskinesias), autonomic dysfunction, and hypoventilation, which can be dangerous and may require intensive care (Dalmau et al. 2011).

Diagnostic Testing

The 2016 diagnostic criteria for anti-NMDAR encephalitis are both sensitive and specific (see Table 14.1) (Graus et al. 2016; Ho et al. 2017).

Diagnostic evaluation of anti-NDMAR encephalitis requires testing for anti-NDMA NR1 antibodies in the serum and CSF, although CSF testing is more sensitive. Most patients with anti-NMDAR encephalitis have other CSF abnormalities, such as lymphocytic pleocytosis, elevated protein, and CSF-unique OCBs. Brain MRI may be normal, but findings can include T2/FLAIR hyperintensity in the medial temporal lobe, cortices, subcortical structures, brainstem, or cerebellum. Although less common, intraparenchymal or meningeal enhancement can occur (Dalmau et al. 2011). EEG is abnormal in 90% of patients with anti-NDMAR encephalitis and typically shows nonspecific focal or diffuse slowing, although epileptic features are present in one-quarter of initial EEGs (Titulaer et al. 2013). Although rare, extreme delta brush is nearly pathognomonic for anti-NMDAR encephalitis (Pollak et al. 2020). Given the association between anti-NDMAR encephalitis and underlying malignancy (usually teratomas), patients should undergo systemic imaging, including full-body CT, PET, or MRI and testicular or transvaginal ultrasound (Abboud et al. 2021).

Management

Acute treatment involves IVMP which may be combined with IVIg, and is often followed by rituximab. Paraneoplastic cases also require tumor treatment (e.g., resection in the case of teratomas). Although patients may still require intensive care, and 2-year mortality rates exceed 5%, most patients show substantial recovery after 2 years (Titulaer et al. 2013).

Anti-LGI1 Encephalitis

Anti-LGI1 encephalitis, which classically presents in older men, is the second most common form of autoimmune encephalitis and is not typically paraneoplastic (Graus et al. 2021). A synaptic antigen secreted by presynaptic neurons in the hippocampus and other regions, LGI1 forms a transsynaptic membrane complex that connects presynaptic voltage-gated potassium channels with postsynaptic AMPA receptors (AMPAR). Anti-LGI antibodies cause AMPAR dysfunction and reduced AMPAR surface density on postsynaptic inhibitory neurons, leading to neuron hyperexcitability (van Sonderen et al. 2017).

History and Presentation

Classically, anti-LGI1 encephalitis presents with subacute limbic encephalitis. Patients may also present with isolated seizures, isolated encephalopathy, or Morvan syndrome (encephalopathy, peripheral nerve hyperexcitability, autonomic dysfunction, and disordered sleep). Encephalopathy in anti-LGI1 encephalitis, which can be more subtle than in anti-NDMAR encephalitis, is characterized by subacute cognitive impairment, often with amnesia, confusion, and visuospatial disorientation. Although multiple seizure types can be seen, faciobrachial dystonic seizures—involving brief, synchronized contractions of ipsilateral facial (often perioral), neck, and upper-extremity muscles—are nearly pathognomonic for anti-LGI1 encephalitis and can occur up to 100 times per day. In the minority of patients who do not develop seizures, new behavioral changes, memory issues, sleep disorders, or hyponatremia should prompt further evaluation (Gadoth et al. 2017; van Sonderen et al. 2017).

Diagnostic Testing

There are no consensus diagnostic criteria for anti-LGI1 encephalitis specifically, so diagnosis is made according to the diagnostic criteria for autoimmune encephalitis (see Table 14.1) (Graus et al. 2016). Anti-LGI1 antibody tests are more sensitive in the serum than CSF but should be performed in both. EEGs are often normal or nonepileptic despite the prevalence of seizures. Although initial MRIs can also be normal, common MRI abnormalities include mesial temporal T2/FLAIR hyperintensity or sclerosis (Gadoth et al. 2017).

Management

Treatment typically involves IVMP for acute presentations and rituximab in cases requiring long-term immunosuppression. Most patients have favorable outcomes at 2 years. Two-year mortality rates are near 20%, however, and surviving patients may have residual cognitive and psychiatric sequela (Gadoth et al. 2017; van Sonderen et al. 2017).

Paraneoplastic Neurologic Syndromes Involving the CNS

Driven by an immunologic response to cancer, *paraneoplastic disorders* differ from metastatic disease, direct tumor invasion, hypercoagulability of malignancy, and treatment side effects. Paraneoplastic neurologic syndromes affect up to 1 in 300 patients with cancer and can affect any part of the nervous system, although this section focuses on CNS involvement. Compared with nonparaneoplastic autoimmune encephalitides, autoantibodies in PNAE tend to target intracellular antigens. However, paraneoplastic autoantibodies that target NSAs or synaptic antigens can develop when tumors express antigens that mimic neuronal antigens (Graus et al. 2021).

Certain neurologic syndromes, autoantibodies, and cancers (e.g., ovarian, testicular, breast, lung, thymic, hematologic, and neuroendocrine) have a higher risk of associated paraneoplastic disease than others (see Table 14.2). Diagnosis of paraneoplastic neurologic syndrome is thus made according to a point-based system that weighs syndrome risk, autoantibody risk, and the presence or absence of malignancy. High-risk CNS syndromes include limbic encephalitis, encephalomyelitis, rapidly progressive cerebellar syndrome, and OMS. Intermediate-risk phenotypes involving the CNS include brainstem and other encephalitides, isolated myelopathy, axonal polyradiculoneuropathies with concurrent CNS involvement, Morvan syndrome, and stiff person syndrome (Graus et al. 2021).

Neurologic symptoms of paraneoplastic disease usually precede cancer diagnosis, although evidence of cancer can usually be found at the time of presentation. It is unusual for paraneoplastic neurologic syndromes to arise during cancer treatment, but other forms of autoimmune encephalitis can develop in association with cancer treatment (e.g., ICI-induced autoimmune encephalitis). A new neurologic syndrome can be a sign of relapse in patients with a history of cancer (Graus and Dalmau 2019).

Accordingly, patients with suspected paraneoplastic disorders should undergo thorough cancer screenings. Because antibody test results can take weeks, cancer workup should not be delayed while awaiting antibody results. Additionally, patients with high-risk syndromes should be evaluated for cancer even if autoantibody testing is negative. Recommended screening usually begins with full-body CT and may also include mammogram or breast MRI and transvaginal or testicular ultrasound. If screening is negative, whole-body PET should be considered. Serum testing for cancer markers may also be indicated in select cases. If initial screening is negative, patients with high- or intermediate-risk phenotypes or autoantibodies should undergo continued cancer surveillance (Abboud et al. 2021; Graus et al. 2021).

PNAE treatment requires interdisciplinary collaboration with oncology teams to coordinate the timing of autoimmune encephalitis immunotherapy relative to cancer treatment, which may include chemotherapy, radiation, and tumor resection. Although treatment responses vary, PNAEs are typically less responsive to immunotherapy than nonparaneoplastic autoimmune encephalitides.

Systemic Rheumatologic Disease With CNS Involvement

Although systemic rheumatologic diseases can affect the CNS and PNS, this section focuses on CNS manifestations. Neuropsychiatric symptoms in patients with rheumatologic disease may be attributable to direct nervous system involvement, secondary complications of rheumatologic disease or its treatments, underlying comorbidities, or disease mimics (e.g., infection, particularly in immunosuppressed patients; malignancy; metabolic disturbances; nutritional deficiencies; and toxin ingestion). Patterns of neurologic involvement vary by disease, although presentations can overlap. Neuropsychiatric manifestations of CNS involvement can mark the first presentation of rheumatologic disease in a patient without a known rheumatologic history. Evaluation often involves serum testing, CSF testing, neuroimaging, vessel imaging, EEG, and neuropsychological testing. Importantly, patients with rheumatologic disease who experience neuropsychiatric events should also undergo standard diagnostic workup for said presentation (e.g., a stroke should prompt evaluation of cardiovascular risk factors, vessel imaging, brain CT and MRI, echocardiogram, and cardiac monitoring). Given the association between NMOSD and several rheumatologic conditions, patients with rheumatologic disease who develop demyelinating syndromes should be tested for anti-AQP4-IgG antibodies. In patients with concern for CNS involvement of a rheumatologic disease but without a known history of rheumatologic disease, providers should also evaluate for signs and symptoms of systemic disease, which may entail serum testing, systemic imaging, and evaluation by ophthalmology, dermatology, or rheumatology. Additional testing may be indicated to measure systemic disease activity, identify contributing factors, and exclude disease mimics.

Neurologic involvement of rheumatologic disease is a major contributor to morbidity and mortality and frequently merits more aggressive treatment than systemic disease alone. Disease driven by neuro-inflammation typically requires a stepwise approach involving conservative management or corticosteroids for mild disease, with consideration of steroid-sparing agents for moderate or severe disease. Given the prevalence of psychiatric comorbidities, screening may be recommended and affected patients should be referred to mental health providers.

Systemic Lupus Erythematosus/ Neuropsychiatric Systemic Lupus Erythematosus

Systemic lupus erythematosus (SLE) affects millions of people worldwide. SLE mainly targets the skin and musculoskeletal systems. Neuropsychiatric symptoms in SLE are prevalent and usually caused by co-occurring conditions or complications of systemic SLE (such as hypertension) but are sometimes caused by primary neuropsychiatric SLE (NPSLE). NPSLE, defined by SLE activity within the nervous system itself, arises via two distinct pathways: one driven by autoantibodies and inflammation, and the other by thrombosis and vasculopathy. NPSLE diagnosis requires the presence of ≥3 systemic SLE criteria and 1 of 19 defined NPSLE syndromes. Cerebrovascular disease, acute confusional states, and seizures are the most common of the 12 defined CNS syndromes, which also include aseptic meningitis, demyelinating syndrome, myelopathy, movement disorder, headache, psychosis, anxiety, mood disorder, and cognitive dysfunction. These syndromes can be nonspecific and most patients with SLE who have nonspecific neuropsychiatric symptoms do not have NPSLE. Patients with SLE without CNS involvement remain at higher risk of psychiatric illness, including anxiety, depression, cognitive dysfunction, phobia, panic disorder, bipolar I disorder, and OCD (Bachen et al. 2009). The presence of antiphospholipid (as seen in associated antiphospholipid antibody syndrome) or antiribosomal P antibodies may increase suspicion for NPSLE in patients with SLE who develop neuropsychiatric symptoms. NPSLE usually occurs in association with systemic SLE flares, so markers of systemic disease activity should be evaluated. Diagnosis of NPSLE should be revisited if systemic disease is quiescent. NPSLE management varies according to the presenting syndrome and its suspected pathophysiology. Immunomodulators treat inflammatory NPSLE. Complications of vasculopathy and hypercoagulability, such as stroke and cerebral venous sinus thrombosis (CVST), are treated with antiplatelet or anticoagulating agents. Symptom management may also require ASMs or psychotropic medications (Hanly 2014).

Behçet Disease/Neuro-Behçet Disease

Most common along the ancient Silk Road, *Behçet disease* is a systemic vasculitis characterized by oral ulcerations, genital ulcerations, and ocular disease (most commonly uveitis). Nearly 10% of patients develop *neuro-Behçet disease* (NBD). NBD predominantly affects the CNS, where it can be driven by neuroinflammation or vasculopathy. NBD diagnosis requires the presence of systemic Behçet disease and at least one NBD syndrome with associated imaging or CSF findings. Brain parenchymal NBD typically follows a relapsing-remitting course and can mimic MS. With a predilection for the brainstem, parenchymal NBD classically manifests with a subacute brainstem syndrome, which can occur in isolation or as a multifocal process involving another recognized cerebral syndrome (e.g., altered mental status, cognitive dysfunction, psychosis, seizure, unilateral numbness or weakness), myelopathy syndrome, or optic neuropathy. Defined nonparenchymal NBD syndromes are usually monophasic and include aseptic meningitis, intracranial hypertension, and CVST. Although nonspecific, headaches are the most common neurologic symptom in Behçet disease and may be attributable to NBD in 10% of cases, so a new or changing headache in patients with Behçet disease should prompt further investigation. In addition to the standard workup, diagnostic evaluation may also include a pathergy (skin prick) test (which supports the diagnosis of NBD in patients without a known history of Behçet disease), HLA-B51, and CSF interleukin-6 (a marker of NBD disease activity) (Kalra et al. 2014).

Sarcoidosis/Neurosarcoidosis

Sarcoidosis is an idiopathic, multiorgan inflammatory disorder characterized by noncaseating granulomas that commonly affect the lungs, skin, eyes, and pulmonary lymph nodes. CNS or PNS involvement, termed *neurosarcoidosis*, occurs in >5% of cases and can develop in isolation or in combination with systemic disease. In fact, neurologic symptoms are the presenting manifestation of sarcoidosis in more than half of patients with neurosarcoidosis, and less than one-third of patients with neurosarcoidosis have systemic sarcoid at first presentation. Recognized neurosarcoidosis syndromes include cranial neuropathy, meningeal disease, cerebral parenchymal disease, hydrocephalus, myelopathy, neuroendocrinopathy (e.g., panhypopituitarism, hypogonadism, syndrome of inappropriate antidiuretic hormone), stroke, and peripheral neuropathy. Multiple cranial neuropathies are common, and neurosarcoidosis should be considered in all patients with sequential or co-occurring cranial neuropathies. Nonspecific fatigue, headaches, and brain fog with symptoms of inattention, impaired concentration, slowed processing, and memory deficits are also frequently reported. Diagnosis of possible neurosarcoidosis requires a suggestive clinical syndrome with supportive diagnostic test results. Probable and definite neurosarcoidosis also require evidence of granulomas on biopsy of systemic or nervous system tissue, respectively. Definite neurosarcoidosis can thus be diagnosed in the absence of systemic disease. Given the diagnostic importance of tissue pathology, workup often involves whole-body PET to identify a biopsy site. Exclusion of tuberculosis and other granulomatous diseases is also critical. Of note, angiotensin-converting enzyme testing is not typically recommended in the serum or CSF given its lack of sensitivity and specificity (Stern et al. 2018).

Sjögren Syndrome

Sjögren syndrome is an idiopathic, systemic autoimmune disorder that classically manifests with sicca symptoms (dry eyes and mouth), muscle pain, joint pain, and fatigue. Approximately 20% of patients have neurologic involvement, which can occur in the CNS or PNS and may be the first presentation of Sjögren syndrome in more than half of such cases. Although the pathophysiology of Sjögren syndrome in the nervous system is incompletely understood, proposed mechanisms invoke a combination of demyelination, vasculopathy, and small-vessel vasculitis. Focal CNS syndromes can mimic MS and present with seizures, language disorders, motor or sensory deficits, movement disorders, cerebellar syndromes, myelopathy, and optic neuropathy. Diffuse CNS involvement can manifest with acute or subacute encephalopathy, cognitive impairment, psychiatric symptoms, and aseptic meningitis. Sjögren syndrome is notably associated with an increased risk of anxiety, depression, and sleep disorders independent of direct CNS involvement. In addition to the standard workup, diagnostic evaluation should include serum testing for anti-SS-A/Ro autoantibodies and other Sjögren-specific testing. Although biopsy is not always indicated, Sjögren syndrome is histologically defined by lymphocytic infiltration within exocrine glands (Margaretten 2017). Treatment involves immunomodulation, and agent selection may be informed by the presence or absence of other co-occurring autoimmune diseases.

Antiphospholipid Antibody Syndrome

Antiphospholipid antibody syndrome (APLAS) causes recurrent thromboses due to anticardiolipin antibodies, anti-2 glycoprotein I antibodies, or lupus anticoagulant. APLAS may be primary or secondary to other autoimmune disorders, most commonly SLE. Examples of venous involvement include deep venous thrombosis of the leg and pulmonary embolism. Examples of arterial involvement include stroke, myocardial infarction, or other organ infarcts. Recurrent miscarriages and livedo reticularis on the skin may also occur.

Rheumatoid Arthritis

Rheumatoid arthritis (RA) is characterized by synovitis but can lead to primary or secondary CNS or PNS complications through small-vessel vasculitis, inflammation, and joint instability. Cervical myelopathy due to atlantoaxial subluxation, the most common CNS complication of RA, classically presents with a myelopathic syndrome and can have devastating complications. Other CNS manifestations include inflammatory transverse myelitis and aseptic meningitis. RA also portends a higher risk of depression, anxiety, sleep dysfunction, and dementia (Figus et al. 2021).

Case Example, Continued

This presentation of a man with a prodromal viral-like illness followed by subacute cognitive and psychiatric symptoms associated with hyponatremia, abnormal movements, and seizures is most concerning for limbic encephalitis. Limbic encephalitis is one of several well-defined syndromes associated with autoimmune encephalitis. The differential diagnosis for limbic encephalitis also includes CNS infection (e.g., HSV encephalitis, HHV-6 encephalitis, neurosyphilis), CNS complications of systemic infection (e.g., HIV, Whipple's disease), CNS involvement of systemic rheumatologic disease, CNS vasculitis, primary malignancy (e.g., glioma), status epilepticus, neurodegenerative disease with associated seizures, toxic-metabolic encephalopathy, toxin ingestion, and medication side effects (Graus et al. 2016).

In this case, the patient's age and sex, subacute emergence of memory deficits, presence of hyponatremia, possibility of EEG-negative faciobrachial dystonic seizures (as suggested by ipsilateral face and arm contractions), and later onset of other seizure semiologies are particularly concerning for anti-LGI1 encephalitis. Diagnostic workup for limbic encephalitis involves serum and CSF testing (including autoimmune encephalitis panels and infectious studies), brain MRI, and EEG. Evaluation for an underlying malignancy may also be recommended. As in this case, brain MRI can be normal, particularly early in the disease course. Imaging should be repeated in such cases when suspicion remains high. EEG is usually abnormal, but may not show epileptiform activity, as autoimmune encephalitis–associated seizures are often EEG-negative.

In this case, repeat brain MRI shows right hippocampal edema, and repeat EEG shows right temporal lobe slowing. The diagnosis of anti-LGI1 encephalitis is later confirmed by serum autoimmune encephalitis panel. Autoimmune encephalitis antibody test results can take weeks, so treatment should not be delayed when suspicion is high. This patient is treated with several days of IV steroids and IVIg followed by a steroid taper, with subsequent improvement.

Key Clinical Points

- Neuropsychiatric symptoms are prevalent across inflammatory disorders of the CNS and can significantly contribute to disease morbidity and mortality. Primary neuropsychiatric symptoms are direct sequelae of CNS inflammation, while secondary neuropsychiatric symptoms are due to extraneural complications of disease or its treatments, comorbidities, or disease mimics.
- Diagnostic evaluation typically includes serum testing, cerebrospinal fluid (CSF) testing, and neuroimaging. Additional workup may be warranted depending on the clinical scenario.
- Careful measures should be taken to rule out alternative etiologies, such as infection, malignancy, cerebrovascular disease, metabolic disturbances, nutritional deficiencies, medication side effects, toxin ingestion, and psychiatric and other co-occurring disorders.
- Treatment varies by disease and presentation but typically involves a combination of symptomatic management and immunomodulation.
- Patients with neuro-inflammatory disorders often benefit from an interdisciplinary, team-based approach to management.

Review Questions

1. The CSF of a patient with multiple sclerosis is most likely to have which of the following findings?

   A. Mild pleocytosis with neutrophil predominance
   B. Low glucose
   C. Atypical cells
   D. CSF-specific oligoclonal bands
   E. Very high protein

2. Which of the following statements about neuropsychiatric lupus (NPSLE) is true?

   A. NSPLE is defined by neurologic or psychiatric symptoms in patients with SLE.
   B. Patients with SLE and migraines meet criteria for NPSLE.
   C. NPSLE typically develops during flares of systemic SLE.
   D. Patients with neuropsychiatric symptoms and elevated ANAs have neuropsychiatric lupus.
   E. All patients with NPSLE should be treated with immunosuppression.

3. Which of the following are NOT included in the 2016 Graus criteria for autoimmune encephalitis?

   A. Seizures
   B. T2/FLAIR hyperintensities in the medial temporal lobes
   C. CSF pleocytosis
   D. EEG slowing or epileptiform activity
   E. Catatonia

Answers

Question 1: C. Although they are not specific for MS, the vast majority of patients with MS have CSF-specific oligoclonal bands (IgG bands present in the CSF but not the serum). CSF-specific OCBs are less prevalent in other neuroinflammatory disorders. Other CSF findings often seen in patients with MS include normal or mild pleocytosis with lymphocytic or monocytic predominance, normal glucose, and normal or mildly elevated protein. The presence of atypical cells is more suggestive of other autoimmune, malignant, or infectious processes.

Question 2: B. NPSLE usually develops during a flare of systemic SLE, so markers of systemic SLE activity should be evaluated in patients with concern for NPSLE. In NPSLE, symptoms develop as a response to direct nervous system involvement of SLE (rather than from systemic SLE, comorbidities, or medication side effects). Although a positive ANA test is required for a diagnosis of SLE, it is not sufficient for the diagnosis of SLE or NPSLE. Migraines and other manifestations of NPSLE are nonspecific—many patients with SLE have migraines, but few have NPSLE. Not all patients with NPSLE (including those with APLAS) require immunotherapy, and treatment varies by presentation and suspected pathophysiology.

Question 3: E. Catatonia can be a presentation of autoimmune encephalitis, especially anti-NMDAR encephalitis, but it is not specific to autoimmune encephalitis. Although a patient does not need to meet every criterion, the rest of the choices are included in the 2016 Graus diagnostic criteria.

References

Abboud H, Probasco JC, Irani S, et al: Autoimmune encephalitis: proposed best practice recommendations for diagnosis and acute management. J Neurol Neurosurg Psychiatry 92(7):757–768, 2021 33649022

Bachen EA, Chesney MA, Criswell LA: Prevalence of mood and anxiety disorders in women with systemic lupus erythematosus. Arthritis Rheum 61(6):822–829, 2009 19479699

Banwell B, Bennett JL, Marignier R, et al: Diagnosis of myelin oligodendrocyte glycoprotein antibody-associated disease: International MOGAD Panel proposed criteria. Lancet Neurol 22(3):268–282, 2023 36706773

Cross A, Riley C: Treatment of multiple sclerosis. Continuum (Minneap Minn) 28(4):1025–1051, 2022 35938656

Dalmau J, Graus F: Antibody-mediated encephalitis. N Engl J Med 378(9):840–851, 2018 29490181

Dalmau J, Tüzün E, Wu HY, et al: Paraneoplastic anti-N-methyl-D-aspartate receptor encephalitis associated with ovarian teratoma. Ann Neurol 61(1):25–36, 2007 17262855

Dalmau J, Lancaster E, Martinez-Hernandez E, et al: Clinical experience and laboratory investigations in patients with anti-NMDAR encephalitis. Lancet Neurol 10(1):63–74, 2011 21163445 de Bruijn MAAM, van Sonderen A, van Coevorden-Hameete MH, et al: Evaluation of seizure treatment in anti-LGI1, anti-NMDAR, and anti-GABABR encephalitis. Neurology 92(19):e2185–e2196, 2019 30979857

Figus FA, Piga M, Azzolin I, et al: Rheumatoid arthritis: extra-articular manifestations and comorbidities. Autoimmun Rev 20(4):102776, 2021 33609792

Flanagan EP, Geschwind MD, Lopez-Chiriboga AS, et al: Autoimmune encephalitis misdiagnosis in adults. JAMA Neurol 80(1):30–39, 2023 36448466

Gadoth A, Pittock SJ, Dubey D, et al: Expanded phenotypes and outcomes among 256 LGI1/CASPR2-IgG-positive patients. Ann Neurol 82(1):79–92, 2017 28628235

Graus F, Dalmau J: Paraneoplastic neurological syndromes in the era of immune-checkpoint inhibitors. Nat Rev Clin Oncol 16(9):535–548, 2019 30867573

Graus F, Titulaer MJ, Balu R, et al: A clinical approach to diagnosis of autoimmune encephalitis. Lancet Neurol 15(4):391–404, 2016 26906964

Graus F, Vogrig A, Muñiz-Castrillo S, et al: Updated diagnostic criteria for paraneoplastic neurologic syndromes. Neurol Neuroimmunol Neuroinflamm 8(4):e1014, 2021 34006622

Hanly JG: Diagnosis and management of neuropsychiatric SLE. Nat Rev Rheumatol 10(6):338–347, 2014 24514913

Ho ACC, Mohammad SS, Pillai SC, et al: High sensitivity and specificity in proposed clinical diagnostic criteria for anti-N-methyl-D-aspartate receptor encephalitis. Dev Med Child Neurol 59(12): 256–1260, 2017 28972277

Kalra S, Silman A, Akman-Demir G, et al: Diagnosis and management of neuro-Behçet's disease: international consensus recommendations. J Neurol 261(9):1662–1676, 2014 24366648

Lancaster E: Continuum: the paraneoplastic disorders. Continuum (Minneapolis, Minn) 21(2 Neuro-oncology):452–475, 2015 25837906

Margaretten M: Neurologic manifestations of primary Sjögren syndrome. Rheum Dis Clin North Am 43(4):519–529, 2017 29061239

Montalban X, Lebrun-Frénay C, Oh J, et al: Diagnosis of multiple sclerosis: 2024 revisions of the McDonald criteria. Lancet Neurol 24(10):850–865, 2025 39058509

Moore P, Methley A, Pollard C, et al: Cognitive and psychiatric comorbidities in neuromyelitis optica. J Neurol Sci 360:4–9, 2016 26723962

Murphy R, O'Donoghue S, Counihan T, et al: Neuropsychiatric syndromes of multiple sclerosis. J Neurol Neurosurg Psychiatry 88(8):697–708, 2017 28285265

Pohl D, Alper G, Van Haren K, et al: Acute disseminated encephalomyelitis: updates on an inflammatory CNS syndrome. Neurology 87(9)(Suppl 2):S38–S45, 2016 27572859

Pollak TA, Lennox BR, Müller S, et al: Autoimmune psychosis: an international consensus on an approach to the diagnosis and management of psychosis of suspected autoimmune origin. Lancet Psychiatry 7(1):93–108, 2020 31669058

Stern BJ, Royal W 3rd, Gelfand JM, et al: Definition and consensus diagnostic criteria for neurosarcoidosis: from the Neurosarcoidosis Consortium Consensus Group. JAMA Neurol 75(12):1546–1553, 2018 30167654

Thompson AJ, Banwell BL, Barkhof F, et al: Diagnosis of multiple sclerosis: 2017 revisions of the McDonald criteria. Lancet Neurol 17(2):162–173, 2018 29275977

Titulaer MJ, McCracken L, Gabilondo I, et al: Treatment and prognostic factors for long-term outcome in patients with anti-NMDA receptor encephalitis: an observational cohort study. Lancet Neurol 12(2):157–165, 2013 23290630

van Sonderen A, Petit-Pedrol M, Dalmau J, et al: The value of LGI1, Caspr2 and voltage-gated potassium channel antibodies in encephalitis. Nat Rev Neurol 13(5):290–301, 2017 28418022

Wingerchuk DM, Lucchinetti CF: Neuromyelitis optica spectrum disorder. N Engl J Med 387(7):631–639, 2022 36070711

15

Sleep Disorders

Khurshid A. Khurshid, M.B.B.S.
Sheldon Benjamin, M.D.

Case Example

A 72-year-old widowed man with a history of hypertension and osteoarthritis is involuntarily admitted to an inpatient psychiatric hospital after being found at night in the middle of a river, having jumped off a bridge. He denied having jumped when found by the police, although he could not explain how he got there. He appears confused. He remembers dreaming about walking to feed his horse. He denies depression, poor concentration, appetite changes, or suicidal ideation but reports missing his wife, who died the year before. A toxicology screen is negative, and he denies using substances. By hospital day 3, he is awake, alert, and fully oriented. He denies sleep disruption and reports sleeping 7–8 hours per night. However, he has been told he snores loudly, and he endorses daytime sleepiness. Many years ago, his wife complained that he had punched her during the night. He is discharged home with an appointment for follow-up in the sleep disorders clinic.

The biological functions of sleep are incompletely understood. Its restorative function may be related to its roles in protein synthesis and clearing of wastes from the brain via the glymphatic system. Sleep has positive effects on memory consolidation, appetite regulation, and cardiovascular and immune functions, and may help protect against dementia. Sleep disorders are associated with medical comorbidity. Hypertension, coronary artery disease, arrhythmias, stroke, and heart failure are more common in patients with untreated sleep disorders than in the general population. Poor sleep from sleep disorders can cause inattention and cognitive impairment.

Sleep is determined in the laboratory by changes in muscle movement, responsiveness to stimuli, breathing, and brain wave patterns. Sleep is divided into non–rapid eye movement (NREM) and rapid eye movement (REM) sleep based on polysomnography (PSG), which includes electroencephalogram (EEG), electrooculogram (EOG), and electromyogram (EMG). The two sleep phases alternate during sleep cycles lasting 90–110 minutes each. NREM sleep, which accounts for 75%–80% of sleep time in adults, is predominant in the first third of the night and is further subdivided into three stages based on EEG characteristics: N1 (light sleep), N2 (intermediate sleep), and N3 (slow wave or deep sleep). REM sleep is predominant in the last third of the night, although it accounts for 50% of the sleep of infants. With aging, total sleep time and slow-wave sleep (N3) decrease, and sleep becomes more fragmented.

Arousal is maintained by the ascending reticular activating system (ARAS) and mediated by acetylcholine. Cholinergic activity in the ARAS decreases to initiate sleep. Raphe nuclei and basal forebrain activity increase in slow-wave sleep, associated with increased serotonergic and GABAergic activity as well as changes in opiate, α-melanocyte stimulating hormone, and somatostatin activity. Neurons in the ventrolateral preoptic area of the hypothalamus secrete GABA, which maintains NREM sleep, and are activated by the sleep-producing substance adenosine. REM sleep is initiated by cholinergic neurons in the pontine tegmentum. Serotonergic, histaminergic, and adrenergic activity are suppressed during REM sleep. The orexin/hypocretin system helps suppress REM and helps maintain wakefulness. The suprachiasmatic nucleus in the hypothalamus is responsible for controlling circadian rhythms.

Sleep disorders are commonly classified according to the *International Classification of Sleep Disorders,* 3rd Edition (ICSD-3) (American Academy of Sleep Medicine 2014) or DSM-5 (American Psychiatric Association 2022). For consistency, this chapter uses the ICSD-3 classification. After reviewing the approach to the patient and the use of sleep laboratory testing, we summarize the neurology of insomnia, sleep-related breathing disorders, hypersomnias, circadian disorders, parasomnias, sleep-related movement disorders, sleep changes in psychiatric disorders, and psychopharmacologic treatment.

Approach to Patients With Sleep Disorders

A detailed sleep history is essential to the diagnosis and treatment of sleep disorders and may require an interview with the patient and their sleep partner. Table 15.1 lists areas of inquiry in gathering the sleep history.

The examination of the patient with sleep complaints begins with noting the level of alertness and observation of body habitus. Truncal obesity with body mass index (BMI) >30, large waist girth, large neck size (>17 inches in men, >16 inches in women), and small oropharyngeal opening may indicate a propensity toward obstructive sleep apnea (OSA). Any craniofacial abnormalities that would decrease oropharyngeal opening size are described. Elevated blood pressure, often associated with OSA, should be noted.

Sleep questionnaires are useful adjuncts to sleep evaluation. For insomnia complaints, the Insomnia Severity Index is often used (Bastien et al. 2001). For complaints of daytime sleepiness, the patient can complete the Epworth Sleepiness Scale (Johns 1991), and for possible OSA, the STOP-BANG questionnaire (Chung et al. 2008) or the Berlin questionnaire (Netzer et al. 1999) is useful to evaluate risk. Other medical causes and the possible effects of other sleep disorders must always be considered before making a sleep diagnosis and initiating treatment. A sleep diary can be a valuable adjunct to the evaluation of insomnia or hypersomnia.

Use of the Sleep Laboratory

Depending on the sleep laboratory, a sleep clinic consultation may be required before testing. Common sleep laboratory modalities include home sleep apnea testing, PSG, multiple sleep latency testing (MSLT), and the maintenance of wakefulness test. Overnight PSG is performed and scored by a sleep technologist, and the results are interpreted by a sleep specialist. The PSG (Figure 15.1) consists of a video recording, limited (2–6 channels) EEG for seizure detection and to determine sleep stages, EOG to detect rapid-eye movements, EMG to detect limb

Table 15.1 Elements of the sleep history

Sleep hygiene	Bedtime/awakening time, arrangement of bedroom (TV, clock position, lighting, noise), regular nighttime ritual, evening exercise, sexual activity, use of stimulants/sedatives, nighttime eating, napping behavior, shift work, circadian demands
Issues that may interfere with sleep or increase risk of sleep disorders	Medical conditions (pain, nocturia, dyspnea, chronic nasal congestion, seizures), medications, psychosocial stressors, mood or anxiety disorders, caffeine intake (amount, time of day), substance use (including any substances used to fall asleep), smoking
History to obtain from sleep partner	Habitual loud snoring; witnessed apnea, gasping; irregular breathing; movements during sleep/acting out dreams; talking in sleep; aggressive or disinhibited behaviors; estimated sleep length and quality; mood changes/performance changes; nocturnal seizures or brief stereotyped events
History of medical conditions that may be exacerbated by sleep disorders	Hypertension, atrial fibrillation, congestive heart failure, obesity, diabetes, attention disorders, depression
Insomnia history	Duration of complaint, sleep latency (time to fall sleep), frequency of awakenings and reasons for awakening, early morning awakening (time), nonrestorative sleep, anxiety about sleep symptoms, daytime napping, caffeine intake, impairment of daytime functioning, work schedule
Hypersomnia history	Irresistible daytime naps, daytime drowsiness, sleep drunkenness, situations in which naps occur (sedentary activity vs. driving, talking, eating, etc.), impairment of daytime functioning
Narcolepsy symptoms	Excessive daytime sleepiness, cataplexy, hypnagogic/hypnopompic hallucinations, sleep paralysis, awaken refreshed in morning or after naps

Table 15.1 Elements of the sleep history (*continued*)

Parasomnia symptoms	Recurrent nightmares, autonomic symptoms, difficulty waking up, awakening confused, awakening out of bed, signs of nocturnal food consumption with no recall, sleep paralysis, perception of loud noise in sleep
Sleep-related movement disorders	Leg discomfort in the evening, daytime sleepiness, holes worn through at base of sheets

and jaw movements, electrocardiogram, pulse oximetry, a nasal airflow sensor, and elastic belts around the abdomen and chest to detect breathing patterns. The MSLT, which consists of in-laboratory monitoring of five daytime nap opportunities 2 hours apart (to assess sleep latency), is used for the diagnosis of narcolepsy or other central hypersomnias and is generally done on the day after the PSG. A home sleep apnea test is a cost-effective and convenient alternative for the initial assessment of a patient in whom there is a high likelihood of obstructive sleep apnea.

Insomnia Disorder

Insomnia is defined as difficulty initiating or maintaining sleep or early morning awakening with difficulty resuming sleep. Insomnia is not diagnosed when the cause is restricted sleep opportunity or the presence of environmental factors that make sleep difficult (e.g., light, noise such as snoring from a bed partner). Insomnia is classified as a disorder when the patient or caregiver reports marked concern about sleep, impairment of daytime functioning, occurrence on at least three nights per week, and presence for at least 3 months (ICSD-3). Symptoms of impaired daytime function include fatigue, irritability, depressed mood, cognitive dysfunction, or impaired social, occupational, or academic performance. ICSD-3 describes two major types of insomnia disorders: chronic insomnia disorder and short-term insomnia disorder, depending on whether the condition has been present for more or less than 3 months (American Academy of Sleep Medicine 2014).

Insomnia is the most common sleep disorder, affecting 10%–15% of the adult population. More than one-third of adults experience

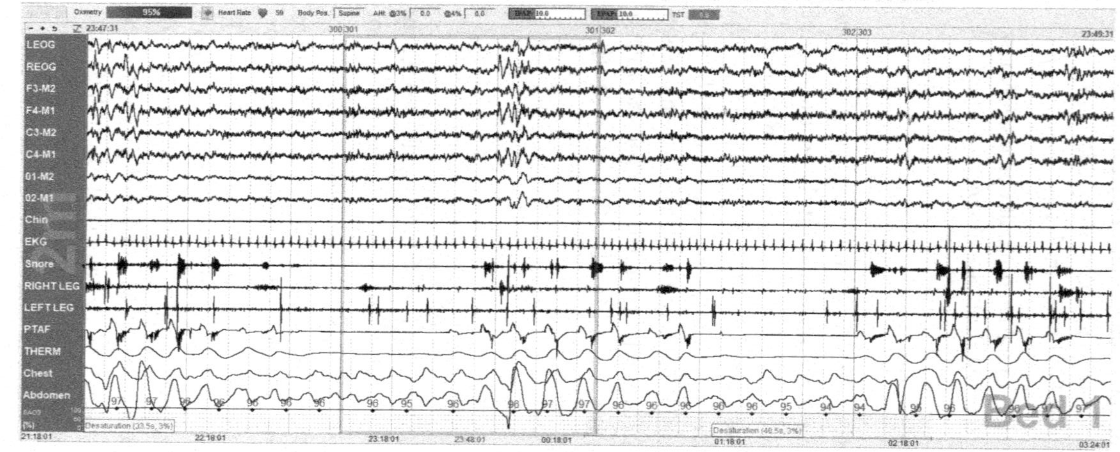

Figure 15.1 **Two-minute epoch of a polysomnogram recording.**

EEG (electroencephalogram) leads help determine sleep stage and arousals. EOG (electrooculogram) helps determine REM sleep by monitoring eye movements. THERM (thermistor) and PTAF (pressure transducer air flow) measure airflow intake and output. Chest and abdomen elastic pressure sensor belts detect chest wall and abdominal movement that can indicate apneic periods. Leg EMG (electromyogram) detects the presence or absence of any limb movements.

LEOG = left electrooculogram; REOG = right electrooculogram; *EEG recordings:* F3-M2 = left frontal-right mastoid, F4-M1 = right frontal-left mastoid, C3-M2 = left central-right mastoid (behind ear), C4-M1 = right central-left mastoid (behind ear), 01-M2 = left occipital-right mastoid, 02-M1 = right occipital-left mastoid; Chin = EMG of chin muscles; EKG = electrocardiogram lead; Snore = microphone recording; SAO_2 = oxygen saturation; (%) = degree of desaturation.

transient insomnia at some point in their lives. The cost to society of untreated insomnia has been estimated at $100 billion per year, adjusting for inflation (Wickwire et al. 2016).

Insomnia is associated with a 27%–45% increased risk of cardiovascular disease or cardiac death (Javaheri and Redline 2017). Insomnia occurs in most people with major depression or chronic pain disorder, and one-third of people with insomnia have comorbid depression. Insomnia also increases the risk of relapse after treatment of depression. It is a risk factor for substance abuse, bipolar disorder, psychotic disorder, and suicide, as well as diabetes, hypertension, obesity, and decreased immune function.

Although there can be some overlap, chronic insomnia disorder should be differentiated from delayed and advanced sleep-wake phase disorders. Chronic insomnia disorder may occur in the setting of comorbid restless legs syndrome (RLS) or sleep apnea. In those settings, insomnia disorder is not diagnosed unless it either predates the comorbid sleep disorder or persists despite adequate treatment of the other disorder.

The precise pathophysiological mechanisms underlying insomnia have not yet been identified, but the leading hypotheses involve sympathetic hyperarousal and increased activity of the hypothalamic-pituitary-adrenal axis across sleep and wakefulness. Insomnia is commonly explained by the interaction of a genetic vulnerability to an imbalance between arousal and sleep-inducing brain activity, combined with medical and psychosocial stress factors and perpetuating factors (e.g. poor sleep hygiene, rumination about lack of sleep). Two processes simultaneously influence the development of insomnia: the length of time awake and the control of circadian cycles by light/dark exposure (Levenson et al. 2015).

Although there can be a role for pharmacologic treatment of chronic insomnia disorder in combination with cognitive-behavioral therapy for insomnia (CBT-I), CBT-I has the stronger evidence base (Morin 2004). Before initiating treatment, a thorough sleep history is obtained (Table 15.1), including substance use and medical comorbidities and their treatments. Sleep laboratory testing is undertaken only if there is suspicion of a co-occurring sleep disorder. Instruction on sleep hygiene is given (Table 15.2) (Bragg et al. 2019). Simple measures to reduce sensory input, control room temperature, and create a sleep-conducive environment can be useful. Other measures to restrict time awake in bed are designed to have the brain associate the bed with sleep. Benzodiazepines and benzodiazepine receptor agonists are approved for the treatment of insomnia but should be avoided if

Table 15.2 Sleep hygiene advice

Sleep hygiene advice
Create environment conducive to sleep (cooler temperature, room-darkening shades, blocked sound)
Set a regular sleep schedule
Avoid daytime napping
Avoid going to bed until drowsy
Get out of bed in 15–20 minutes if not asleep
Avoid caffeine, nicotine, alcohol, or stimulants within 6 hours of bedtime
Exercise regularly, but avoid exercise within 4 hours of bedtime
Use bed only for sleep or sex; read, work, or watch TV elsewhere
Develop a nighttime ritual
Turn luminous clock faces so that they are not visible from bed

possible because of their side effects and dependency profiles unless other approaches have failed. Orexin receptor antagonists and melatonin agonists may be used. Antiseizure medications, over-the-counter agents such as L-tryptophan and melatonin, and especially quetiapine, are not recommended, the latter because of its side effect profile. For short-term insomnia disorder only, the above pharmacologic agents are sometimes used during adjustment to the precipitating stressful event or other precipitating factors.

Sleep-Related Breathing Disorders

The term *sleep-disordered breathing* (SDB) encompasses a spectrum of abnormalities, including snoring, OSA, central sleep apnea (CSA), respiratory-related arousals, and hypoventilation. In some cases, respiration is abnormal during both wakefulness and sleep. OSA can be due to partial or complete obstruction of the upper airway predominantly due to loss of muscle tone, whereas CSA is due to a lack of central respiratory effort. In complex sleep apnea, the two causes are combined.

Obstructive Sleep Apnea

Upper-airway collapse in OSA results in oxygen desaturation, nocturnal arousals, and fragmented sleep. OSA both co-occurs with and is a risk factor for hypertension, coronary artery disease, and type 2 diabetes. Patients with atrial fibrillation often have comorbid OSA; they are more likely to remain in normal sinus rhythm if their sleep apnea is treated. Treatment of OSA in patients with heart failure improves cardiac function and quality of life. Patients with OSA are also at risk for motor vehicle accidents. OSA occurs with increased frequency in middle-age men, postmenopausal women, African Americans, and Latinx/Hispanic, Native American, and South Asian people.

OSA is diagnosed by a combination of symptoms and the apnea-hypopnea index (AHI). Apneas are indicative of complete airway collapse, and hypopneas are due to partial collapse. The AHI is determined by PSG in a sleep laboratory or by a portable device at home. Home devices are less sensitive to mild OSA and less reliable in patients with co-occurring disorders or complex forms of SDB. The total number of apneas and hypopneas lasting at least 10 seconds divided by the number of hours of sleep recorded yields the AHI. An AHI of 5–14 indicates mild OSA, 15–29 is considered moderate, and 30 or greater is seen in severe OSA. The degree of oxygen desaturation with events is also noted.

The STOP-BANG questionnaire is a mnemonic that predicts OSA risk: snoring, tiredness, observed apnea, and high blood pressure, combined with BMI, age, neck circumference, and gender (Chung et al. 2008). OSA is diagnosed if there is a positive sleep study and at least one of the following: excessive daytime sleepiness, nonrestorative sleep, fatigue, or insomnia; nocturnal awakenings due to breath holding, gasping, or choking; report by sleep partner of snoring or breathing interruptions; and the presence of hypertension, stroke, coronary artery disease, congestive heart failure, atrial fibrillation, type 2 diabetes, mood disorder, or cognitive impairment. An AHI of 15 or greater is diagnostic in the absence of other symptoms.

Management of OSA starts with a thorough sleep history including evaluation of risk factors and comorbidities (Table 15.1) to address. In the setting of obesity, weight loss is a critical component of therapy. Depending on the oropharyngeal abnormality, otorhinolaryngological surgical assessment may be indicated. For mild cases of OSA, conservative therapies such as weight loss, decongestants, and avoiding factors that may worsen sleep apnea (such as supine position, sedatives, and CNS depressants) may be helpful.

In most cases, the cornerstone of treatment is continuous positive airway pressure (CPAP) therapy (Pavlova and Latreille 2019). CPAP devices deliver air under defined pressure through a facial interface to prevent airway collapse in sleep. Bilevel PAP devices allow both inspiratory and expiratory pressure to be specified. Automatic PAP devices automatically determine the pressure needed. In addition to improvement in symptoms and daytime functioning, CPAP treatment improves blood pressure and glycemic control. Oral appliances such as mandibular advancement devices may be helpful in patients with mild to moderate OSA unassociated with significant medical comorbidities or in patients who cannot tolerate CPAP. Surgical treatments such as correction of nasal or craniofacial abnormalities contributing to obstruction, adenotonsillectomy, or implantation of hypoglossal nerve stimulators are sometimes used.

Central Sleep Apnea

The symptoms of CSA are similar to those of OSA; however, the PSG shows a lack of ventilatory effort rather than obstruction. CSA may be seen in congestive heart failure (CHF), brainstem lesions, opioid use, obesity hypoventilation syndrome, neuromuscular disease, neurodegenerative disorders, or at high altitudes. The mechanism of CSA is thought to be dysregulated sensitivity of medullary chemokines to CO_2 shifts. Cheyne-Stokes respiration may be seen in patients with CSA related to CHF. Treatment of CSA consists of PAP therapy, supplemental oxygen, respiratory stimulant medications, and treatment of underlying medical disorders, particularly CHF (Foldvary-Schaefer and Waters 2017).

Sleep-Related Hypoventilation and Hypoxemia

In this disorder, the partial pressure of CO_2 is elevated during sleep owing to either obesity hypoventilation syndrome or central alveolar hypoventilation. The latter may be caused by hypothalamic dysfunction or congenital or idiopathic conditions.

Hypersomnias

The cardinal feature of *hypersomnias* is excessive daytime sleepiness despite adequate sleep at night. Hypersomnias are not diagnosed if due to untreated primary sleep disorders such as OSA or to misaligned sleep as in delayed sleep phase disorder. Disorders causing central hypersomnia include narcolepsy, idiopathic hypersomnia, and Kleine-Levin syndrome.

Narcolepsy

Narcolepsy is a disorder of REM sleep regulation characterized by the tetrad of excessive daytime sleepiness, sleep paralysis, hypnagogic hallucinations, and cataplexy (a brief loss of muscle tone in response to strong emotional expressions such as laughter, surprise, or anger). Cataplexy is sometimes limited to head drops and rarely may include facial weakness or dysarthria but does not involve respiratory muscles. Narcolepsy is classified as either type 1 (with hypocretin deficiency) or type 2 (without hypocretin deficiency). The former classification of sleep disorders divided narcolepsy into cases with or without cataplexy. About 90% of those with cataplexy have decreased cerebrospinal fluid (CSF) hypocretin levels, and only 10% of those without cataplexy are deficient. In addition, type 1 narcolepsy is strongly associated with a particular human leukocyte antigen (HLA) haplotype, DQB1*0602, found in 85% of patients. HLA typing is not a standard screening test, however, since the same haplotype can be present in one-third of individuals without narcolepsy. The risk of narcolepsy is increased 10 to 40 times in first-degree relatives of patients with the disorder. An autoimmune etiology is strongly suspected due to the combination of typical age of onset in the second decade, the HLA haplotype, the loss of hypothalamic hypocretin neurons, and hypocretin deficiency (Barateau et al. 2022; Kumar and Sagili 2014).

ICSD-3 diagnostic criteria for narcolepsy type 1 include 1) daytime sleep attacks or irrepressible need to sleep over at least 3 months and 2) cataplexy with a positive sleep study or hypocretin deficiency as measured by low CSF hypocretin-1 levels or both. The daytime sleepiness is characterized by frequent 15- to 40-minute refreshing naps, especially when doing monotonous activities. The positive sleep study may be an average sleep latency of ≤8 minutes combined with two or more episodes of sleep-onset REM on MSLT or with only one episode of sleep-onset REM if an episode also occurred on the PSG the night before. Various forms of dysregulated REM, such as hypnagogic or hypnopompic hallucinations and sleep paralysis, are frequently present, as is nighttime sleep disruption. If cataplexy is absent and CSF hypocretin is normal, narcolepsy type 2 is diagnosed.

The treatment of narcolepsy is generally directed at the daytime sleepiness with wakefulness-promoting medications such as modafinil, armodafinil, pitolisant, or solriamfetol (Barateau et al. 2022). Methylphenidate can be used if these agents do not help or are not tolerated. If cataplexy persists despite the use of wakefulness-promoting agents, venlafaxine or clomipramine may be used. Sodium oxybate is effective for excessive daytime sleepiness, cataplexy, and middle insomnia, but its use is highly regulated due to its abuse potential. Prescribers must complete an online education program, and the drug is dispensed from a single U.S. pharmacy.

Idiopathic Hypersomnia

Patients with *idiopathic hypersomnia* present with excessive daytime sleepiness that, like narcolepsy, is not due to another disorder or insufficient sleep. They do not fulfill the other criteria for narcolepsy, however, and patients take frequent nonrefreshing naps. MSLT shows decreased sleep latency of ≤8 minutes and fewer than two episodes of sleep-onset REM. Alternatively, PSG may show 12–14 hours of total sleep time. Treatment is symptomatic with wakefulness-promoting agents.

Kleine-Levin Syndrome

Kleine-Levin syndrome is a relatively rare disorder of unknown etiology that typically presents in adolescence and consists of periodic hypersomnolence associated with abnormal behavior while awake during episodes. The disorder is more common in males and people of Jewish descent. Hypersomnolent episodes occur at least every 18 months and last from 2 days to 5 weeks, with an average duration of 10 days. During episodes, the patient will sleep 16–20 hours per day. Cognitive dysfunction, confusion, derealization, disordered eating, or disinhibited behaviors may occur when awake during episodes. Cognitive function and behavior are completely normal between hypersomnolence episodes. Treatment with wakefulness-promoting agents has been tried for the hypersomnia, and there are a few reports of lithium use to decrease episode frequency, although no treatment has high-level evidence (Arnulf 2015).

Insufficient Sleep Syndrome

Patients with *insufficient sleep syndrome* suffer from excessive daytime sleepiness due to insufficient sleep at night. Sleep is usually curtailed by such measures as an alarm clock or being woken up. Sleep history, sleep logs, and actigraphy show decreased total sleep times compared with age-expected sleep duration norms. Improving sleep time leads to resolution of symptoms.

Circadian Rhythm Sleep-Wake Disorders

Circadian disorders are characterized by misalignment between the time required for occupational, social, or educational activities and the internal circadian rhythms that regulate the sleep-wake cycle. Symptoms may include excessive daytime sleepiness and/or insomnia. Circadian rhythm sleep-wake disorders include delayed and advanced sleep-wake phase disorder, irregular sleep-wake rhythm disorder, non-24-hour sleep-wake rhythm disorder, shift work disorder, and jet lag. A 7- to 14-day sleep log is useful in making circadian rhythm disorder diagnoses.

Delayed Sleep-Wake Phase Disorder

Delayed sleep-wake phase disorder is characterized by sleep times that are consistently delayed, usually more than 2 hours, relative to conventional or socially acceptable sleep times for a period of at least 3 months. These patients have trouble initiating sleep when needed for social or occupational obligations but sleep normally once asleep. They have trouble waking up at socially acceptable times and may appear confused upon awakening. This disorder is more common in adolescents. Bright-light therapy upon awakening in the morning is sometimes used for treatment, as are melatonin or melatonin agonists.

Advanced Sleep-Wake Phase Disorder

Advanced sleep-wake phase disorder occurs more commonly in the elderly. Sleep onset is typically at least 2 hours earlier than desired or socially acceptable, and the patient wakes up earlier than planned for a period of at least 3 months. When able to sleep according to their own biological clock, sleep quality and duration gradually improve. Advanced sleep phase does not impair function if the patient is able to sleep on their own schedule. If light therapy is used, it is used in the afternoon or evening. Sleep agents are not used.

Other Circadian Sleep-Wake Disorders

Irregular sleep-wake rhythm disorder is characterized by a chronic pattern of irregular sleep and wake episodes throughout the 24-hour period without a clear circadian pattern. This disorder may be seen more often in people with dementia or developmental disabilities. *Non-24-hour sleep-wake rhythm disorder* reflects a failure to entrain one's circadian rhythm to the usual visual cues, resulting in a circadian pattern of less than or greater than 24 hours. This occurs most frequently in blind or developmentally disabled people.

Shift work disorder involves insomnia or sleepiness due to working in shifts that coincide in part with the typical hours of sleep. Twenty percent of labor in industrialized countries involves shift work, and up to 38% of night-shift workers are symptomatic. *Jet lag* results from temporary misalignment between one's internal circadian clock and that required by a change in time zone, generally of at least 2 hours. Eastward travel requiring advancing circadian sleep-wake hours is more difficult to adjust to than westward travel.

Parasomnias

Parasomnias are abnormal behaviors and movements that occur during REM sleep, NREM sleep, or transition to or from sleep. Parasomnias are common. The lifetime prevalence of different parasomnias is 4%–67% (Singh et al. 2018). Depressive mood has been associated with confusional arousal, sleep terror, sleep-related injury, and nightmare disorder. About 12% of respondents in one study reported having five or more parasomnias (Bjorvatn et al. 2010).

NREM Parasomnias

NREM parasomnias include confusional arousals, sleepwalking, and sleep terrors, all of which involve incomplete arousal from slow-wave sleep and no or limited response to attempted intervention by others. None are caused by psychiatric disorders or brain damage. All are associated with minimal cognitive function during and amnesia for the episode. NREM parasomnias typically occur in the first half of the night when slow-wave sleep is more prominent and do not typically occur during naps. They are more common in children than in adults and occur equally in males and females. Stress, sleep deprivation, use of sedative hypnotics, and OSA or other respiratory events during sleep may be predisposing factors. Attacks may be precipitated by sensory stimuli, such as a pager going off or a phone ringing, especially in the setting of sleep deprivation. If the brevity and stereotyped nature of the episodes raise a question of nocturnal seizures, PSG and sometimes an additional sleep EEG study are indicated.

Treatment of NREM parasomnias consists of creating a safe sleeping environment, addressing any causes of sleep fragmentation, treating co-occurring sleep disorders, and avoiding sedative hypnotics.

Confusional Arousals

Confusional arousals, sometimes called sleep inertia or sleep drunkenness, occur while the patient is still in bed. The patient fully or partially awakens confused and irritable but does not manifest the heightened autonomic response and fearful affect seen in sleep terrors and does not move out of the bed as seen in sleepwalking. Sometimes the patient will speak out loud, shout, or engage in automatic behavior during the episodes, which can last from a few minutes to as long as half an hour. Confusional arousals may be precipitated by stress, insufficient sleep, or too much sleep and occur more frequently in people with a family history of parasomnias.

Sleepwalking (Somnambulism)

Sleepwalking often begins with confusional arousal but includes ambulation or other behaviors out of bed. Sometimes the sleepwalker will bolt out of bed. Episodes tend to last several minutes and end by either returning to bed or ending precipitously in another location. A sleepwalking patient may perform complex behaviors, sometimes dangerous to the patient or others, and can appear superficially to be awake. Adult sleepwalkers may become violent when attempts are made to restrain them. Lifetime prevalence has been estimated to be 6.9%, but the disorder is most common in children (Stallman and Kohler 2016).

Sleep Terrors

Sleep terrors are also known as "pavor nocturnus" or night terrors. They begin with an abrupt terror arousal, usually accompanied by a loud scream or alarming vocalization. The person appears intensely frightened and manifests signs of autonomic arousal including tachycardia, tachypnea, diaphoresis, and mydriasis. During an episode, the person sits up in bed, eyes wide open, but is unresponsive to external stimuli, sometimes muttering incoherently. Episodes tend to be brief but can last as long as 30–40 minutes and may be followed by the patient appearing inconsolable. They are difficult to arouse and, if they do wake up, they are confused and disoriented and can become violent if attempts are made to restrain them. After an episode, the person usually goes back to sleep and is amnestic for the episode upon awakening.

Sleep-Related Eating Disorder

Sleep-related eating disorder consists of recurrent episodes of dysfunctional eating and drinking during arousals from sleep. During these episodes, the patient may consume peculiar forms or combinations of food or inedible or toxic substances, perform potentially injurious behaviors in seeking and cooking food, or suffer adverse health consequences from nocturnal eating. Like other NREM parasomnias, there is impaired consciousness during the episode and impaired recall of it afterward. Episodes may begin with sleepwalking.

REM Parasomnias

REM Sleep Behavior Disorder

The most common *REM parasomnias* are REM sleep behavior disorder, sleep paralysis, and nightmare disorder. Symptoms of *REM sleep behavior disorder* (RBD) include vocalizations and complex behaviors that occur during REM sleep that can even result in injury to the patient or bed partner. Reports of apparent acting out of dreams or PSG indicate that the behaviors occur during REM sleep owing to loss of usual muscle atonia. RBD tends to occur in the latter half of a night's sleep, when REM sleep is predominant. In contrast to NREM parasomnias, the patient's eyes are typically closed. Patients regain orientation rapidly if awakened. Although it can occur in either sex or at any age, RBD typically occurs in men older than 50. RBD may be a harbinger of synucleinopathies (Parkinson disease, dementia with Lewy bodies, and multiple system atrophy). RBD can also occur in people with narcolepsy type 1. Several agents have been found to trigger RBD, including selective serotonin reuptake inhibitors (SSRIs), serotonin-norepinephrine reuptake inhibitors (SNRIs), beta-blockers, and anticholinesterase agents. Treatment consists of creating a safe sleep environment and starting clonazepam or melatonin, with the latter often used in older people at risk of falling (Roguski et al. 2020; Wang and Salas 2021).

Recurrent Isolated Sleep Paralysis

Recurrent isolated sleep paralysis produces episodes of inability to move the trunk or limbs at sleep onset or on awakening. Episodes last for a few seconds to a few minutes and cause significant anxiety and distress, as the person is awake and remembers the episodes. Hallucinations frequently occur during the paralysis. Although a form of sleep paralysis may occur in narcolepsy, recurrent isolated sleep paralysis is not diagnosed in people with narcolepsy. The episodes may terminate with sensory stimulation. Sleep deprivation and irregular sleep-wake schedules are predisposing factors. Onset is typically in adolescence and may persist into adulthood.

Nightmare Disorder

Patients with *nightmare disorder* have repeated awakenings from sleep with recollection of lengthy, terrifying dreams, usually involving threats to survival, safety, or physical integrity of oneself or loved ones. The nightmares cause significant distress, as manifested by mood disturbance; sleep resistance; impaired concentration or recall; disruption of family or parental sleep; behavioral problems in children; daytime sleepiness, fatigue, or anergia; or impaired occupational, educational, interpersonal, or social functioning. Nightmares occur most frequently in the final third of the night, when REM sleep is predominant. Upon awakening from a nightmare, the person is alert and able to recall the dream in detail. In the morning, children often recall the arousal. Very common in children, nightmare disorder can persist into adulthood as well.

Other Parasomnias

Exploding Head Syndrome

Exploding head syndrome is characterized by the perception of a sudden, loud noise or sense of explosion in the head while transitioning to sleep or awakening during sleep. In response, the individual is suddenly aroused and fearful but does not experience pain. The patient may describe their symptoms as a cymbal crash, a bomb exploding, or the sound of a loud bang, and it may occasionally be accompanied by a flash of light or a myoclonic jerk. Episodes last only a second or two, and the frequency varies from infrequent to several times per night. Episodes may occur in clusters of several days' duration. Patients may develop anticipatory insomnia. Reportedly more common in women than in men, the mean age at onset is 58. In some cases, attacks appear to be precipitated by stress or sleep deprivation. Exploding head syndrome is a rare side effect of SSRIs as well.

Sleep Talking (Somniloquy)

Talking with variable degrees of comprehensibility can occur in either REM or NREM sleep. Sleep talking is common, with a lifetime prevalence of up to 66% (Bjorvatn et al. 2010). It may be associated with other parasomnias, or it may be normal behavior. Sleep talking can be problematic if it is loud enough to disturb the bed partner or roommate, but the person is typically unaware that they are speaking aloud. The symptom is generally idiopathic but can be seen in confusional arousal or RBD as well. In the context of dementia, sleep talking is more common in dementia with Lewy bodies than in Alzheimer disease.

Sleep-Related Movement Disorders

Sleep-related movement disorders involve simple, usually stereotyped, movements that occur during sleep or transition to sleep (Avidan 2009). The exception is RLS, in which the person walks or moves their legs in a nonstereotyped fashion to reduce leg discomfort. Sleep-related movement disorders cause sleep disturbances, daytime sleepiness, or fatigue. Patients with sleep-related movement disorders should be screened for iron deficiency.

Restless Legs Syndrome and Periodic Limb Movements of Sleep

See Chapter 9 ("Movement Disorders") for a description of RLS. *Periodic limb movements of sleep* (PLMS) occur in 80%–90% of patients with RLS. The presence of PLMS is also supportive of the diagnosis of RLS. PLMS can be a normal finding, an incidental finding on PSG, or part of periodic limb movement disorder.

Periodic Limb Movement Disorder

Patients with *PLMD* show PSG evidence of PLMS that occurs 15 or more times per hour (5 times per hour in children) and complain of sleep disturbance and daytime impairment of cognitive, social, occupational, or educational functioning. PLMD is not common in adults and is not diagnosed in the presence of other sleep disorders. All other causes of insomnia or hypersomnia must be ruled out before making this diagnosis.

Sleep-Related Leg Cramps

Sleep-related leg cramps occur at night in sleep or wakefulness. Sudden intense painful muscle contractions and hardness, usually in calf muscles, are the hallmarks of this disorder. The cramps last from seconds to minutes, can vary in frequency, and can be idiopathic or occur in relation to stress, dehydration, neuropathy, or any of several metabolic disorders. Leg muscle tightness and pain can persist for minutes to hours after an episode. The pain can sometimes be relieved by gentle stretching or massage of the limb muscles.

Sleep-Related Bruxism

Sleep-related bruxism is characterized by the combination of audible nocturnal tooth grinding with craniofacial pain and wearing down of molars. Bruxism can cause jaw pain, temporomandibular spasm, and morning temporal headaches. Sleep bruxism is common and can lead to dental erosion. Differential diagnosis includes faciomandibular myoclonus, RBD, sleep apnea, confusional arousals, and focal dystonias. Wearing a mouth guard during sleep can help protect teeth from wear and tear. Improved sleep hygiene and relaxation training may be helpful.

Sleep in Psychiatric Disorders

Sleep complaints are common to nearly all psychiatric disorders. Abnormalities of sleep continuity, sleep efficiency (percentage of time asleep while in bed), sleep latency, and total sleep time are frequently seen. Abnormalities of REM sleep occur in depression, schizophrenia, substance use disorders, eating disorders, and other conditions. Long recognized as a symptom secondary to psychiatric disorders, sleep quality itself may also contribute to the cause of or exacerbate psychiatric disorders. A number of lines of evidence, for example, point to an increased risk of psychotic symptoms in people who report sleep symptoms (Freeman et al. 2020).

Abnormalities of sleep are well known to occur in mood disorders, particularly depression. In untreated depression, PSG findings include increased sleep latency, paucity of slow-wave sleep, increased REM sleep in the first third of the night, decreased REM latency, increased REM sleep density (frequency of rapid eye movements during REM sleep), and increased percentage of time spent in REM sleep (Sutton 2014). Nearly 75% of patients seen by primary care physicians for anxiety report insomnia or shortened sleep time. Data are similar in PTSD. Insomnia and circadian rhythm abnormalities are reported in half of people with schizophrenia, and worsening insomnia can be a hallmark of the prodrome to a psychotic exacerbation. A sleep history is therefore an important adjunct in evaluating all psychiatric presentations.

In addition to sleep symptoms either due to or contributing to psychiatric disorders, primary sleep disorders often co-occur with mental illness (Khurshid 2018). Patients with depression, for example, have a higher prevalence of insomnia disorder, OSA, and RLS. Conversely, a higher prevalence of depression is found in people with sleep-disordered breathing in clinical and community samples. Untreated sleep disorders, such as OSA, can cause or worsen depressive symptoms (Ettensohn et al. 2016). As many as 44% of people with ADHD have RLS, and up to 26% of people with RLS meet criteria for ADHD (Snitselaar et al. 2016).

Effects of Psychiatric Medications on Sleep

Many agents used in psychiatric treatment are known to affect the sleep-wake cycle. Benzodiazepines can increase daytime sleepiness and precipitate depression. Psychostimulants decrease both N3 and REM sleep. Chronic use can increase daytime sleepiness. Antidepressants including monoamine oxidase inhibitor therapies, tricyclic antidepressants, SSRIs, and SNRIs generally decrease total REM sleep and increase REM latency. SSRIs have been implicated in insomnia and increased sleep fragmentation, as well as increased eye movements in non-REM sleep. Antidepressants, however—especially those with higher anticholinergic load—can increase daytime sleepiness. Antidepressants are also known to cause or exacerbate RBD. The nonserotonergic antidepressant bupropion has fewer effects on the sleep-wake cycle, including not tending to cause sleep fragmentation, daytime sleepiness, or

RBD. Lithium increases total sleep time and tends to decrease REM sleep. Opioid analgesics decrease N3 slow-wave sleep. Antipsychotic agents tend to suppress REM and increase N3 sleep. They increase the risk of metabolic syndrome and high BMI, with resulting increased risk or severity of OSA. Antidepressants and antipsychotics can trigger or aggravate RLS and PLMS. Atypical antipsychotics, particularly sedating agents such as quetiapine, can cause or worsen excessive daytime sleepiness. When evaluating a patient with a sleep disorder, it is important to weigh the contribution of psychopharmacologic agents (Schweitzer and Randazzo 2017).

Case Example, Continued

The patient's evaluation in the sleep clinic includes an Epworth Sleepiness Scale score of 16 (scale 0–24 with score >10 consistent with excessive daytime sleepiness). On oropharyngeal exam, he has a small oropharyngeal opening. A PSG examination reveals moderate obstructive sleep apnea as well as absence of atonia during REM sleep. Despite this, no episodes of RBD were captured on PSG. In hindsight, RBD is thought to explain how he was found in the river and how he previously punched his wife at night without memory. His symptoms improved with CPAP, and no further episodes of RBD occurred in the following 6 months. In addition to being an early symptom of α-synucleinopathies, RBD can occur secondary to OSA.

Key Clinical Points

- Sleep not only serves a restorative function but also helps with memory consolidation and disease prevention.
- Sleep disorders increase the risk of cardiovascular disease, hypertension, stroke, diabetes, and obesity. Treatment of sleep disorders can prevent the onset or worsening of these disorders.
- A sleep history should be part of every psychiatric or neurological evaluation.
- Always consider the effects of psychopharmacologic agents on the sleep-wake cycle.
- Use sleep evaluation questionnaires as part of sleep disorder evaluations.

Review Questions

1. A person complaining of daytime sleepiness is referred for a multiple sleep latency test (MSLT). The person is not known to snore or stop breathing during sleep and has had a consistent bedtime for years. The average sleep latency was 10 minutes, and REM sleep was not detected immediately upon falling asleep. Which of the following treatments would be most helpful for this individual?

   A. Sodium oxybate
   B. Sleep hygiene instruction
   C. Armodafinil
   D. CPAP
   E. Morning bright light therapy

2. A man hospitalized after arrest for attempted murder is alleged to have suddenly awoken following a loud noise outside and begun to strangle his partner. After a major struggle, she was able to escape and call the police, who entered the bedroom and found him sleeping and snoring loudly. When the police arrested him, he insisted, despite the marks on his partner's throat, that he had no recall of choking her. Which of the following sleep disorders is most likely to be present in the assailant?

   A. Obstructive sleep apnea
   B. Narcolepsy
   C. Sleep drunkenness
   D. Nightmare disorder
   E. Sleep terrors

3. A young adult who lives alone presents with recurrent episodes of awakening from sleep, unable to move their extremities for more than a minute while at the same time hearing someone yelling at them. The person feels very anxious that they will remain paralyzed in a future occurrence. Recently, there have been a few episodes that occurred during the transition to sleep as well. There are no complaints of daytime sleepiness or episodes of loss of muscle tone. Which of the following sleep disorders is most likely to be present?

A. Recurrent isolated sleep paralysis
B. Confusional arousal
C. REM behavior disorder
D. Narcolepsy
E. Exploding head syndrome

Answers

Question 1: B. An average sleep latency of more than 8 minutes is not consistent with narcolepsy or idiopathic hypersomnia. The absence of sleep-onset REM is also inconsistent with narcolepsy. The history does not suggest obstructive sleep apnea or sleep phase disorder. The most likely etiologies are poor sleep habits, inadequate sleep, or poor sleep quality, so the treatment begins with sleep hygiene instruction.

Question 2: C. A person with sleep drunkenness (confusional arousal) may respond to being suddenly awoken by becoming confused and agitated. This behavior does not occur spontaneously and is not limited to REM sleep. It is not caused by nightmares or sleep terrors and is not seen with increased frequency in narcolepsy or obstructive sleep apnea.

Question 3: A. Recurrent isolated sleep paralysis occurs during transition to sleep or wakefulness and can be associated with hallucinations. It can be a major source of anxiety. The absence of movements or agitation and presence during sleep onset as well as awakening make REM behavior disorder and confusional arousal less likely. Sleep paralysis can occur in narcolepsy, but this patient has no other symptoms consistent with that diagnosis. Exploding head syndrome includes a hallucination of a loud noise but does not include paralysis.

References

American Academy of Sleep Medicine: International Classification of Sleep Disorders, 3rd Edition. Darien, IL, American Academy of Sleep Medicine, 2014

American Psychiatric Association: Diagnostic and Statistical Manual of Mental Disorders, 5th Edition, Text Revision. Washington, DC, American Psychiatric Association, 2022

Arnulf I: Kleine-Levin syndrome. Sleep Med Clin 10(2):151–161, 2015 26055863

Avidan AY: Parasomnias and movement disorders of sleep. Semin Neurol 29(4):372–392, 2009 19742413

Barateau L, Pizza F, Plazzi G, et al: Narcolepsy. J Sleep Res 31(4):e13631, 2022 35624073

Bastien CH, Vallières A, Morin CM: Validation of the Insomnia Severity Index as an outcome measure for insomnia research. Sleep Med 2(4):297–307, 2001 11438246

Bjorvatn B, Grønli J, Pallesen S: Prevalence of different parasomnias in the general population. Sleep Med 11(10):1031–1034, 2010 21093361

Bragg S, Benich JJ, Christian N, et al: Updates in insomnia diagnosis and treatment. Int J Psychiatry Med 54(4–5):275–289, 2019 31269837

Chung F, Yegneswaran B, Liao P, et al: STOP questionnaire: a tool to screen patients for obstructive sleep apnea. Anesthesiology 108(5):812–821, 2008 18431116

Ettensohn M, Soto Y, Bassi B, et al: Sleep problems and disorders in patients with depression. Psychiatr Ann 46(7):390–395, 2016

Foldvary-Schaefer NR, Waters TE: Sleep-disordered breathing. Continuum 23(4):1093–1116, 2017

Freeman D, Sheaves B, Waite F, et al: Sleep disturbance and psychiatric disorders. Lancet Psychiatry 7(7):628–637, 2020 32563308

Javaheri S, Redline S: Insomnia and risk of cardiovascular disease. Chest 152(2):435–444, 2017 28153671

Johns MW: A new method for measuring daytime sleepiness: the Epworth sleepiness scale. Sleep 14(6):540–545, 1991 1798888

Khurshid KA: Comorbid insomnia and psychiatric disorders: an update. Innov Clin Neurosci 15(3–4):28–32, 2018 29707424

Kumar S, Sagili H: Etiopathogenesis and neurobiology of narcolepsy: a review. J Clin Diagn Res 8(2):190–195, 2014 24701532

Levenson JC, Kay DB, Buysse DJ: The pathophysiology of insomnia. Chest 147(4):1179–1192, 2015 25846534

Morin CM: Cognitive-behavioral approaches to the treatment of insomnia. J Clin Psychiatry 65(Suppl 16):33–40, 2004 15575803

Netzer NC, Stoohs RA, Netzer CM, et al: Using the Berlin Questionnaire to identify patients at risk for the sleep apnea syndrome. Ann Intern Med 131(7):485–491, 1999 10507956

Pavlova M, Latreille V: Sleep disorders. Am J Med 132(3):292–299, 2019 30292731

Roguski A, Rayment D, Whone AL, et al: A neurologist's guide to REM sleep behavior disorder. Front Neurol 11:610, 2020 32733361

Schweitzer PK, Randazzo A: Drugs That Disturb Sleep and Wakefulness, 6th Edition. Philadelphia, Elsevier, 2017

Singh S, Kaur H, Singh S, et al: Parasomnias: a comprehensive review. Cureus 10(12):e3807, 2018 30868021

Snitselaar MA, Smits MG, Spijker J: Prevalence of restless legs syndrome in adult ADHD and its subtypes. Behav Sleep Med 14(5):480–488, 2016 26418664

Stallman HM, Kohler M: Prevalence of sleepwalking: a systematic review and meta-analysis. PLoS One 11(11):e0164769, 2016 27832078
Sutton EL: Psychiatric disorders and sleep issues. Med Clin North Am 98(5):1123–1143, 2014 25134876
Wang Y, Salas RME: Approach to common sleep disorders. Semin Neurol 41(6):781–794, 2021 34826879
Wickwire EM, Shaya FT, Scharf SM: Health economics of insomnia treatments: the return on investment for a good night's sleep. Sleep Med Rev 30:72–82, 2016 26874067

16

Neurovascular Disorders

Howard S. Kirshner, M.D.
Matthew Schrag, M.D., Ph.D.

Case Example

An 80-year-old man is brought to the emergency department after awakening with left hemiplegia (National Institutes of Health [NIH] Stroke Scale 19). Blood pressure is 150/90. Cranial CT scan reveals a large right frontal lobe hemorrhage (see Figure 16.1). He had at least two prior strokes. Six years earlier, he had had another right frontal hemorrhage that presented with headache, vomiting, and paucity of speech (not frank aphasia) following a single brief episode of atrial fibrillation during central line placement. Although his memory had worsened after that hemorrhage, he regained his baseline and was able to engage in his usual recreational activities of golf and bowling. Cognitive screening at the time was otherwise intact, but he required category prompts to recall three words on memory testing. Nine months after his first stroke, he suffered a small left temporal hemorrhage, and his cognition declined. He had developed attention dysfunction; no longer benefited from category prompts in trying to recall three words; and had significant deficits in verbal fluency in both semantic (animal) and phonemic (letter) word generation. His language gradually deteriorated in the

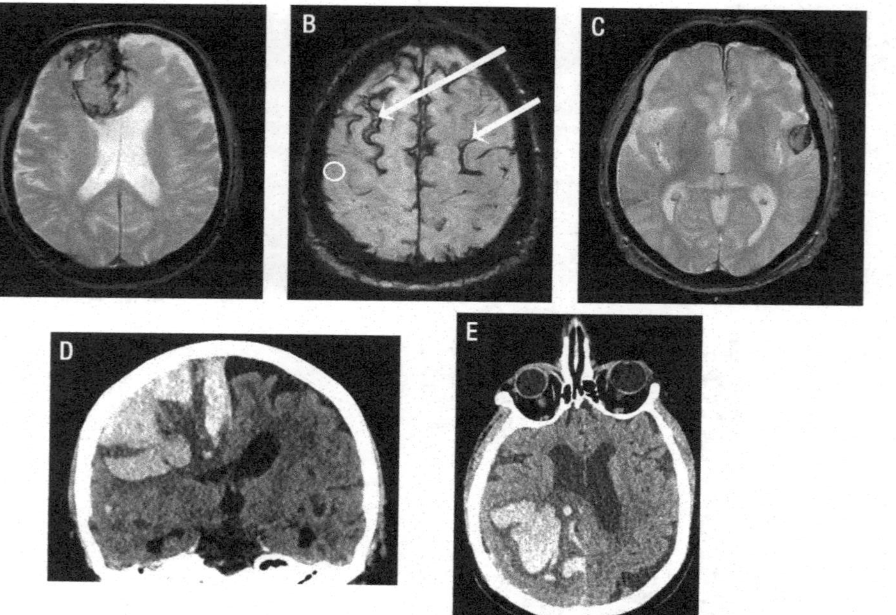

Figure 16.1 Neuroimaging results characteristic of cerebral amyloid angiopathy.

A) T2 gradient echo showing initial right frontal intracerebral hemorrhage at age 74. B) Susceptibility-weighted imaging (SWI) showing "tram track" sign (arrow) and microhemorrhage (circle) consistent with cerebral amyloid angiopathy (CAA) at age 74. C) T2 gradient echo showing left temporal intracerebral hemorrhage at age 75. D) Coronal CT image showing large right frontal intracerebral hemorrhage at age 80. E) Axial CT image showing large right parieto-occipital intracerebral hemorrhage at age 80.

ensuing 2 years, and he began to defer most conversation to his wife. He was asked to check his own BP regularly and was treated with transdermal rivastigmine.

Stroke is a focal abnormality of brain function caused by ischemia, from obstructed blood flow or hemorrhage from a ruptured vessel. The presentation of a focal deficit in a conscious patient, especially an older one with known risk factors, is instantly recognizable as a stroke.

Stroke is the most common serious neurological disorder and the most common cause of neurological disability in adults. Stroke is the fifth leading cause of death in the United States and the second worldwide. Over 800,000 strokes occur every year in the United States. Roughly 80%–85% of strokes are ischemic, while 15%–20% are hemorrhagic. Despite accounting for a minority of strokes, approximately half of stroke-related mortality is attributable to hemorrhages. From MRI evidence (Leary and Saver 2003), as many as 11 million "silent" strokes occur annually in the United States, contributing to dementia.

In this chapter, the following conditions are discussed: transient ischemic attack (TIA), ischemic stroke, intracranial hemorrhage, cerebral venous sinus thrombosis, hypertensive encephalopathy, and posterior reversible encephalopathy syndrome (PRES). Then, poststroke deficits such as aphasia, alexia, agraphia, apraxia, agnosia, depression, and dementia are also reviewed.

Approach to Patients With Neurovascular Disorders

As in all of neurology, the management of stroke begins with clinical diagnosis, based on symptoms and signs. First, one considers the patient's risk factor profile and prior history of transient ischemic attack or stroke. Next, one reviews the temporal evolution of the symptoms. In an acute stroke, critical data include the time the patient was last known as being well or time of symptom onset, the patient's baseline functional status, and contact information for the family.

Several rapid tools for the diagnosis of an acute stroke have been developed. In the Think FAST acronym, F stands for facial weakness, A for arm drift or weakness, S for slurred speech or aphasia, and T for time. A recent modification, BE FAST, adds B for balance issues and E for eye signs (visual field loss or extraocular movement difficulty). These tools can be useful, especially in a pre-hospital setting.

On arrival at a hospital, the NIH Stroke Scale (NIHSS) is measured to quantify the stroke deficit. The NIHSS has no gait measure, and truncal ataxia can be missed, so it should not replace a competent neurological exam. Another common stroke scale, the Modified Rankin Score (mRS), quantifies pre- and postmorbid disability. Further examinations, performed later, include cognitive batteries.

The history and examination suggest the location and mechanism of the stroke, but the diagnosis is usually confirmed by imaging studies. For an acute stroke, an urgent CT and CTA are obtained to evaluate for hemorrhage and vessel occlusions. The CT scan of the patient in the Case Example is shown in Figure 16.1.

Transient Ischemic Attacks

Transient ischemic attacks (TIAs), the "warning signs" of stroke, involve temporary focal ischemia. Carotid distribution TIAs include loss of vision in one eye (transient monocular blindness or amaurosis fugax), or symptoms of speech or language difficulty and contralateral weakness or numbness. TIAs in the vertebrobasilar artery distribution are associated with dizziness, diplopia, dysarthria, numbness, weakness, or somnolence. TIA symptoms resolve within 24 hours; longer syndromes are strokes. If an MRI shows an acute stroke, the diagnosis is stroke, not TIA, even if symptoms are transient.

Acute Ischemic Stroke

Symptoms and Signs

Presenting stroke symptoms are the same as those of TIAs. The TOAST criteria classify stroke mechanisms (Publications Committee 1998). First, *large artery strokes* occur in either the carotid or vertebrobasilar territory, often preceded by TIAs and evolving in a stepwise or waxing and waning manner, typically during early morning hours. Second, *small artery strokes* ("lacunes") occur in the white matter, basal ganglia, brainstem, or cerebellum, with infarction diameter less than 15–20 mm. *Lacunar strokes* may evolve gradually or wax and wane; sometimes flurries of TIAs herald the onset. Third, *embolic strokes*, usually of cardiac origin, occur suddenly, typically with maximal deficits at the onset of the event. The fourth category comprises rare, known causes (such as mitochondrial encephalopathy, lactic acidosis, and stroke-like episodes

[MELAS], cerebral autosomal dominant arteriopathy with subcortical infarcts and leukoencephalopathy [CADASIL], and Fabry disease), and the fifth are of unknown (cryptogenic) cause. Strokes that appear embolic (sudden onset with maximal deficit) without a known source of embolus are "embolic strokes of unknown source," an important subset of cryptogenic strokes.

Differential Diagnosis

The differential diagnosis of TIA includes other causes of transient neurological symptoms, including migraine, seizures, and transient alterations of consciousness. Other disorders such as subdural hematomas, tumors, abscesses, or multiple sclerosis can also present relatively acutely. A history of abrupt onset usually favors stroke; the less clear the history, as in the patient was "found down," the more likely another diagnosis will emerge. About 15% of initial stroke diagnoses prove to be stroke mimics (Kirshner 2000).

Laboratory and Radiological Investigation

Once the patient is assessed clinically, brain imaging is obtained. The CT scan is usually the first test; it detects hemorrhage early, but ischemic stroke can be invisible for 2–3 days. Occasionally, a clot in the middle cerebral artery is visible on CT (*hyperacute MCA sign*). The ASPECTS score quantifies the extent of early infarction (Aviv et al. 2007). CT angiography (CTA) images the cerebral and cervical arteries to evaluate for stenosis, occlusions, dissections, or malformations. Sometimes, a CT perfusion map is obtained to distinguish areas of irreversible infarction from reversible ischemia. If the infarct core is small and the hypoperfused area is large (*ischemic penumbra*), mechanical thrombectomy can prevent damage.

The magnetic resonance versions of the CT/CTA and CT perfusion scans are the MRI/MRA and perfusion weighted image (PWI). Acute ischemia shows up on magnetic resonance as hyperintensity on the diffusion weighted image (DWI) and corresponding hypointensity on the apparent diffusion coefficient (ADC). MRI also reveals hemorrhages as hypointensity on T2* weighted images such as susceptibility-weighted imaging (SWI) and gradient echo sequences (GRE).

Doppler ultrasound images of the carotid bifurcations analyze blood flow. Transcranial Doppler (TCD) visualizes the major intracranial arteries. Finally, catheter arteriography is the gold standard, as it can detect small aneurysms or vasculitis, but it is invasive with some risk.

Evaluation of a stroke also involves cardiac investigations: electrocardiography and heart rhythm monitoring to detect atrial fibrillation. Echocardiography can be performed as a transthoracic study (TTE) or, for more accuracy but more invasively, transesophageal (TEE). Echocardiography can image thrombus in the left atrium or ventricle, poor ventricular contractility, valve pathology, or a right-to-left shunt. Atrial septal defects or the more common patent foramen ovale (PFO) occur in up to 25% of the general population. This condition allows clots from the venous circulation to cross from right to left and embolize to the brain (*paradoxical embolization*). A bubble study, involving the injection of agitated saline, can detect a septal defect when bubbles cross from the right to left atrium. TCD, with intravenous injection of agitated saline, detects microemboli.

Blood tests are also important. A complete blood count detects increased red blood cell counts, thrombocytosis, or thrombocytopenia, a cause of bleeding. Clotting tests such as the prothrombin time (PT) and partial thromboplastin time (PTT) detect clotting defects associated with cerebral hemorrhage. Testing for a hypercoagulable state is performed in young patients without stroke risk factors. The lupus anticoagulant and anticardiolipin antibody are most often associated with arterial strokes. To detect modifiable risk factors, all patients generally should have an A1C and a lipid panel.

Treatment

Stroke treatment includes acute interventions, such as tissue plasminogen activator (tPA), an intravenous clot dissolver, and preventive therapies. With active stroke treatment, rapid diagnosis is essential. Mobile stroke units, using CT-equipped ambulances, shorten the time to tPA treatment and improve outcomes (Ebinger et al. 2021). In the National Institute of Neurological Disorders trial, intravenous tPA within 3 hours of onset improved excellent outcomes by about 30%, with an OR of 1.7:1 (National Institute of Neurological Disorders 1995). A European trial demonstrated a persistent benefit of tPA treatment out to 4.5 hours with additional patient selection criteria (Hacke et al. 2008). tPA increases the risk of hemorrhage but improves outcomes. Recently, tPA has been given to "wake up" strokes, within 4.5 hours of deficit discovery if the MRI shows a diffusion-weighted but minimal FLAIR lesion

(Thomalla et al. 2018). Thrombolytic therapy is avoided in patients with stroke mimics (Kirshner 2000). In mild strokes (Khatri et al. 2018), tPA was not superior to aspirin. Another thrombolytic agent, tenecteplase, is noninferior to tPA and easier to administer as a single bolus without the 1-hour infusion. Tenecteplase is gradually replacing tPA in the United States.

A new era in stroke treatment began with mechanical thrombectomy, and early detection of large vessel occlusions with transfer to thrombectomy-ready facilities is crucial. In 2015, five studies showed improved outcomes in patients with internal carotid or middle cerebral artery (M1) occlusions who were treated within 6 hours (Goyal et al. 2016). Perfusion studies distinguish areas of infarcted tissue from areas of reversible ischemia (*penumbra*), and the treatment time window has been extended to as much as 24 hours (Nogueira et al. 2018). Intravenous tPA before mechanical thrombectomy may or may not add benefit. Recent studies suggested that acute endovascular therapy for basilar artery occlusion, as in anterior circulation stroke, has definite benefit (Alemseged et al. 2023; Langezaal et al. 2021).

For patients with large strokes despite acute therapy, measures to reduce intracranial pressure with intravenous mannitol or hypertonic saline can prevent cerebral herniation and death. In large MCA or cerebellar strokes, decompressive craniectomy is lifesaving (Jüttler et al. 2011), especially in patients younger than 60.

After acute treatment, the next steps are secondary stroke prevention and rehabilitation. Speech/language pathologists assess swallowing before permitting oral intake. Prevention of deep vein thrombosis by sequential compression devices or subcutaneous heparin or enoxaparin reduces pulmonary emboli. Physical and occupational therapists prevent contractures and begin active exercises to regain function.

In secondary prevention, antiplatelet therapy is given for most strokes; anticoagulation is recommended for patients with atrial fibrillation and other cardioembolic sources. Studies have suggested that a period of dual antiplatelet therapy with aspirin and clopidogrel (Johnston et al. 2018), aspirin and ticagrelor (Johnston et al. 2020), or aspirin and cilostazol (Toyoda et al. 2019) reduces recurrent strokes with a low risk of hemorrhage. Dual antiplatelet therapy has not proved beneficial for long-term use. For patients with stroke or TIA secondary to an intracranial artery stenosis, aggressive medical therapy with dual antiplatelet therapy and statins is superior to angioplasty and stenting (Zaidat et al. 2015). Statin therapy helps prevent recurrent strokes. Other treatment measures include smoking cessation, hypertension management, a healthy diet, and treatment of sleep apnea. Patients with >70% carotid artery stenosis are offered surgery or stenting. In patients with PFO, closure benefits patients younger than 60, especially with few traditional stroke risk factors and with a large PFO or associated atrial septal aneurysm (Kent et al. 2021). For patients with a definite cardiac source of embolism, especially atrial fibrillation, anticoagulation is indicated with warfarin or a direct oral anticoagulant (DOAC) such as apixaban. DOACs are easy to manage, have minimal drug interactions, and cause fewer cerebral hemorrhages than warfarin. However, patients with valvular heart disease still require warfarin. Indications for anticoagulation in stroke are limited to patients with cardiac sources of embolism, cerebral venous sinus thrombosis, and hypercoagulable states. Carotid or vertebral artery dissections are treated with antiplatelet therapy (Markus et al. 2019).

Course and Prognosis

About 10% of strokes are fatal, and many survivors are disabled. Almost a third of patients with strokes become cognitively impaired in the year following the stroke. The risk of recurrent stroke is greatest during the first few months.

Intracranial Hemorrhage

Intracranial hemorrhage can occur in the epidural, subdural, subarachnoid, and intracerebral spaces (ICH). Acute intracranial hemorrhages typically present with severe headache, nausea, and vomiting, while a more insidious headache onset may be seen in subdural hematomas. Only ICH will be discussed here, but Table 16.1 summarizes the major types of intracranial hemorrhages.

ICH is bleeding in the brain parenchyma that mimics an ischemic stroke (Qureshi et al. 2001). The most common cause is hypertension. The small arteries that arise directly from larger arteries such as the MCA or basilar artery are the most vulnerable. As such, these hemorrhages have a predilection for deep brain structures such as the putamen and basal ganglia, followed by the thalamus, brainstem, and cerebellum. Cerebellar hemorrhage is the most amenable to neurosurgical treatment; hence, acute diagnosis is critical. Cerebellar hemorrhage causes nonspe-

Table 16.1 Intracranial hemorrhage

Type	Location	Usual shape of blood on imaging	Common mechanism
Epidural	Between dura and skull	Lentiform	Trauma to middle meningeal artery from skull fracture
Subdural	Between dura and arachnoid	Crescent	Trauma to bridging veins
Subarachnoid	Between arachnoid and pia	Tracks sulci, fissures, cisterns	Trauma, or rupture of aneurysm or other vascular malformation
Intracerebral	Inside brain parenchyma	Various but often rounded	Trauma, hypertension, arteriovenous malformation, tumor

cific symptoms such as dizziness, nausea, vomiting, and headache. A key to diagnosis is gait ataxia. Hemorrhages in the brainstem, usually the pons, often cause quadriparesis and coma. The prognosis is poor unless the hemorrhage is small. Occasional pontine hemorrhages may present with less severe deficits than expected, which should prompt the examiner to look for the presence of a cavernous malformation. Hemorrhages into the basal ganglia usually cause hemiparesis. Those in the caudate nucleus or thalamus can rupture into the ventricles, resulting in increased intracranial pressure due to obstructive hydrocephalus. Hemorrhages into cortical-subcortical brain regions, "lobar hemorrhages," may be caused by either cerebral amyloid angiopathy or hypertension.

The management of ICH is supportive, emphasizing control of blood pressure (Schrag and Kirshner 2020). A target blood pressure of 140–160 mmHg is recommended as both high and low blood pressure can be detrimental. Neurosurgical techniques to evacuate cerebral hemorrhage have had limited success except in cerebellar hemorrhages (Mendelow et al. 2005), but new, less invasive devices for hemorrhage evacuation have recently shown benefits in lobar hemorrhages (Pradilla, et al. 2024).

Less Common Vascular Syndromes

Cerebral Venous Sinus Thrombosis

Cerebral venous sinus thrombosis (CVST) produces symptoms of headache and confusion. Occasionally, hemorrhage or associated infarction, caused by venous outflow obstruction, produces focal neurological deficits suggestive of stroke. Treatment involves anticoagulation, even in cases associated with hemorrhage. CVST with associated thrombocytopenia has been described in patients with COVID-19, and rarely after coronavirus vaccines (Ebinger et al. 2021; See et al. 2021).

Hypertensive Encephalopathy and Posterior Reversible Encephalopathy Syndrome

Hypertensive encephalopathy has been known for decades. A variant involving posterior, often symmetric T2 hyperintense signal in the cerebral white matter called *hypertensive encephalopathy and posterior reversible encephalopathy syndrome* (PRES) has been described (Hinchey et al. 1996). However, this may be a misnomer because the syndrome is not always posterior, restricted to white matter, or reversible.

Reversible Cerebral Vasoconstriction Syndrome

A *reversible cerebral vasoconstriction syndrome* (RCVS) of acute thunderclap headache, followed by ischemic lesions or intracerebral or subarachnoid hemorrhages, has also been described (Call et al. 1988). The hemorrhages may be small, cortical rather than deep, and not in locations associated with ruptured aneurysms. The cerebral arteries show segmental narrowing on CTA, and more often on arteriography. The syndrome occurs in the postpartum period, after carotid endarterectomy, or in association with drugs and substances. Calcium channel blockers such as verapamil or nimodipine provide benefit (Burton and Bushnell 2019). The prognosis is variable with rare recurrence, and most patients improve.

Poststroke Problems

Aphasia

Aphasia is a disorder of language caused by brain disease. A mute patient cannot be presumed to have aphasia. Normal writing and comprehension make aphasia unlikely; signs of left hemisphere dysfunction, such as right hemiparesis, make aphasia more likely. Aphasias are often divided into two groups of syndromes: expressive versus receptive, motor versus sensory, nonfluent versus fluent, or anterior versus posterior. Aphasia is classified into eight syndromes (see Tables 16.2 and 16.3).

Broca Aphasia

The patient with *Broca aphasia* has articulatory difficulty but relatively intact comprehension. There is little speech—often single words and phrases, articulated effortfully—and the production may be agrammatic or telegraphic. Naming is impaired; the patient may produce the beginning syllable (tip-of-the-tongue phenomenon). Like speech, repetition is hesitant and effortful. Auditory comprehension is less affected, but complex grammatical sentences cause difficulty. Most patients have right hemiparesis and are aware of and concerned about their deficits.

Strokes associated with Broca aphasia classically involve the posterior two thirds of the left inferior frontal gyrus, Brodmann areas 44 and 45. Patients with strokes restricted to this area often recover well (Mohr et al. 1978). Patients with chronic Broca aphasia typically have larger infarctions of the frontoparietal operculum and subcortical areas, with an initial global aphasia that recovers toward Broca aphasia. Mild, transient Broca aphasia, with normal comprehension and usually intact writing, is called *aphemia*.

Wernicke Aphasia

In contrast to the nonfluent Broca aphasia, the patient with *Wernicke aphasia* speaks effortlessly, with normal or increased numbers of words (*logorrhea*). Speech content seems nonsensical, containing few meaningful nouns and verbs. The patient makes paraphasic errors of both literal (phonemic) and verbal (semantic) type; speech may be incomprehensible (*jargon aphasia*). Naming is impaired, and repetition is disrupted by paraphasic substitutions. Auditory and reading comprehension are poor, but occasionally patients may comprehend better in one modality

Table 16.2 Language features of common types of aphasia

Feature	Broca	Wernicke	Global	Conduction	Anomic
Spontaneous speech	Nonfluent	Fluent and paraphasic	Nonfluent	Fluent	Fluent with pauses
Naming	Impaired	Paraphasic	Poor	Variable	Most impaired
Comprehension	Intact except complex grammar	Poor	Poor	Intact	Intact
Repetition	Impaired	Impaired	Impaired	Impaired	Intact
Reading	May be impaired	Impaired	Poor	May be intact	Intact
Writing	Impaired	Impaired	Poor	May be intact	Intact
Approximate lesion location	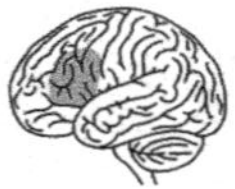	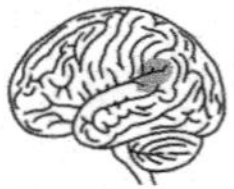	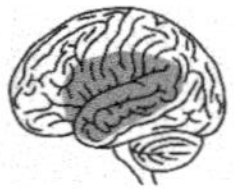	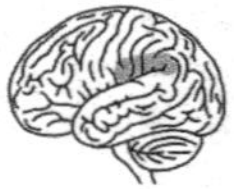	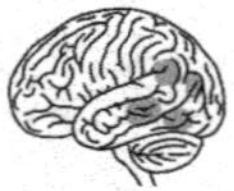

The gray-shaded areas indicate approximate locations of the left-hemisphere lesions causing each aphasia type. Note that anomic aphasia may be caused by lesions in several different locations as shown in the diagram.

Table 16.3 Characteristics of transcortical aphasias

Feature	Transcortical motor aphasia	Transcortical sensory aphasia	Mixed transcortical aphasia
Speech	Nonfluent	Fluent	Nonfluent
Naming	Impaired	Impaired	Impaired
Repetition	Preserved	Echolalic	Echolalic
Comprehension	Preserved	Impaired	Impaired
Reading	Preserved	Impaired	Impaired
Writing	Impaired	Paragraphic	Impaired
Associated signs	Right leg > arm weakness, abulia	Variable, often none	Right or bilateral hemiparesis
Approximate lesion location			

The gray-shaded areas indicate approximate locations of the left-hemisphere lesions causing each aphasia type. Note that mixed transcortical aphasia is caused by simultaneous anterior and posterior lesions as shown in the diagram.

versus the other (Kirshner et al. 1989). The patient writes well-formed letters but with misspellings and nonwords. Most patients have no motor or sensory deficits. Because of the lack of associated paralysis, Wernicke aphasia may be mistaken for psychosis or confusion. Patients seem unaware of their deficits and may even be angry or paranoid at not being understood.

Strokes causing Wernicke aphasia involve the left superior temporal gyrus, supplied by the inferior division of the left MCA; some extend into the inferior parietal lobule (supramarginal and angular gyri). Destruction of Wernicke's area predicts lasting loss of word comprehension (Naeser et al. 1987). Incomplete damage permits recovery toward conduction or anomic aphasia.

Pure Word Deafness

Pure word deafness results in poor auditory comprehension and impaired repetition, but otherwise intact language and hearing functions. Some patients have paraphasic speech and impaired naming. Pure word deafness can be caused by bitemporal lesions that disconnect Wernicke's area from the auditory cortices. Occasionally, the cause is a unilateral left temporal lesion.

Global Aphasia

In *global aphasia,* the patient speaks with a Broca aphasia and comprehends with a Wernicke aphasia, the worst of both worlds. Some produce stereotyped sounds. Milder cases are called *mixed aphasia.* Most patients with global aphasia have right hemiparesis. The etiology is usually a large stroke in the left MCA or ICA territory or a left basal ganglia hemorrhage. The patient usually improves toward Broca aphasia.

Conduction Aphasia

Conduction aphasia involves a loss of repetition. Auditory comprehension is intact, and speech is relatively fluent, with literal paraphasic errors. Most patients have right-sided motor and sensory deficits. The lesions involve the left superior temporal lobe, with sparing of Wernicke's area, or the inferior parietal region. Broca's and Wernicke's areas are intact but "disconnected." Patients with parietal damage may have apraxia (Benson et al. 1973; Damasio and Damasio 1980). Damage to the supramarginal gyrus causes phoneme production errors, along with literal paraphasic errors (Démonet et al. 1992).

Anomic Aphasia

Anomic aphasia involves naming difficulty. Spontaneous speech is fluent, and other language functions are relatively intact. Associated deficits are variable or absent. Almost all aphasia includes some anomia, and many patients recover toward anomic aphasia. Associated lesions vary; the damage lies outside the perisylvian language circuit.

Transcortical Aphasias

Transcortical aphasia spares repetition, indicating preservation of the perisylvian language circuit. The three traditional transcortical aphasia syndromes are described in Table 16.3.

Transcortical motor aphasia (TCMA) resembles Broca aphasia, with preserved repetition. Strokes involve the ACA territory in the anterior frontal lobe, the deep subcortical frontal white matter, or the supplementary motor cortex. ACA strokes feature leg more than arm and shoulder more than hand weakness, often with an involuntary grasp reflex. *Transcortical sensory aphasia* (TCSA) resembles Wernicke aphasia, with spared repetition. TCSA is an uncommon stroke syndrome, with lesions near the temporo-occipital junction. Mixed transcortical aphasia resembles global aphasia, but with preserved repetition or even echolalia.

Subcortical Aphasias

Strokes in the left basal ganglia and deep white matter cause *subcortical aphasias*. In *thalamic aphasia*, first described with left thalamic hemorrhage, the patient speaks fluently, with paraphasic errors, but partially preserved comprehension. Language impairment is worse in drowsy states.

Lesions of the caudate nucleus, putamen, and adjacent white matter cause aphasia. *Anterior subcortical aphasia syndrome* involves the caudate head, anterior limb of the internal capsule, and anterior putamen, in the territory of lenticulostriate MCA branches. Patients have dysarthria, dysfluency, mild comprehension deficits, and intact repetition, usually with right hemiparesis. Other subcortical aphasia syndromes also occur.

Alexia and Agraphia

Pure Alexia Without Agraphia

Alexia is an acquired loss of reading, and *agraphia* is an acquired loss of writing. Pure alexia without agraphia occurs in left posterior cerebral artery strokes resulting in left occipital lobe and splenium lesions. The syndrome is a "linguistic blindfolding": patients can write but not read their own writing. Other language modalities are normal, but naming is affected, especially colors. Patients cannot read; over time, they learn to read slowly, letter by letter. They understand words spelled aloud, and they can spell normally. Most have a right visual field defect; many have memory difficulties. Dejerine postulated a disconnection between the right visual cortex and left hemisphere language centers (Dejerine 1892).

Alexia With Agraphia

This syndrome is an acquired illiteracy. Oral speech modalities are preserved, except for paraphasic speech and impaired naming. Associated deficits include right hemianopia and, in addition to agraphia, other elements of Gerstmann syndrome: acalculia, right-left confusion, and finger agnosia. The lesions involve the inferior parietal lobule, especially the angular gyrus.

Agraphia

As in reading, strokes may affect writing. Prominent cases of agraphia have been reported with strokes in the left frontal or parietal regions.

Apraxia

Apraxia is a disorder of learned motor acts, in the absence of paralysis, incoordination, sensory deficit, or lack of understanding. The patient cannot carry out skilled actions on command but understands the command and performs the same action in a different context (Geschwind 1975). Liepmann described three types of apraxia: ideomotor, ideational, and limb kinetic (Liepmann 1900).

Ideomotor Apraxia

Ideomotor apraxia is an inability to perform a motor act on command despite intact comprehension and the ability to perform the same act in a different context. The idea of the movement is disconnected from its execution. A patient with ideomotor apraxia cannot perform the requested action on command, improves with imitation, and improves further with the actual object. This apraxia often accompanies aphasia (De Renzi et al. 1980; Geschwind 1975). By the Liepmann model, in Broca and conduction aphasia, ideomotor apraxia interferes with following commands on either side of the body. Apraxia may be mistaken for a comprehension deficit. Asking yes/no questions establishes normal comprehension. *Callosal apraxia* disturbs movement of the left limbs only and is caused by a corpus callosum lesion that prevents information from reaching the right hemisphere motor area. The left hemisphere seems dominant for learned actions as well as for speech.

Ideational Apraxia

Ideational apraxia has two separate definitions. First, it can mean apraxia for real objects. In one case, a patient was described who could name objects but not indicate how to use them; he had lost the concept of tool use (Ochipa et al. 1989). The second definition involves the loss of the ability to carry out a multistep activity, such as making a cup of coffee. Failure to perform a series of actions may reflect motor planning difficulties seen with frontal lobe lesions. By either definition, ideational apraxia is associated with left hemisphere lesions, often with severe aphasia.

Limb-Kinetic Apraxia

The third apraxia syndrome is *limb-kinetic apraxia,* a fine motor deficit of one hand. Stroke patients with mild hemiparesis may have grossly normal strength but difficulty with fine finger movements. Heilman called this apraxia a "loss of deftness" (Heilman et al. 2000).

Other Apraxias

Constructional apraxia and dressing apraxia, associated with right parietal strokes, are discussed in the next section. *Gait apraxia* refers to an inability to walk, not explained by motor weakness or ataxia. These are not primarily motor deficits; hence, they are not true apraxias.

Agnosia

Agnosias are disorders of recognition. Most affect a single sensory system (visual, auditory, or tactile agnosia) or a specific class of items (e.g., prosopagnosia is an agnosia for faces). The diagnosis of agnosia requires normal sensory perception, normal naming, and no general cognitive deterioration. For example, a patient with visual agnosia fails to recognize keys by sight but identifies them by palpation or by sound.

Most agnosias require bilateral cortical lesions, cutting off input from the sensory cortex to left hemisphere language centers.

Visual Agnosia

Bilateral occipital lesions may cause complete "cortical" blindness, or *visual agnosia*. Partial lesions permit some visual perception; a patient may be able to draw the item but fail to identify it. For example, the patient sees the two circles in a drawing of a bicycle but misidentifies it as eyeglasses. Agnosia can be selective for subsets of items, such as faces.

Auditory Agnosia

Auditory agnosias overlap with cortical deafness, resulting from bilateral temporal lesions. Patients have preserved pure tone hearing but cannot understand spoken language (pure word deafness), interpreted by Geschwind as a disconnection of both auditory cortices from Wernicke's area (Geschwind 1970). Other auditory agnosias include *auditory nonverbal agnosia* and *phonagnosia* (for voices).

Tactile Agnosia

Strokes involving the parietal lobe can cause *astereognosis*, or the inability to identify objects by feel; or *agraphesthesia*, the inability to recognize letters or numbers drawn on the hand. These cortical sensory deficits can be thought of as *tactile agnosias*.

Neglect

Just as aphasia commonly accompanies left hemisphere strokes, spatial deficits and neglect accompany right hemisphere injury. Syndromes include constructional and dressing deficits, spatial and topographical disorientation, inattention to the left side of the body and of space, neglect and denial of neurological deficits, and disrupted emotional aspects of communication. *Constructional impairment* is usually localized to the right parietal lobe. *Dressing apraxia* reflects an inability to conceptualize the spatial relationships of clothing to parts of the body. Right-hemisphere stroke patients may become lost traveling familiar routes. They have difficulty drawing maps or locating cities on a map. Damage to the right retrosplenial area causes *topographical deficits* (inability to orient oneself in surroundings).

Unilateral neglect and inattention are striking abnormalities in right-hemisphere stroke patients. The patient lies on the right side, head turned to the right. They may eat only from the right side of a plate or shave only the right side of the face. Neglect can include denial of the stroke deficit itself (*anosognosia*), and the patient may acknowledge the deficit but seem unconcerned about it (*anosodiaphoria*). In severe neglect, patients may deny that the left limbs are theirs when confronted.

Poststroke Depression

Depression develops in many stroke patients; estimates range from 18% (Kim and Choi-Kwon 2000) to 40% (Robinson et al. 2000). Depression limits stroke rehabilitation and recovery. Goldstein described the *catastrophic reaction,* in which patients recovering from left hemisphere strokes become withdrawn or agitated and refuse to participate. Many patients with aphasia become anxious when confronted with a difficult language task. The lack of concern after right-hemisphere strokes has been called the *indifference reaction.* Gainotti associated depression with left hemisphere strokes and indifference with right hemisphere strokes (Gainotti 1972). The implication was that poststroke depression is not simply a psychological reaction but is caused by the stroke itself.

Recent studies have confirmed the common occurrence of depression after stroke, but the anatomy is complex. Depressed mood correlates with anterior left-hemisphere lesions (Robinson et al. 1984), a finding confirmed in only some studies. The association between depression and left hemisphere stroke was later found to be a phenomenon of timing (Aström et al. 1993; Robinson et al. 2000); studies carried out at least 4 months poststroke found equal incidence of depression after right- and left-hemisphere strokes. Neglect of or indifference to a right hemisphere deficit eventually resolves; depression accompanies awareness of the deficits.

Treatment of poststroke depression with several antidepressant drugs has been shown to be beneficial. SSRI antidepressants are preferred because of their lower side effects. Controversy surrounds the use of antidepressants in stroke rehabilitation. In the FLAME study, patients taking fluoxetine 20 mg daily for 3 months showed better motor arm recovery than those on placebo (Chollet et al. 2011). The larger FOCUS trial found no benefit in a 6-month trial, but it required no specific deficit and defined improvement as a 1-point reduction on the mRS (FOCUS Trial Collaboration 2019), and thus may have had lower sensitivity to detect treatment effects. The general consensus is to have a low threshold to treat stroke patients for depression.

Another poststroke mood state, especially with bilateral strokes, is *pseudobulbar affect* (PBA), also called emotional lability, pathological laughter and crying, or emotional incontinence. Patients manifest a profound emotional reaction, more often crying than laughing, due to failure to control the expression of affect. In PBA, the patient may deny feeling depressed or experience only fleeting sadness accompanied by a disproportionate prolonged crying reaction. Pseudobulbar affect is a failure to control the expression of one's affects. These patients cannot play poker; they reveal their hands in their facial expressions. PBA can occur in unilateral as well as bilateral strokes. PBA was found to be more common than depression, especially with subcortical strokes (Kim and Choi-Kwon 2000). PBA may respond to antidepressant therapy with an SSRI (Mukand et al. 1996). The combination of dextromethorphan and quinidine is approved for PBA as well (Panitch et al. 2006).

Apathy is another psychiatric sequela of stroke. Apathy overlaps with depression and involves a loss of interest and initiative, with blunted emotional response (van Dalen et al. 2013). Apathy is associated with both depression and cognitive decline and is found in approximately one third of stroke survivors. There is no specific association with stroke location, but involvement of the basal ganglia or frontal lobe is common. Treatment is unproved, but antidepressants or stimulants are often tried.

Mania or psychosis is a rare consequence of stroke, compared with depression. Mania has been reported in approximately 1% of 300 stroke patients (Starkstein et al. 1987). Lesions were usually right-sided or bilateral. Cortical lesions have been associated with unipolar mania, while subcortical lesions have been associated with bipolar mania (Starkstein et al. 1991).

Vascular Dementia

Vascular cognitive impairment (VCI) and vascular dementia are common sequelae of stroke and contributors to late-life cognitive decline. The term *multi-infarct dementia* has been replaced by *vascular dementia,* because single strokes in strategic locations can cause dementia. Additionally, strokes can impair cognitive functions without dementia, which would be categorized as VCI. See Chapter 4, "Dementia."

As many as 30% of stroke survivors develop dementia within a year (Pohjasvaara et al. 2000). Features associated with dementia include number and volume of infarctions, associated cortical and hippocampal atrophy, and involvement of the thalamus or of the left hemisphere corona radiata (Stebbins et al. 2008; Szirmai et al. 2002). White matter disease and silent strokes contribute to cognitive impairment.

The neuropsychological deficits of vascular cognitive impairment differ from those of degenerative dementias such as Alzheimer disease. Whereas memory impairment is the hallmark of Alzheimer disease, executive function and processing speed bear the brunt of vascular cognitive impairment. VCI patients have difficulty with generating word lists starting with a specific letter; Alzheimer disease patients have more difficulty producing lists of words in a semantic category such as animals.

Case Example, Continued

Because he has had at least three hemorrhagic strokes, the neurovascular component of the patient's cognitive decline is apparent. However, his progressive memory loss and gradual decline in verbal fluency may also be consistent with Alzheimer disease. Imaging results play a crucial role in determining that the cause of his recurrent hemorrhages is cerebral amyloid angiopathy (CAA). Because of his clear end-of-life preferences to forego intubation or resuscitation if confronting an irreparable injury, comfort-oriented care was provided, and he died in the company of his wife and daughter.

Key Clinical Points

- Stroke is an acute syndrome, recognized by the sudden onset of a focal neurological deficit.
- Causes of stroke include ischemia from thrombosis or embolism, or cerebral hemorrhage.
- Stroke can be diagnosed at the bedside, with confirmatory testing usually by CT scan and CT angiography, and may also involve CT perfusion and MRI.
- Stroke is a treatable disorder, especially if the patient is diagnosed promptly.
- Stroke causes neurological deficits that may improve with rehabilitation and supportive care.
- Stroke may cause depression, cognitive impairment, and dementia.

Review Questions

1. The CT of a patient reveals a crescent-shaped hyperdensity between the brain and skull. Which of the following is the most likely mechanism of this hemorrhage?

   A. Skull fracture injuring the middle meningeal artery
   B. Rupture of an aneurysm
   C. Severe hypertension
   D. Trauma to bridging veins
   E. Hemorrhage within a tumor

2. A 27-year-old woman presents to the emergency room for a sudden-onset headache, stating it is the "worst headache of my life." Initial CT and MRI of the brain are normal. MRA shows alternating tapered narrowing and dilated segments in the cerebral arteries. Which of the following is the most likely diagnosis?

   A. Ischemic stroke
   B. Hemorrhagic stroke
   C. Cerebral venous sinus thrombosis (CVST)
   D. Posterior reversible encephalopathy syndrome (PRES)
   E. Reversible cerebral vasoconstriction syndrome (RCVS)

3. A patient who had a stroke is able to write full sentences but is unable to read even their own writing. Where is the lesion for this patient?

   A. Left occipital lobe and splenium
   B. Left frontal lobe and genu of the corpus callosum
   C. Left temporal lobe and anterior commissure
   D. Left insula and thalamus
   E. Left cerebellum and vermis

Answers

Question 1: D. A crescent-shaped hyperdensity on CT is likely a subdural hematoma, which is caused by injury to the bridging veins. Rupture of the middle meningeal artery causes an epidural hematoma, and rupture of an aneurysm causes subarachnoid hemorrhage. Severe hypertension often results in intracerebral hemorrhage. Tumors might hemorrhage, and the location will depend on the location of the tumor.

Question 2: E. The initial CT and MRI in RCVS may be normal or may show small strokes or hemorrhages, but the cerebral angiography of multifocal segmental constriction, known as "sausages on a string," is diagnostic in this clinical context. Ischemic and hemorrhagic strokes have characteristic appearances on the CT/MRI. CVST would be seen as a filling defect or absence of flow due to a clot on venography. PRES is classically seen as symmetric T2 hyperintensities on MRI.

Question 3: A. A left posterior cerebral artery stroke can result in left occipital lobe and splenium lesions that result in alexia without agraphia. The patient often has a right hemianopsia (due to the left occipital lesion). The intact right occipital lobe is able to see the left visual field but is unable to communicate with the left side of the brain (where language centers are) owing to the lesion of the splenium of the corpus callosum.

References

Alemseged F, Nguyen TN, Coutts SB, et al: Endovascular thrombectomy for basilar artery occlusion: translating research findings into clinical practice. Lancet Neurol 22(4):330–337, 2023 36780915

Aström M, Adolfsson R, Asplund K: Major depression in stroke patients. A 3-year longitudinal study. Stroke 24(7):976–982, 1993 8322398

Aviv RI, Mandelcorn J, Chakraborty S, et al: Alberta Stroke Program Early CT Scoring of CT perfusion in early stroke visualization and assessment. AJNR Am J Neuroradiol 28(10):1975–1980, 2007 17921237

Benson DF, Sheremata WA, Bouchard R, et al: Conduction aphasia. A clinicopathological study. Arch Neurol 28(5):339–346, 1973 4696016

Burton TM, Bushnell CD: Reversible Cerebral Vasoconstriction Syndrome. Stroke 50(8):2253–2258, 2019 31272323

Call GK, Fleming MC, Sealfon S, et al: Reversible cerebral segmental vasoconstriction. Stroke 19(9):1159–1170, 1988 3046073

Chollet F, Tardy J, Albucher JF, et al: Fluoxetine for motor recovery after acute ischaemic stroke (FLAME): a randomised placebo-controlled trial. Lancet Neurol 10(2):123–130, 2011 21216670

Damasio H, Damasio AR: The anatomical basis of conduction aphasia. Brain 103(2):337–350, 1980 7397481

De Renzi E, Motti F, Nichelli P: Imitating gestures. A quantitative approach to ideomotor apraxia. Arch Neurol 37(1):6–10, 1980 7350907

Dejerine J: Contribution à l'étude anatomo-pathologique et clinique des différentes variétés de cécité verbale. C R Seances Soc Biol Fil 44:61–90, 1892

Démonet JF, Chollet F, Ramsay S, et al: The anatomy of phonological and semantic processing in normal subjects. Brain 115(Pt 6):1753–1768, 1992 1486459

Ebinger M, Siegerink B, Kunz A, et al; Berlin_PRehospital Or Usual Delivery in stroke care (B_PROUD) study group: Association Between Dispatch of Mobile Stroke Units and Functional Outcomes Among Patients With Acute Ischemic Stroke in Berlin. JAMA 325(5):454–466, 2021 33528537

FOCUS Trial Collaboration: Effects of fluoxetine on functional outcomes after acute stroke (FOCUS): a pragmatic, double-blind, randomised, controlled trial. Lancet 393(10168):265–274, 2019 30528472

Gainotti G: Emotional behavior and hemispheric side of the lesion. Cortex 8(1):41–55, 1972 5031258

Geschwind N: The organization of language and the brain. Science 170(3961):940–944, 1970 5475022

Geschwind N: The apraxias: neural mechanisms of disorders of learned movement. Am Sci 63(2):188–195, 1975 1115438

Goyal M, Menon BK, van Zwam WH, et al; HERMES collaborators: Endovascular thrombectomy after large-vessel ischaemic stroke: a meta-analysis of individual patient data from five randomised trials. Lancet 387(10029):1723–1731, 2016 26898852

Hacke W, Kaste M, Bluhmki E, et al; ECASS Investigators: Thrombolysis with alteplase 3 to 4.5 hours after acute ischemic stroke. N Engl J Med 359(13):1317–1329, 2008 18815396

Heilman KM, Meador KJ, Loring DW: Hemispheric asymmetries of limb-kinetic apraxia: a loss of deftness. Neurology 55(4):523–526, 2000 10953184

Hinchey J, Chaves C, Appignani B, et al: A reversible posterior leukoencephalopathy syndrome. N Engl J Med 334(8):494–500, 1996 8559202

Johnston SC, Easton JD, Farrant M, et al; Clinical Research Collaboration, Neurological Emergencies Treatment Trials Network, and the POINT Investigators: Clopidogrel and Aspirin in Acute Ischemic Stroke and High-Risk TIA. N Engl J Med 379(3):215–225, 2018 29766750

Johnston SC, Amarenco P, Denison H, et al: Ticagrelor and aspirin or aspirin alone in acute ischemic stroke or TIA. THALES Investigators. N Engl J Med 383(3):207–217, 2020 32668111

Jüttler E, Bösel J, Amiri H, et al; DESTINY II Study Group: DESTINY II: DEcompressive Surgery for the Treatment of malignant INfarction of the middle cerebral arterY II. Int J Stroke 6(1):79–86, 2011 21205246

Kent DM, Saver JL, Kasner SE, et al: Heterogeneity of Treatment Effects in an Analysis of Pooled Individual Patient Data From Randomized Trials of Device Closure of Patent Foramen Ovale After Stroke. JAMA 326(22):2277–2286, 2021 34905030

Khatri P, Kleindorfer DO, Devlin T, et al; PRISMS Investigators: Effect of Alteplase vs Aspirin on Functional Outcome for Patients With Acute

Ischemic Stroke and Minor Nondisabling Neurologic Deficits: The PRISMS Randomized Clinical Trial. JAMA 320(2):156–166, 2018 29998337

Kim JS, Choi-Kwon S: Poststroke depression and emotional incontinence: correlation with lesion location. Neurology 54(9):1805–1810, 2000 10802788

Kirshner H, Casey P, Henson J, Heinrich J: Behavioural features and lesion localization in Wernicke's aphasia. Aphasiology 3(2):169–176, 1989

Kirshner HS: Stroke mimicry. Four cases eligible for tPA therapy. Neurologist 6:220–223, 2000

Langezaal LCM, van der Hoeven EJRJ, Mont'Alverne FJA, et al; BASICS Study Group: Endovascular Therapy for Stroke Due to Basilar-Artery Occlusion. N Engl J Med 384(20):1910–1920, 2021 34010530

Leary MC, Saver JL: Annual incidence of first silent stroke in the United States: a preliminary estimate. Cerebrovasc Dis 16(3):280–285, 2003 12865617

Liepmann H: Das Krankheitsbild der apraxie ("motorischen asymbolie"). Monatschr Psychiatr Neurol 8:15–44, 102–132, 182–197, in: Rottenberg DA, Hochberg FH (Eds.): Neurological Classics in Modern Translation 1977. Hafner, New York: pp. 155–181, 1900

Markus HS, Levi C, King A, et al; Cervical Artery Dissection in Stroke Study (CADISS) Investigators: Antiplatelet Therapy vs Anticoagulation Therapy in Cervical Artery Dissection: The Cervical Artery Dissection in Stroke Study (CADISS) Randomized Clinical Trial Final Results. JAMA Neurol 76(6):657–664, 2019 30801621

Mendelow AD, Gregson BA, Fernandes HM, et al; STICH investigators: Early surgery versus initial conservative treatment in patients with spontaneous supratentorial intracerebral haematomas in the International Surgical Trial in Intracerebral Haemorrhage (STICH): a randomised trial. Lancet 365(9457):387–397, 2005 15680453

Mohr JP, Pessin MS, Finkelstein S, et al: Broca aphasia: pathologic and clinical. Neurology 28(4):311–324, 1978 565019

Mukand J, Kaplan M, Senno RG, Bishop DS: Pathological crying and laughing: treatment with sertraline. Arch Phys Med Rehabil 77(12):1309–1311, 1996 8976317

Naeser MA, Helm-Estabrooks N, Haas G, et al: Relationship between lesion extent in 'Wernicke's area' on computed tomographic scan and predicting recovery of comprehension in Wernicke's aphasia. Arch Neurol 44(1):73–82, 1987 3800725

National Institute of Neurological Disorders and Stroke rt-PA Stroke Study Group: Tissue plasminogen activator for acute ischemic stroke. N Engl J Med 333(24):1581–1587, 1995 7477192

Nogueira RG, Jadhav AP, Haussen DC, et al; DAWN Trial Investigators: Thrombectomy 6 to 24 Hours after Stroke with a Mismatch between Deficit and Infarct. N Engl J Med 378(1):11–21, 2018 29129157

Ochipa C, Rothi LJ, Heilman KM: Ideational apraxia: a deficit in tool selection and use. Ann Neurol 25(2):190–193, 1989 2465733

Pradilla G, Ratcliff JJ, Hall AJ, et al: Trial of early minimally invasive removal of intracerebral hemorrhage. N Engl J Med 2024;390:1277–1289, 2024

Panitch HS, Thisted RA, Smith RA, et al; Psuedobulbar Affect in Multiple Sclerosis Study Group: Randomized, controlled trial of dextromethorphan/quinidine for pseudobulbar affect in multiple sclerosis. Ann Neurol 59(5):780–787, 2006 16634036

Pohjasvaara T, Mäntylä R, Salonen O, et al: How complex interactions of ischemic brain infarcts, white matter lesions, and atrophy relate to poststroke dementia. Arch Neurol 57(9):1295–1300, 2000 10987896

Publications Committee for the Trial of ORG 10172 in Acute Stroke Treatment (TOAST) Investigators. Low molecular weight heparinoid, ORG 10172 (danaparoid), and outcome after acute ischemic stroke: a randomized controlled trial. JAMA 279(16):1265–1272, 1998 9565006

Qureshi AI, Tuhrim S, Broderick JP, et al: Spontaneous intracerebral hemorrhage. N Engl J Med 344(19):1450–1460, 2001 11346811

Robinson RG, Kubos KL, Starr LB, et al: Mood disorders in stroke patients. Importance of location of lesion. Brain 107(Pt 1):81–93, 1984 6697163

Robinson RG, Schultz SK, Castillo C, et al: Nortriptyline versus fluoxetine in the treatment of depression and in short-term recovery after stroke: a placebo-controlled, double-blind study. Am J Psychiatry 157(3):351–359, 2000 10698809

Schrag M, Kirshner H: Management of Intracerebral Hemorrhage: JACC Focus Seminar. J Am Coll Cardiol 75(15):1819–1831, 2020 32299594

See I, Su JR, Lale A, et al: US Case Reports of Cerebral Venous Sinus Thrombosis With Thrombocytopenia After Ad26.COV2.S Vaccination, March 2 to April 21, 2021. JAMA 325(24):2448–2456, 2021 33929487

Starkstein SE, Fedoroff P, Berthier ML, Robinson RG: Manic-depressive and pure manic states after brain lesions. Biol Psychiatry 29(2):149–158, 1991 1995084

Starkstein SE, Pearlson GD, Boston J, Robinson RG: Mania after brain injury. A controlled study of causative factors. Arch Neurol 44(10):1069–1073, 1987 3632381

Stebbins GT, Nyenhuis DL, Wang C, et al: Gray matter atrophy in patients with ischemic stroke with cognitive impairment. Stroke 39(3):785–793, 2008 18258824

Szirmai I, Vastagh I, Szombathelyi E, Kamondi A: Strategic infarcts of the thalamus in vascular dementia. J Neurol Sci 203–204:91–97, 2002 12417364

Thomalla G, Simonsen CZ, Boutitie F, et al; WAKE-UP Investigators: MRI-Guided Thrombolysis for Stroke with Unknown Time of Onset. N Engl J Med 379(7):611–622, 2018 29766770

Toyoda K, Uchiyama S, Yamaguchi T, et al; CSPS.com Trial Investigators: Dual antiplatelet therapy using cilostazol for secondary prevention in patients with high-risk ischaemic stroke in Japan: a multicentre, open-label, randomised controlled trial. Lancet Neurol 18(6):539–548, 2019 31122494

van Dalen JW, Moll van Charante EP, Nederkoorn PJ, et al: Poststroke apathy. Stroke 44(3):851–860, 2013 23362076

Zaidat OO, Fitzsimmons BF, Woodward BK, et al; VISSIT Trial Investigators: Effect of a balloon-expandable intracranial stent vs medical therapy on risk of stroke in patients with symptomatic intracranial stenosis: the VISSIT randomized clinical trial. JAMA 313(12):1240–1248, 2015 25803346

Index

Page numbers printed in **boldface type** *refer to tables and figures.*